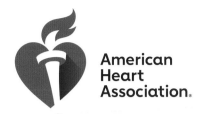

Advanced Cardiovascular Life Support

INSTRUCTOR MANUAL

ISBN 978-1-61669-773-0
Printed in the United States of America

First American Heart Association Printing October 2020
10 9 8 7 6 5 4 3 2

i

Acknowledgments

The American Heart Association thanks the following people for their contributions to the development of this manual: Elizabeth Sinz, MD, MEd; Kenneth Navarro, MEd, LP; Adam Cheng, MD; Elizabeth A. Hunt, MD, MPH, PhD; Sallie Johnson, PharmD, BCPS; Steven C. Brooks, MD, MHSc; Susan Morris, RN; Brian K. Walsh, PhD, RRT; Julie Crider, PhD; and the AHA ACLS Project Team.

To find out about any updates or corrections to this text, visit
www.heart.org/courseupdates.

Contents

Part 1
General Concepts   1

About This Instructor Manual   1

Critical Role of the Instructor   2

Instructor Needs and Resources   3
    Science Update Information   3
    Instructor Network   3

Course Planning and Support Materials   4
    Notice of Courses   4
    Ordering Materials   4
    Copyright of AHA Materials   4
    Smoking Policy   4
    Course Completion Cards   4

Course Equipment   6
    High-Fidelity vs Low-Fidelity Simulation   6
    Infection Control   6
    Equipment and Manikin Cleaning   7

Course Materials   8
    Templates   8
    Lesson Plans   8
    Using the Provider Manual   8

Tailoring to the Audience   9
    Determining Course Specifics   9
    Course Flexibility   9
    Non-AHA Content   9
    Students With Special Needs   10

Implementing Resuscitation Education Science in Training   11
    Importance of High-Quality CPR   12
    High-Performance Teamwork   12
    The Role of a CPR Coach in a Resuscitation Team   13
    Calculating CCF   15
    Prebriefing   15
    Feedback and Coaching   15

Contents

Debriefing   15

Contextual Learning   18

Testing for Course Completion   19

Skills Testing   19

Skills Testing of Blended-Learning Students   19

Exam   19

Exam Security   20

Remediation   21

Provider Course Student Remediation   21

Remediation Concepts for Instructors   21

Steps to Successful Remediation   22

After the Course   23

Program Evaluation   23

Issuing Provider Course Completion Cards   23

Continuing Education/Continuing Medical Education Credit for Courses   23

Provider Renewal   24

Renewal Timeline   24

Instructor Training   25

Recruiting and Mentoring Instructors   25

Instructor Candidate Selection   25

Instructor Course Prerequisites   25

Receiving an Instructor Card   25

Instructor Renewal Criteria: Advanced Cardiovascular Life Support   25

Special Exceptions to Teaching Requirements   26

Part 2
Preparing for the Course   27

Course Overview   27

Course Overview and Design   27

Course Description   27

Course Goal   28

Course Objectives   28

Educational Design   28

Instructor-Led Training   29

Blended Learning (HeartCode)   29

Preparing to Teach Blended-Learning Courses   30

Understanding HeartCode   30

Validation of Online Course Certificates   30

Course Audience   31

Course Prerequisites   31

BLS Provider Course Completion Card   32

ACLS Student Resources 32
ACLS Course Flexibility 33
Creating Additional Case Scenarios 33
ACLS Case Scenario Template 34
Students Obtaining BLS Cards in an ACLS Course 35

Instructor Requirements **36**
Who Can Teach the Course 36
Lead Instructor 36
Faculty Requirements 36
Instructor-to-Student Ratio 36
Student-to-Manikin Ratio 37

Instructor Preparation **38**
Preparing to Teach 38

Course Planning and Support Materials **39**
Determining Course Specifics 39
Templates 39
Sample Precourse Letter to Students (ACLS Course) 40
Sample Precourse Letter to Students (ACLS Traditional Course) 41
Sample Precourse Letter to Students (HeartCode ACLS) 42
Room Requirements 43
Core Curriculum 43
Course Equipment 46
Equipment List 46

Part 3
Teaching the Course
51

Interacting With Students **51**
Greeting Students 51
During the Course 51

Learning Stations and Skills Practice **52**
Introduction 52
Preparing for Learning Stations 53
Conducting Learning Stations 53
Case Scenarios for the Learning Stations 58

Instructor Teaching Materials **61**
Understanding Icons 61
Understanding Lesson Plans 61
Using Lesson Plans 62

Course Outlines and Agendas **63**

Part 4
Testing   81

Testing for Course Completion   81
Course Completion Requirements   81
Skills Testing   82
High-Quality BLS Skills Testing   82
High-Quality BLS Test Scenario   82
Airway Management Skills Testing   82
Mandatory Audiovisual Feedback Device   82
Skills Testing of Blended-Learning Students   83
Using the Skills Testing Checklist and Critical Skills Descriptors   84
Skills Testing Checklist Rules   85
Adult High-Quality BLS Skills Testing Checklist   86
Adult High-Quality BLS Skills Testing Critical Skills Descriptors   87
Retesting Students   88

High-Performance Teams: Megacode   89
Assessment and Testing Guidelines   89
Passing the Megacode Test   89
Objective and Uniform Testing of Students   90
ACLS Megacode Cases: General Information   91

Part 5
Appendixes   93

A. Learning Station Scenarios, Megacode Scenarios,
and Debriefing Tool   95
ACLS Case Scenarios   97
Megacode Scenarios   209

B. Testing Checklists, Learning Station Checklists,
and Other Tools   221
Adult High-Quality BLS Skills Testing Checklist   222
Airway Management Skills Testing Checklist   223
Megacode Testing Checklist: Scenarios 1/3/8   224
Megacode Testing Checklist: Scenarios 2/5   225
Megacode Testing Checklist: Scenarios 4/7/10   226
Megacode Testing Checklist: Scenarios 6/11   227
Megacode Testing Checklist: Scenario 9   228
Megacode Testing Checklist: Scenario 12   229
Adult Cardiac Arrest Learning Station Checklist (VF/pVT)   230
Adult Cardiac Arrest Learning Station Checklist (Asystole/PEA)   231
Adult Bradycardia Learning Station Checklist   232
Adult Tachycardia With a Pulse Learning Station Checklist   233

Adult Post–Cardiac Arrest Care Learning Station Checklist   234

Adult Cardiac Arrest Learning Station Checklist (VF/pVT/Asystole/PEA)   235

Cardiac Arrest in Pregnancy In-Hospital ACLS Learning Station Checklist 236

Adult Ventricular Assist Device Learning Station Checklist   237

ACLS Code Timer/Recorder Sheet   239

Drug Boxes   241

Science Summary Table   247

Part 6
ACLS Lesson Plans   1-68

Abbreviations

Abbreviation	Definition
ACLS	Advanced Cardiovascular Life Support
ACS	acute coronary syndromes
AED	automated external defibrillator
AHA	American Heart Association
AV	atrioventricular
BLS	Basic Life Support
CCF	chest compression fraction
CE	continuing education
CME	continuing medical education
CPR	cardiopulmonary resuscitation
CPSS	Cincinnati Prehospital Stroke Scale
CT	computed tomography
ECC	emergency cardiovascular care
ECG	electrocardiogram
EMS	emergency medical services
IO	intraosseous
IV	intravenous
MET	medical emergency team
MI	myocardial infarction
NPA	nasopharyngeal airway
NSTE	non–ST-segment elevation
OPA	oropharyngeal airway
PCI	percutaneous coronary intervention
PEA	pulseless electrical activity
pVT	pulseless ventricular tachycardia
ROSC	return of spontaneous circulation
RRT	rapid response team
RV	right ventricular
STEMI	ST-segment elevation myocardial infarction
VF	ventricular fibrillation

ACLS Instructor Resources

Available on the AHA Instructor Network at **www.ahainstructornetwork.org**.

ACLS courses include precourse online video lessons. ACLS traditional courses do not include precourse online video lessons. All courses include the mandatory precourse self-assessment.

Precourse Materials

Equipment List

Sample Agenda for ACLS Course

Sample Agenda for ACLS Update Course

Sample Agenda for ACLS Traditional Course

Sample Agenda for ACLS Traditional Update Course

Sample Outline for HeartCode ACLS Hands-On Skills, Option 1

Sample Outline for HeartCode ACLS Hands-On Skills, Option 2

Sample Agenda for ACLS Course Plus BLS Card

Sample Agenda for ACLS Update Course Plus BLS Card

Sample Precourse Letter to Students, ACLS Course

Sample Precourse Letter to Students, ACLS Traditional Course

Sample Precourse Letter to Students, HeartCode ACLS

ACLS Case Scenario Template

Course Materials

2020 Science Summary Table

ACLS Code Timer/Recorder Sheet

ACLS Medication Sheets

ACLS Learning Station Checklists

Adult High-Quality BLS Skills Testing Checklist

Airway Management Skills Testing Checklist

ACLS Megacode Testing Checklists

ACLS Megacode Testing Scenarios

Part 1

General Concepts

About This Instructor Manual

We have reorganized our instructor manuals to provide an introductory section that discusses the science and educational principles of resuscitation training as well as the basic logistics for conducting any American Heart Association (AHA) course. For new instructors, Part 1 provides essential and practical tools to help launch them as AHA Instructors. For more seasoned instructors, Part 1 offers insights into the science and educational principles that go into the design of all AHA courses. Although some of this information applies mostly to the AHA advanced resuscitation courses, Basic Life Support (BLS) Instructors may find it useful. The remaining Parts of this instructor manual cover course-specific information.

Critical Role of the Instructor

The ultimate goal of AHA courses is to improve outcomes for people with cardiovascular disease, especially those who need cardiopulmonary resuscitation (CPR) or emergency cardiovascular care (ECC). AHA Instructors have a unique opportunity to impact the survival of real people by helping to enhance student skills through learning and practice. Instructors should use the educational design of ECC courses to simulate events that are as close to real emergencies as possible. In this way, AHA courses can prepare students to function optimally for their next emergency.

As an AHA Instructor, your role is to help your students by

- Demonstrating effective case management consistent with the current *AHA Guidelines for CPR and ECC*
- Modeling high-quality principles of care
- Facilitating discussions with a focus on desired outcome
- Listening to students' responses and providing feedback to ensure that they understand the learning concepts
- Observing students' actions and coaching them as necessary
- Providing positive or corrective feedback
- Managing discussions and simulations to optimize classroom time and maximize learning
- Leading, modeling, and promoting prebriefing sessions before each simulation and structured debriefing sessions after each simulation

Some AHA Instructors will also teach blended-learning courses. These courses combine eLearning, in which a student completes part of the course online, with a hands-on instructor-led session. You'll learn more about blended-learning courses later in this manual.

Instructor Needs and Resources

Science Update Information

Science and education updates occur periodically. The AHA provides the following resources so that you can access these updates as they are released:

- The AHA Instructor Network, which includes the *ECC Beat*; for instructions on how to access, visit **www.ahainstructornetwork.org**.
- The AHA website (**cpr.heart.org**)

For full details of all changes that were made to the resuscitation guidelines, the AHA strongly recommends that each instructor access the guidelines, available at **eccguidelines.heart.org**.

Instructor Network

The AHA provides the Instructor Network as a resource to instructors. Here, instructors can access up-to-date resources and reference information about the AHA ECC programs and science.

AHA Instructor Registration
www.ahainstructornetwork.org

All AHA Instructors are required to register with the AHA to be aligned with a Training Center. For instructions on how to register, visit **www.ahainstructornetwork.org**. Alignment must be approved by that Training Center before access to content is available. Acceptance of the user agreement is required during registration.

Once registered and approved, you will receive an instructor identification number. This number will be placed on your instructor card and is the same for all disciplines. This number stays the same if you change Training Centers. It is used on all course completion cards for classes that you teach.

The AHA reserves the right to delete or deny alignments.

Course Planning and Support Materials

Before teaching a classroom course or hands-on session, please take the time to read and review in detail the instructor manual and lesson plans, provider manual and any additional student resources, and videos. Your preparation is key to a successful and rewarding teaching experience.

As you view the videos and the lesson plans (Part 6), note how the course is organized and the expectations for you and the students. Make notes on your lesson plans as needed.

This important preparation will enable you to teach the course more effectively and anticipate what you will need to do as the course unfolds. This is especially true for those parts of the course that require you to organize the students for practice or testing, present the video to give information, facilitate discussions, distribute equipment, conduct debriefings, and give exams or hands-on tests.

Notice of Courses

For US-based instructors aligned with the AHA Instructor Network, the AHA offers the My Courses tool, where instructors can enter and maintain the classes they offer to the general public. These are displayed to customers searching for scheduled classes on the AHA's CPR and First Aid website, **cpr.heart.org**. Before entering classes, check with your Training Center to determine what policies that center may have regarding instructors entering their classes. As an instructor, you can still add your classes for display through My Courses even if your Training Center is not participating in listing through My Courses.

For instructors based outside the United States, inform your International Training Center of courses open to the public so that they can send inquiries for classes to you.

Ordering Materials

As an instructor, you can order books and other support materials through your Training Center or directly from the AHA at **ShopCPR.Heart.org**. There are also distributors available for AHA Instructors outside the United States (**https://international.heart.org/en/how-to-buy**). However, only a Training Center Coordinator can order course completion cards. Work with your Training Center Coordinator to ensure that your students receive their cards.

Copyright of AHA Materials

The AHA owns the copyright to AHA books and other training materials. These materials may not be copied, in whole or in part, without the prior written consent of the AHA.

For more information and to request permission to reprint, copy, or use portions of ECC textbooks or other materials, go to **copyright.heart.org**.

Smoking Policy

The Training Center must prohibit smoking in classrooms and training facilities during all AHA ECC training programs.

Course Completion Cards

Only a Training Center Coordinator, or another authorized Training Center representative designated by the Training Center Coordinator, can use the confidential security code to order course completion cards (eCard or printed) for approved disciplines. The Training Center Coordinator should keep this code confidential. Training Center Coordinators cannot order course completion cards without this code.

The Training Center Coordinator has final responsibility to the AHA for the security code. The Training Center Coordinator must notify ECC Customer Support immediately if the security code is suspected as lost, stolen, disclosed, or used without authorization.

The AHA may change the code if deemed necessary to maintain the confidentiality of the code.

Misuse of the confidential security code could result in termination of the Training Center Agreement.

For more information on course completion cards, refer to the *ECC Course Card Reference Guide* on the Instructor Network and at **cpr.heart.org**.

Course Equipment

All AHA ECC courses require that manikins and equipment allow demonstration of the core skills (eg, airway management, correct hand placement, compression depth, chest recoil). The AHA requires the use of an instrumental directive feedback device or manikin in all AHA courses that teach the skills of adult CPR.

The AHA neither endorses nor recommends a particular brand of manikin or other equipment. The decision on which brand or model of equipment to use is the responsibility of the Training Center.

You can find a detailed equipment list for your course or hands-on session in Part 2 of this instructor manual.

High-Fidelity vs Low-Fidelity Simulation

Simulators have been used in AHA courses for decades. They give students the opportunity to practice and improve the clinical skills needed for resuscitating real patients.

Because of improvements in technology, healthcare professionals can more easily observe pathophysiologic signs. The variety of simulators has expanded considerably. Some are as simple and old-fashioned as using an orange to practice intramuscular injections. Others are more sophisticated, such as computer-guided mechanical devices that make practicing specific procedures look and feel more real. Improved plastics have made task trainers (eg, airway practice models) more versatile and realistic, and many manikins have lifelike features and enhancements.

While the term *high fidelity* has been used as a synonym for *high technology*, *fidelity* actually refers to the level of realism as this relates to specific learning objectives. Thus, *high fidelity* implies a very realistic simulation, while *low fidelity* implies that the student must use his or her imagination to fill in the gaps. These definitions are based on the experience of the student rather than on the device itself.

While advanced technology and high-fidelity simulation are appealing and may result in higher student satisfaction, they increase costs substantially without necessarily enhancing learning compared with more basic simulators. In fact, none of the available products is truly realistic compared with real human beings.

You may find high-fidelity manikins useful for teamwork and skills integration, but it is not certain which specific aspects of the scenario are improved by a higher degree of realism. Having a relevant case and setting for students—or matching the equipment to what the students use in their practices—may be more important than a high-fidelity manikin for translating the learning process to clinical practice. As an instructor, you can tailor your approach by using the resources available to create a high-fidelity environment that both satisfies students and achieves the desired learning objectives.

Feedback devices can accurately measure rate, depth, and recoil of compressions and rate and volume of ventilation. This feedback should be used throughout the course and for testing so that students are able to practice until they can do it without having to think about it (ie, automatically). Because you are trying to build automaticity, it is important for students to perform these skills correctly and consistently and for Team Leaders and team members to recognize correct performance by others.

Infection Control

It is your responsibility as an instructor to ensure that a safe, clean environment is maintained in your class. Inform your students in advance that training sessions involve close physical contact with manikins and that they will be close to other students.

In your welcome letter that is sent with course materials, tell students not to attend class if they know they have an infectious disease, feel sick, or have open sores or cuts on their hands, mouth, or areas around their mouth. Participants and instructors should postpone CPR training if they are in the active stages of an infectious disease or have reason to believe they have been exposed to an infectious disease.

Equipment and Manikin Cleaning

To reduce the risk of potential disease transmission, all manikins and training equipment need to be thoroughly cleaned after each class. Manikins used for CPR practice and testing require special actions to be taken between each student. The AHA strongly recommends that you follow manufacturers' recommendations for manikin use and maintenance. In the absence of manufacturers' recommendations, the following guidelines may be used during and after class:

During Class

- Students and instructors should practice good hygiene with proper handwashing techniques.
- When individual protective face shields are used, continue to follow all decontamination recommendations listed for cleaning manikins during and after a course. In addition, to reduce the risks to each user for exposure to contaminants, ensure that all students consistently place the same side of the face shield on the manikin during use.
- If you are not using face shields during the course, clean the manikins after use by each student with a manikin wipe that has an antiseptic with 70% ethyl alcohol.
  - Open the packet, and take out and unfold the manikin wipe.
  - Rub the manikin's mouth and nose vigorously with the wipe.
  - Wrap the wipe snugly over the mouth and nose.
  - Keep the wipe in place for 30 seconds.
  - Dry the manikin's face with a clean paper towel or something similar.
  - Continue with the ventilation practice.

After Class

- Take apart the manikins as directed by the manufacturer. Anyone taking apart and decontaminating manikins should wear protective gloves and wash their hands when finished.
- As soon as possible after each class, clean any part of the manikin that comes into contact with potentially infectious body fluids during training to prevent contaminants from drying on manikin surfaces.
- If manikins are stored for more than 24 hours before cleaning, follow these steps:
  - Wash all surfaces, reusable protective face shields, and pocket masks thoroughly with warm, soapy water and brushes.
  - Moisten all surfaces with a sodium hypochlorite solution having at least 500 ppm free available chlorine (one quarter cup of liquid household bleach per gallon of tap water) for 10 minutes. Make this solution fresh for each class and discard after each use. Using a concentration higher than one quarter cup has not been proven to be more effective and may discolor the manikins.
  - Rinse all surfaces with fresh water and air dry before storing.
  - Because some manufacturers have recommendations for cleaning manikin parts in a dishwasher, check with the manufacturer of the manikins being used to determine if this is an acceptable method. Some manikin materials could be damaged in a dishwasher.
- Replace disposable airway equipment at the end of each class.
- Clean manikin clothing and the manikin carrying case periodically or when soiled.
- Maintain other equipment used in class according to hospital policy. Wipe surfaces touched by students with antiseptic solution.

Course Materials

Templates

As a registered instructor, you can log in to your account to find templates for letters, forms, and other materials to help you prepare to teach the course. You will need to customize some of these materials, including the precourse letter, which tells students what they need to do to prepare for the course or hands-on session.

Lesson Plans

All AHA ECC instructor manuals include lesson plans that are intended to

- Help you as an instructor to facilitate your courses
- Ensure consistency from course to course
- Help you focus on the main objectives for each lesson
- Explain your responsibilities during the course

Your lesson plans were created to be used before and during courses and during skills practice and testing sessions, as noted in Table 1.

Table 1. How to Use Lesson Plans

When	How to use
Before the course	Review your lesson plans, making notes of anything you want to emphasize on the basis of your students' roles and environment. • Identify objectives for each lesson. • Define your role for each lesson plan. • Gather the resources needed for each lesson.
During the course	• Follow each lesson plan as you conduct the course. • Remind students what each video segment covers. • Make sure you have all the resources, equipment, and supplies ready for each lesson. • Help all students achieve the objectives identified for each lesson. • Encourage students to work in teams and to help each other. • Create an atmosphere that encourages peak performance and improvement that will carry over into clinical practice.
During practice before a skills test	A student may have a question about a certain part of skills they will be tested on. The lesson plans serve as a resource for you when answering those questions.

Using the Provider Manual

Students must have their own copy of the current provider manual to read before and to use as a resource during and after the course. The lesson plans tell you when to refer students to specific sections of the provider manual during the course.

The provider manual is designed for individual use and is an integral part of the student's education. Students may reuse their manuals during renewals or updates until new science guidelines are published.

Students taking a blended-learning course have access to the provider manual and other reference materials within the online portion. They may access the reference materials for up to 2 years from the date they activate their online portion. Students should be allowed to bring electronic devices into the classroom to access these electronic materials.

Tailoring to the Audience

Determining Course Specifics

Before you teach a course, determine the course specifics:

- Student audience
- Number of students
- Special needs or local protocols
- Room requirements
- Course equipment

Details specific for the type of course or hands-on session that you will be conducting are located in Part 3.

Course Flexibility

The AHA allows instructors to tailor their courses to meet audience-specific needs. One example of this course flexibility is local CPR protocols used within the learning and testing stations. For specific examples, refer to Part 2.

Any changes to the course are in addition to the basic course contents as outlined in this manual and will add to the length of the course. Instructors may not delete course lessons or course components. Any additions or alterations to the course must be specifically identified as *non-AHA* material (refer to the Non-AHA Content section). Some evidence suggests that *adding content* to the course may actually decrease learning and retention. Although it is not considered a best practice to insert additional material into this course, instructors may add related topics, as long as none of the required lessons or course content is eliminated or shortened.

Non-AHA Content

As an instructor, you can best serve your students when you can adapt to meet the needs of a specific audience. If you find that your students will be better served by adding location-specific information, equipment, or specialty-specific content and you plan to discuss that non-AHA content in class or distribute handouts, follow these rules:

- None of the required AHA lessons or course content can be eliminated or shortened.
- Any changes to the course are in addition to the basic content as outlined in your instructor manual.
- Adding additional content will add time to the course.
- Additional topics or information should be covered at the *beginning or end* of the course to avoid disrupting the flow of the required lessons.
- Any location-specific protocols or procedures that do not comply with AHA processes (eg, substituting new medications, specialized techniques) should be identified to the audience as *location-specific*.
- Any non-AHA content must be identified as *not approved or reviewed by the AHA*, and the source of the information must be provided to the students.
- Supplementary materials that you use need to be approved by the Lead Instructor or the Course Director for advanced courses, as well as by your Training Center Coordinator.
- A copy of a revised agenda and any print material shared in class must be part of the permanent course file.
- Your students cannot be tested on non-AHA content. If they complete the AHA-defined course completion requirements, they must be issued an AHA course completion card.

Students With Special Needs

- The AHA does not provide advice to Training Centers on Americans With Disabilities Act requirements or any other laws, rules, or regulations. Training Centers must determine accommodations necessary to comply with applicable laws. The AHA recommends consultation with legal counsel.
- A student must be able to successfully complete all course completion requirements to receive a course completion card. Reasonable accommodations may be made, such as manikin positioning, use of a text reader, or reading the exam to the student.
- If a student is unable to successfully complete skills testing because of a disability, he or she should be given written documentation of class attendance, with a listing of what testing was not successfully completed.

Implementing Resuscitation Education Science in Training

According to research reviewed in the 2018 AHA Scientific Statement "Resuscitation Education Science: Educational Strategies to Improve Outcomes From Cardiac Arrest," providers' skills can begin to decay only weeks after taking standardized resuscitation courses, which can lead to poor clinical care and survival outcomes for cardiac arrest patients. The Resuscitation Education Statement presented evidence supporting the following strategies to improve how well providers learn and retain these critical skills.

- Mastery learning: To increase the likelihood that a student will truly learn key resuscitation skills, have students practice until they demonstrate mastery. AHA courses are designed to give students time to practice with video demonstration, scenarios, and group activities. As an AHA Instructor, your role is to provide the feedback and coaching to make students' practice time meaningful and effective.

- Perfect practice makes perfect: Use a mastery learning model that requires students to demonstrate key skills, and set a minimum passing standard for mastery. Video demonstrations in AHA courses allow students to observe accurate and consistent resuscitation skills and to practice with the video and in group scenarios. Give students time to practice until they are comfortable with the skills and feel ready to take the skills test.

- Measuring performance to motivate students: Set performance standards on the basis of observable behaviors. Determine the most important measures for patient outcomes and process standards such as time, accuracy, and best practices. The skills testing checklists in all AHA courses define the passing standard for critical skills and allow instructors to measure and document student performance.

- Deliberate practice: Use skill repetition paired with feedback and exercises, known as *deliberate practice,* to teach behaviors that are difficult to master or should be performed automatically.

- Use of overlearning to improve retention: Train students beyond the minimum standard, known as *overlearning*, for behaviors that are likely to decay and would require effort to retrain someone to a level of mastery.

- Spaced learning: Students who participate in more frequent, shorter learning sessions have a better chance of retaining new knowledge and procedures. Strategies like eLearning, rolling refresher events, and other ways to increase learning outside of scheduled training can reinforce training after the class. Resuscitation Quality Improvement® is an example of low-dose, high-frequency training that providers can use to regularly practice skills and reinforce learning at their workplace. Instructors may offer periodic skills refreshers between course events.

- Contextual learning: Training that applies directly to students' scope of practice can engage students and make them eager to expand their expertise. Ensure that team composition, roles, and contexts are right for each group activity, and consider implementing appropriate levels of stress and cognitive load.

- Prebriefing, feedback, and debriefing:
  - Prebriefing: Briefing before a learning event creates a safe environment for students by setting their expectations. Prebriefing builds rapport between instructor and student, which can make students more receptive to feedback after the event.
  - Using data in feedback and debriefing: Students need performance data to improve. This includes data from instructors, other students, and devices.
  - Debriefing tools: Debriefing tools or scripts improve instructors' debriefing effectiveness by providing direction and content that is focused on improving learning outcomes.

- Assessment: Assessment of student competence is a critical part of developing efficient resuscitation teams. Plan for various, high-quality assessments throughout each course to get a broader picture of each student's knowledge and skills.

- Innovative educational strategies: New methods of accessing up-to-date information can improve laypeople's willingness to act, provider performance, and survival rates.

For example, gamified learning can improve engagement, and social media delivers information quickly to large audiences.

- Faculty development: Initial instructor training is crucial, but empowering instructors to commit to lifelong learning creates a culture of training excellence, inspires students, and enhances the classroom experience.
- Knowledge translation and implementation strategies: The best evidence evaluation won't improve patient survival if providers aren't able to apply the knowledge gained to clinical practice. According to the Resuscitation Education Statement, improving methods for translating scientific knowledge into clinical practice is an ongoing field of study that could save more lives than a new breakthrough in managing cardiac arrest. AHA courses teach resuscitation skills as well as team skills and use tools like debriefing so that students learn not only how to perform the critical skills but how to assess and analyze behaviors in real resuscitation events to help their teams improve performance.

Importance of High-Quality CPR

High-quality CPR, comprising manual chest compressions and ventilation, is the foundation of lifesaving resuscitation for cardiac arrest victims. Maintaining blood flow to the heart and brain is the first priority, ahead of other interventions, such as administering medications. Individuals and teams should focus on maintaining cardiac output at all times during an attempted resuscitation for cardiac arrest.

Too often, CPR either is not performed or is performed with too many interruptions during both out-of-hospital and in-hospital arrests. Studies of CPR skills retention have shown patterns of significant erosion of CPR skills in the days, weeks, and months after CPR training. CPR should be performed in real time with an audiovisual feedback device guiding each student's performance in all learning stations where CPR is required. This is critical for a high-performance team. In addition, chest compression fraction (CCF), the proportion of time that chest compressions are performed during a cardiac arrest, should drive increased performance in learning stations and cannot be measured unless compressions are conducted in real time. Ventilation should also be timed or have real-time audiovisual feedback to help ensure optimal performance. This is true in practice, in testing, and in real-life emergencies.

All students will have the opportunity to practice high-quality CPR and then to demonstrate these lifesaving skills during the course assessment.

Components of high-quality CPR for adult cardiac arrest victims include the following:

- Push hard (at least 2 inches [5 cm]), using an automated feedback device to assist with performance improvement.
- Push fast, compressing at a rate of 100 to 120 per minute.
- Minimize interruptions in compressions to 10 seconds or less.
- Achieve a CCF that is ideally greater than 80%.
- Allow for complete chest recoil between compressions (ie, do not lean on the chest between compressions).
- Avoid excessive ventilation, delivering breaths over 1 second that produce visible chest rise.
- Switch compressors about every 2 minutes or earlier if fatigued.

High-Performance Teamwork

With resuscitation teams, high-performance teamwork is a critical element of providing high-quality CPR and increasing survival rates. Resuscitation skills competency is most often verified on an individual basis despite the fact that successful patient outcome from cardiac arrest depends on a team. Students will learn about high-performance teamwork and will practice it in the classroom.

High-performance teams effectively incorporate timing, quality, coordination, and administration of the appropriate procedures during a cardiac arrest (Figure 1). These 4 key areas of focus include the following specifics:

- **Timing:** time to first compression, time to first shock, CCF ideally greater than 80%, minimizing preshock pause, and early emergency medical services (EMS) response time
- **Quality:** rate, depth, complete recoil; minimizing interruptions; switching compressors every 2 minutes or sooner if fatigued; avoiding excessive ventilation; and using a feedback device
- **Coordination:** team dynamics; team members working together, proficient in their roles
- **Administration:** leadership, measurement, continuous quality improvement, and number of participating code team members

Teams function differently in different facilities and in all out-of-hospital settings. Knowing the policies and procedures and the local protocols of your classroom audience is essential to instructor preparation.

Figure 1. Key areas of focus for high-performance teams to increase survival rates.

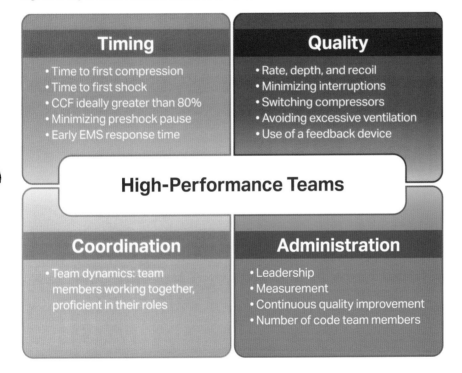

The Role of a CPR Coach in a Resuscitation Team

When caring for a cardiac arrest victim, the resuscitation team must perform many important tasks. Efficiently coordinating these tasks is critical to improving patient outcome. The Team Leader is typically responsible for monitoring the performance of BLS skills in addition to overseeing many other critical tasks. Coordinating so much at once is difficult and can lead to delays and errors in treatment.

For these reasons, many resuscitation teams now include the role of CPR Coach. The CPR Coach supports performance of high-quality BLS skills, allowing the Team Leader to focus on other aspects of clinical care. Studies have shown that resuscitation teams with a CPR Coach perform higher-quality CPR with higher CCF and shorter pause durations compared with teams that don't use a CPR Coach.

The CPR Coach does not need to be a separate role; they can be blended into the current responsibilities of the Monitor/Defibrillator. The CPR Coach's responsibilities begin with the start of CPR. A primary focus is to coach team members in performing high-quality BLS skills and help them minimize pauses in chest compressions. Below is a brief summary of specific responsibilities:

Coordinate the start of CPR: As soon as the patient is identified as pulseless, the CPR Coach prompts action by saying, "I am the CPR Coach. There is no pulse, so let's start compressions." The CPR Coach then prepares the environment to optimize compressions. This may include lowering the bed and bed rails, getting a step stool, or rolling the victim to place the backboard and defibrillator pads. These actions help prevent Compressor fatigue and ensure high-quality compressions.

Coach to improve the quality of chest compressions and ventilation: The CPR Coach does the following to help improve the quality of chest compressions and ventilation:

- Convey objective data from a CPR feedback device to help the Compressor improve performance. Team members' visual assessment of CPR quality is commonly inaccurate
- Coach performance of compressions (ie, depth, rate, and chest recoil) and ventilation (ie, ventilation rate, volume and if needed, compression-to-ventilation ratio)
- State the specific midrange targets to help team members perform compressions and ventilation within the recommended range (eg, tell them to compress at a rate of 110/min instead of a rate between 100 and 120/min)
- Give corrective feedback and reinforce positive performance of CPR skills with specific acknowledgment (eg, good job with compression depth)

Coordinate provider switches and defibrillation: The CPR Coach helps minimize the length of pauses during provider switches and defibrillation. The goal is to pause for less than 5 seconds.

Here is an example of a CPR Coach's dialogue: "Team Leader, we have 30 seconds until the next rhythm check. Next Compressor, please come stand by the current Compressor. I'll precharge the defibrillator, and then I'll give a 5-second countdown. The Compressor will stop compressions at 1 second. Then, the Compressors will switch and hover over the chest. We'll check a pulse, and the Team Leader will assess the rhythm. If it's a shockable rhythm, we'll shock immediately and then resume compressions."

Coordinate the placement of an advanced airway: The CPR Coach coordinates the placement of an advanced airway to minimize interruptions in compressions. First, the CPR Coach ensures that the Team Leader and Airway provider have a shared understanding: "My understanding is that we'll attempt intubation without stopping compressions. If that doesn't work, we can pause for up to 10 seconds for the intubation attempt. Is that correct?" Then, the CPR Coach announces the start of the intubation attempt and coordinates a pause if needed. Once the pause duration reaches 10 seconds, the CPR Coach directs the Compressor to start compressions again.

Instructor Tips

- Any healthcare professional can be a CPR Coach. This person must have a current BLS Provider card, understand the responsibilities of a CPR Coach, and demonstrate the ability to coach Compressors and Airway providers effectively to improve performance.
- The CPR Coach should be positioned next to the Defibrillator and in the direct line of sight of the Compressor.
- Because the CPR Coach must continually talk to give ongoing coaching, they must modulate their voice's tone and volume so that they do not disrupt other aspects of patient care.
- The CPR Coach should respect the Team Leader's role and not be perceived as trying to take over leadership. They should keep the Team Leader informed, share their understanding with the Team Leader, and ask for verification of key tasks and decisions.

Calculating CCF

Healthcare providers can calculate CCF mechanically by using a feedback device or manually by using 2 timers. One timer measures the total code time from code start until code stop or the return of spontaneous circulation (ROSC), and a second timer measures the total chest compression time. To measure chest compression time, the second timer is started each time compressions begin or resume and is stopped during each pause in compressions. The chest compression time is then divided by the total code time to equal CCF:

CCF = actual chest compression time/total code time

Prebriefing

Effective briefing before a learning event, known as *prebriefing*, helps establish a safe environment for learning.

Educators can build a sense of psychological safety by prebriefing to let students know that mistakes are expected and serve as sources of learning and that interpersonal risk-taking is encouraged. Effective prebriefing builds rapport between students and instructors and encourages feedback receptivity by clarifying performance targets and explicitly outlining aspects of performance feedback relevant for the session so that students know what to expect: timing, sources, purpose (training or assessment), for example.

- Prebriefing should establish a supportive learning environment where it is safe to make mistakes and learn from them.
- This includes highlighting key performance goals and performance expectations, emphasizing the importance of ongoing practice, actively preparing students for the feedback they will receive, and describing when and how the debriefing will occur.
- Set rules and realism for the simulation.
- The high-performance team should establish goals and then discuss if those goals were met in the structured debriefing afterward.

Feedback and Coaching

At times, you will need to help a student master a skill. This may require expertise in communication and educational creativity. The fundamental principle of AHA courses is that students who are not able to master the required skills during the course can practice until they do. Instructors should be committed to finding and using the proper techniques that will be effective for a particular student. Adult learning principles coupled with debriefing techniques usually make for an effective combination. Here are some suggestions:

- Review the objectives for a particular scenario or skills station with the student.
- Give positive feedback when desired actions are observed; ask open-ended questions when nonpreferred actions are observed to determine the student's thought process.
- Use the same scenario repeatedly if necessary until the student accomplishes the objectives.

Debriefing

Debriefing is an organized, evidence-based, student-focused process that takes place in a nonthreatening environment. It is a method of assisting students in thinking about what they did, when they did it, why and how they did it, and how they can improve.

In an effective debriefing session, instructors ask questions and encourage students to analyze their own performance rather than offer only the instructor's perspective. Because this approach is focused on what the student thinks and does rather than on the instructor's viewpoint, students are more likely to remember and apply the lessons in their practice.

Feedback vs Debriefing

Simple feedback is typically geared toward correcting student actions the instructor has observed—an approach that can sometimes have the unintended consequence of fixing one mistake only to create others. Effective debriefing, on the other hand, focuses more on understanding why students acted a certain way, which allows correction of their thinking. Students typically do things for a reason that makes sense to them. Good debriefing helps students review their own performance and achieve a deeper understanding.

Although debriefing takes longer than simply giving feedback, reframing students' understanding will make the lesson more applicable to real life and will have a more lasting impact on future performance.

Effective Debriefing Characteristics

Effective debriefings must be fit for the purpose and focus on how to achieve performance standards. Specifically, instructors should attend to the established debriefing processes, tailor debriefings to context, use debriefing scripts to promote debriefing effectiveness, and view training as an opportunity to model debriefing practice and to prepare students for the process of a debriefing after actual clinical events.

Students need performance data to improve; these data should be included in debriefings whenever possible. Quantitative data provided during resuscitation education should come from several sources, including instructors, CPR devices, and data from simulators. Some data may be available in real time; other data, during debriefings.

Feedback and debriefing should be part of a larger curriculum design and should not occur in isolation. These powerful educational interventions are integral elements to overarching curriculum design considerations.

The characteristics of an effective debriefing session include

- Active participation
- Student discussion
- Self-analysis
- Application
- Thorough processing of information

With effective debriefing, students should

- Analyze and evaluate what happened
- Recognize how tools can help them manage situations
- Develop the habit of self-critique

We recommend using structured and supported debriefing, a learner-centered debriefing model that focuses on what the student knows and thinks. This approach draws on evidence-based findings from behavioral science to focus on critical thinking and encourage students to analyze their motivations and performance. It is an efficient and organized process to help students think about what they did—why, how, and when they did it—and how they can improve.

Structured and supported debriefing follows a simple 3-step format to achieve a comprehensive and effective debriefing:

- *Gather* information about the events.
- *Analyze* the information by using an accurate record.
- *Summarize* the attainment of objectives for future improvement.

Structured elements include the 3 specific phases described in Table 2, while supported elements include both interpersonal support and the use of protocols, algorithms, and best evidence. Be sure to allow enough time to conduct a debriefing session after each case scenario.

Table 2. Structured and Supported Debriefing Process

Phase	Goal	Actions
Gather	Ask what happened during the case, to develop a shared mental model of the events. Listen to students to understand what they think and how they feel about the simulation.	• Request a narrative from the Team Leader. • Request clarifying or supplementary information from the high-performance team.
Analyze	Facilitate students' reflection on and analysis of their actions.	• Review an accurate record of events. • Report observations (both correct and incorrect steps). • Assist students in thoroughly reflecting on and examining their performance during the simulation as well as in reflecting on their perceptions during the debriefing. • Direct and redirect students during the debriefing to ensure continuous focus on session objectives.
Summarize	Facilitate identification and review of the lessons learned that can be taken into actual practice.	• Summarize comments or statements from students. • Have students identify positive aspects of their high-performance team or individual behaviors. • Have students identify areas of their high-performance team or individual behaviors that require change or correction.

You should view yourself as a facilitator whose goals are to enhance learning during the training session and encourage students to critique themselves and reflect on future clinical encounters. This promotes continued self-improvement and will have a long-lasting effect well beyond any individual course.

A good facilitator effectively uses the key skills of listening, genuine inquiry, and open-ended questions to determine how the student understood the situation and what he or she was thinking. Correcting a particular action will have an impact on only a single behavior; correcting an approach will affect the student's actions in a variety of situations.

Appropriate pauses and silence can give students the time they need to formulate their thoughts. Demonstrating the usefulness of protocols and algorithms is also part of an effective facilitation.

Structured and supported debriefing can help facilitate learning the skills and techniques needed for clinical practice. It is also important that you model and encourage good debriefing techniques because debriefing of actual resuscitation events can be a useful strategy to help healthcare providers improve future performance in clinical practice.

Contextual Learning

Another core concept for resuscitation training is to use training experiences that apply to students' real-world scope of practice.

- Consider that different students find relevance in different things and tailor the learning experience for the types of students, their settings, and the resources available in their environment.
- When simulating resuscitation, acknowledge that manikin fidelity is not enough and use manikin features that matter. These features should engage students and be relevant to the learning objectives.
- Enhance realism for team training by ensuring that team composition, roles, and contexts are right for your student groups.
- Don't be afraid to stress your students (to a certain extent). The right amount of stress can enhance experiential learning by maximizing student engagement.

Testing for Course Completion

The AHA requires successful completion of skills tests, as well as an exam in instructor-led courses or successful completion of the online portion of HeartCode, for a student to receive a provider course completion card.

The prompt and accurate delivery of provider skills and knowledge is critically important for patient survival. Accurate, objective, and uniform testing reinforces these lifesaving skills and knowledge and is critical for the consistent delivery of content by all instructors.

All AHA Instructors are expected to maintain high standards of performance for all skills tests, as discussed in the following sections.

Skills Testing

During skills testing, students must demonstrate competency in all skills without any assistance, hints, or prompting from the instructor.

Instructors of the appropriate discipline will evaluate each student for his or her didactic knowledge and proficiency in all core psychomotor skills of the course. No AHA course completion card is issued without the required skills testing by either an AHA Instructor for that discipline or an AHA-approved computerized manikin in an AHA eLearning course.

Students in advanced life support courses are not required by the AHA to have a current BLS Provider card, but they are expected to demonstrate proficiency in BLS skills. Training Centers do have the option to require a current BLS Provider card, but requiring the card does not mean that BLS content and testing may be omitted from advanced courses.

Skills Testing of Blended-Learning Students

Instructors may need to conduct skills practice and testing during the hands-on session of a blended-learning course. The lesson plans in Part 6 will help facilitate these sessions. The skills testing portion of the hands-on session should be conducted the same as in an instructor-led course. Some skills tests may require that additional students be present while the tests are being conducted (refer to Part 4 for further details).

Exam

The exam measures the mastery of cognitive knowledge in ECC instructor-led healthcare courses. Each student must score at least 84% on the exam to meet course completion requirements.

The AHA has adopted an open-resource policy for exams administered through an eLearning course or in a classroom-based course. Open resource means that students may use resources as a reference while completing the exam. Resources could include the provider manual, either in printed form or as an eBook on personal devices, any notes the student took during the provider course, the *2020 Handbook of ECC for Healthcare Providers*, the *AHA Guidelines for CPR and ECC*, posters, etc. Open resource does not mean open discussion with other students or the instructor. Students may not interact with each other during the exam.

In the welcome letter you send to students with their course materials, emphasize the importance of bringing their books to class to use during the exam. Students using the eBook version should download the manual to their device's eReader app and bring it with them in case there is no Internet connection.

Exams are administered online, though there may be an occasional need to administer a paper exam. More information about online exams can be found on the Instructor Network.

If you use a paper exam, grade the exam and answer any questions as soon as the student returns it. Students who score less than 84% will need to take a second exam or receive verbal remediation to confirm knowledge and understanding. If you give a student a second exam, review the first exam with the student, allowing them time to study the questions they got wrong. If you provide verbal remediation, ask the student to verbally answer the questions that he or she answered incorrectly, and document on the answer sheet whether the student correctly answered each question. You must document on the answer sheet that the remediation was successful, and that the student achieved a passing score.

If a student has difficulty reading or understanding the written questions, you may read the exam to the student. You must read the exam as written and in a manner that does not indicate the correct answer. You may verbally translate the exam if needed.

ECC blended-learning healthcare courses have a cognitive assessment incorporated into the online portion, so an exam does not need to be given to students when they attend the classroom portion.

Exam Security

Exam security is of the utmost importance:

- Ensure that all exams are kept secure and not copied or distributed outside the classroom.
- Exams are copyrighted; therefore, Training Centers or instructors may not alter them in any way or post them to any learning management systems such as Internet or intranet sites. This includes precourse self-assessments.*
- When a paper exam must be used, always print the most current version from the online exam platform for the course you are teaching.
- Each paper exam should be accounted for and returned to the instructor at the end of the testing period.

*Exams are translated into multiple languages. If a translated exam is needed for a course you are teaching, have your Training Center Coordinator contact ECC Customer Support to find out if the needed translation is available.

Remediation

Provider Course Student Remediation

At times, you will have to provide remediation to a student who is unable to perform satisfactorily in portions of the course. This is often resource-intensive and may require considerable expertise in communication and educational creativity.

The fundamental principle is that every student who is not able to master the required skills during the course is still able to benefit from remediation. The instructor should be committed to finding and using the proper techniques that will be effective for a student. Adult learning principles coupled with debriefing techniques usually make for an effective combination. Here are some suggestions:

- Review the objectives for a scenario or skills station with the student.
- Give positive feedback when desired actions are observed; ask open-ended questions when nonpreferred actions are observed to determine the student's thought process.
- Use the same scenario repeatedly if necessary until the student accomplishes the objectives.

Consider using another instructor to provide remediation because that instructor might be able to offer an alternative approach that will be helpful for the student.

At the time of the course, remediation for some students might not be successful within certain sections of the course (or exam or skills tests). When this happens, the student may arrange for a separate remediation session. A student must meet all learning objectives to the satisfaction of the Course Director or Lead Instructor before receiving a course completion card.

Students must complete all remediation sessions, including exams, skills tests, and skills stations, within 30 days after the last day of the original course. The remediation date will be listed as the issue date on the course completion card.

If a student does not successfully complete all course requirements within 30 days, the course is considered incomplete and a course completion card will not be issued.

Remediation Concepts for Instructors

Remediation is a learning process in which the instructor provides additional opportunities for the student to master the required skills of the course.

Informal remediation occurs throughout the course and is part of the learning process. When a student is having difficulty mastering a skill, he or she can be placed last in line for performing skills for practice and/or testing. This gives the student additional time to observe and learn from other students.

Formal remediation occurs after a student has been formally tested in a skills or core case testing station and has been unable to demonstrate mastery. Have the student work one-on-one with an instructor during breaks, lunchtime, or at the end of the day to assess areas for improvement in performing a skill. Then, encourage the student to practice and, when ready, to indicate when he or she wishes to be tested.

It is important to communicate the need for formal remediation in a private, sensitive, and objective debriefing immediately after the testing has taken place by using the scenario critical action objectives as a guide.

- Every student, with rare exceptions, should be able to benefit from remediation.
- Commit to providing remediation for students who have difficulties learning the skills and principles in the course the first time through.
- Instructor styles of facilitating and student styles of learning may not match; therefore, a change of instructor may be necessary.
- Don't assume that poor performance is associated with a lack of knowledge. There may be other factors (eg, personal or work-related issues) that are influencing the student's performance.
- If a student is still having difficulty after receiving remediation, you may need to examine the student's style of learning and make adjustments.
- The role of the instructor is to facilitate learning. Always be respectful, courteous, positive, professional, and diplomatic when providing remediation to a student.

Additional materials to assist in remediation will be provided in a later section of the manual.

Steps to Successful Remediation

You may find these steps helpful when providing remediation:

- Review the critical action steps that the student did not perform satisfactorily.
- Using open-ended questions (debriefing tool), assess the student's thought process, and correct it if necessary.
- Identify whether other factors might have affected the student's performance (eg, performance anxiety).
- Use the same or a similar scenario for retesting the student (eg, if the initial scenario was a respiratory case, use a respiratory case again for the retest).
- Use other students who need remediation or other instructors to help form a high-performance team to manage the case scenario.
- If performance anxiety or an instructor-student personality clash is a factor, ask another instructor to conduct the remediation.

Instructors should make every effort to correct knowledge and skills deficits during the course. Doing so can help minimize the chances that students will require formal remediation at the end of the course.

After the Course

Program Evaluation

Ongoing evaluation and improvement of AHA materials and instructors are important to the AHA. Each student should have an opportunity to evaluate the class. As an instructor, it is your responsibility to provide that opportunity. There are several options for how a course evaluation can be provided.

- Paper evaluation: A template for a written evaluation is available on the Instructor Network. Make enough copies so all your students can complete the evaluation at the end of the course and return it to you. Review the feedback, and then send the completed forms to your Training Center Coordinator.
- eCard survey (United States): If you are an instructor with a US Training Center and your Training Center is issuing eCards, your students will complete an online evaluation before they claim their course completion card. eCard surveys are another important way to gain valuable feedback from your students on their overall satisfaction of the course. eCard Reports are available on the Instructor Network.
- Online evaluation (international): If you are an instructor with an International Training Center, your students are encouraged to complete an evaluation online before they can claim their CPRverify™ course completion card (eCard); in addition, instructors can have students complete the paper evaluation located on CPRverify.

Issuing Provider Course Completion Cards

Each student who successfully completes the course requirements will be issued an AHA course completion card (eCard or printed).

No AHA course completion card is issued without hands-on manikin skills practice and testing by an AHA-approved computerized manikin as part of an AHA eLearning course or by an AHA Instructor for that discipline.

Continuing Education/Continuing Medical Education Credit for Courses

Most ECC online and blended courses offer continuing education (CE)/continuing medical education (CME) credit and are designed to meet CE criteria. The CE/CME certificate is automatically generated when students complete a course and claim their credit. This may not be the same as the certificate of completion.

Some classroom courses also offer credit for EMS professionals. The AHA is contracted to offer all EMS students CE hours through the Commission on Accreditation for Prehospital Continuing Education (CAPCE). Because there are contractual obligations to make CAPCE credit available to all EMS professionals completing a qualifying course, your Training Center and you, as an instructor, are required to collect and submit the information requested: first name, last name, and email address. The submission is done through the Instructor Network. Each student is then sent an email invitation to provide the additional needed information and claim his or her credit. While the information for all EMS students must be submitted, students are not obligated to accept or claim their certificates.

CAPCE accreditation does not represent that the content of a course conforms to any national, state, or local standard or best practice of any nature.

If you would like to offer CE credit to other professionals who attend your instructor-led courses, you will need to work with your Training Center or employer to apply for credit through the appropriate authorizing body.

Visit the Instructor Network to learn which courses offer CE/CME credit and to find more information and updates.

Provider Renewal

Renewal Timeline

The current recommended timeline for renewal of an AHA course completion card is every 2 years. Although there is insufficient evidence to determine the optimal method and timing of retaking a course, research on skills retention and training show the following:

- There is growing evidence that BLS knowledge and skills decay rapidly after initial training.
- Studies have demonstrated the deterioration of BLS skills in as little as months after initial training.
- Studies examining the effect of brief, more frequent training sessions demonstrated improvement in chest compression performance and shorter time to defibrillation.
- Studies also found that students reported improved confidence and willingness to perform CPR after additional or high-frequency training.

Given how fast BLS skills decay after training, and with the observed improvement in skills and confidence among students who train more frequently, students should be encouraged to periodically review their provider manuals and practice skills whenever possible. In addition, instructors and Training Centers may offer opportunities for students to practice and test their skills between course events.

Instructor Training

Recruiting and Mentoring Instructors

You may have students in your course who want to become AHA Instructors. The AHA encourages you, as a current AHA Instructor, to take a moment to pass along this information to all students who are interested in becoming an instructor after they successfully complete the provider course.

An AHA Instructor course teaches the methods needed to effectively teach others. The AHA requires that instructors be at least 18 years of age to attend an AHA Instructor course.

Instructor Candidate Selection

The ideal instructor candidate

- Is motivated to teach
- Is motivated to facilitate learning
- Is motivated to ensure that students acquire the skills necessary for successful course completion
- Views student assessment as a way to improve individual knowledge and skills

Instructor Course Prerequisites

Prospective participants in an AHA Instructor course must

- Have current provider status in the discipline they wish to teach
- Have completed an Instructor Candidate Application (obtained from the Training Center Coordinator)

Receiving an Instructor Card

Your instructor card for your discipline is issued by your primary Training Center. This may not be the same Training Center where you took your training or monitoring.

All instructor cards are valid for 2 years.

If you are a new instructor:

- You must be monitored teaching your first course within 6 months after completing the classroom portion of your training. A current Training Faculty member for your discipline must monitor you while you teach an initial provider course or an update or renewal course. It is your responsibility to schedule this monitoring, working with the Training Faculty member who conducted your course or with the Training Center Coordinator of your Training Center.
- You will receive your instructor card from your Primary Training Center once you have successfully completed all monitoring requirements. The expiration date will be 2 years from the month you completed all requirements, including monitoring.
- You must register on the Instructor Network with your Primary Training Center so that you receive your instructor ID number. This number is placed on the back of your card, so you need it before your card can be issued. Any questions about receiving your instructor card should be directed to your Training Center Coordinator.

Instructor Renewal Criteria: Advanced Cardiovascular Life Support

Your instructor status must be renewed by a Training Faculty member. You can renew your Advanced Cardiovascular Life Support (ACLS) instructor status by meeting all of the following criteria or by successfully completing all requirements for a new instructor.

- Maintain current provider status. You can do this by maintaining a current provider card or by demonstrating exceptional provider skills to a Training Faculty member and by successfully completing the provider exam.
- If you choose the demonstration route, successful completion must be documented on the Instructor/Training Faculty Renewal Checklist. A new provider card may be issued at the discretion of the Training Center or if you request one, but it is not required by the AHA.

- You will need to earn 4 credits during each 2 years of your instructor recognition by doing any combination of the following:
  - Teach an instructor-led ACLS class (1 credit per class).
  - Conduct the hands-on session of a HeartCode® ACLS blended-learning course. Each day of HeartCode ACLS hands-on sessions counts as 1 credit.
  - If you are also an ACLS for Experienced Providers Instructor, the ACLS for Experienced Providers classes you teach count toward your ACLS Instructor renewal.
- Attend updates as required within the previous 2 years. Updates may address new course content or methodology and review Training Center, regional, and national ECC information.
- Be monitored while teaching before your instructor status expires. The first monitoring after the Instructor Essentials Course does not satisfy this requirement.

Special Exceptions to Teaching Requirements

The requirement for instructors to teach a minimum of 4 courses in 2 years to renew instructor status may be waived or extended under special circumstances. These circumstances include, but are not limited to, the following:

- Call to active military duty (for an instructor who is in the military reserve or National Guard). Monitoring during duty may be waived if Military Training Network Faculty members are not available
- Illness or injury that has caused the instructor to take a leave from employment or teaching duties
- A limited number of courses offered in an area because of lack of audience or delay of course materials

The Training Center Coordinator, in consultation with the assigned Training Faculty, may decide to waive the teaching requirements for the discipline in question. Consideration should be given to the amount of time an instructor is away from normal employment, the length of delay in release of materials, and the number of courses taught in relation to the number of teaching opportunities. Documentation supporting the decision must be maintained in the instructor's file. All other requirements for renewal must be met as stated previously.

Part 2

Preparing for the Course

Course Overview

Course Overview and Design

Scientific evidence has pointed the way toward better content, while educational research has led to improved design of the Advanced Cardiovascular Life Support (ACLS) Provider Course. Both the design and the content of the AHA ACLS Provider Course are evidence based.

The ACLS Provider Course emphasizes 3 major concepts:

- The crucial importance of early high-quality CPR and early defibrillation to patient survival
- The integration of effective BLS with ACLS interventions
- The critical importance of effective high-performance team interaction, timing, and communication during resuscitation

The course is designed to give students the opportunity to practice and demonstrate proficiency in the following skills used in resuscitation:

- Systematic approach (assessment)
- High-quality BLS
- Airway management
- Rhythm recognition
- Defibrillation
- Intravenous (IV)/intraosseous (IO) access (information only)
- Use of medications
- Cardioversion
- Transcutaneous pacing
- High-performance teams

Students will practice applying these and other skills in simulated cases and will practice in both Team Leader and team member roles.

Course Description

The ACLS Provider Course is designed for healthcare providers who either direct or participate in the management of cardiopulmonary arrest or other cardiovascular emergencies. Through instruction and active participation in simulated cases, students will enhance their skills in the recognition and intervention of cardiopulmonary arrest, post–cardiac arrest care, acute arrhythmia, stroke, and acute coronary syndromes (ACS).

Course Goal

The goal of the ACLS Provider Course is to improve outcomes for adult patients of cardiac arrest and other cardiopulmonary emergencies through early recognition and interventions by high-performance teams.

Course Objectives

After successfully completing this course, students should be able to

- Define *systems of care*
- Apply the BLS, Primary, and Secondary Assessments sequence for a systematic evaluation of adult patients
- Discuss how the use of a rapid response team (RRT) or medical emergency team (MET) may improve patient outcomes
- Discuss early recognition and management of ACS, including appropriate disposition
- Discuss early recognition and management of stroke, including appropriate disposition
- Recognize bradycardias and tachycardias that may result in cardiac arrest or complicate resuscitation outcome
- Perform early management of bradycardias and tachycardias that may result in cardiac arrest or complicate resuscitation outcome
- Model effective communication as a member or leader of a high-performance team
- Recognize the impact of team dynamics on overall team performance
- Recognize respiratory arrest
- Perform early management of respiratory arrest
- Recognize cardiac arrest
- Perform prompt, high-quality BLS including prioritizing early chest compressions and integrating early automated external defibrillator (AED) use
- Perform early management of cardiac arrest until termination of resuscitation or transfer of care, including post–cardiac arrest care
- Evaluate resuscitative efforts during a cardiac arrest through continuous assessment of CPR quality, monitoring the patient's physiologic response, and delivering real-time feedback to the team

Educational Design

The ACLS Course uses a variety of teaching methods and adult learning principles in an environment that, in some cases, will mimic (simulate) or actually be a real healthcare setting (eg, the back of an ambulance, an emergency department bed). **From an educational perspective, the closer the simulated emergency is to a real-life case (eg, setting, equipment), the better the transfer of skills.** Cognitive, psychomotor, and some affective domains will be accomplished through small-group teaching and case scenario practice on a manikin as Team Leader and team members (ie, hands-on learning).

Simulation has been the fundamental educational model for ACLS for more than 20 years. Although the technology is more sophisticated and the science of simulation education continues to expand, the fundamentals remain the same. Simulation offers students the opportunity to learn and practice their cognitive and psychomotor skills before applying them to real patients. There is ample evidence from many disciplines to support the effectiveness of such simulation-based education in improving participant knowledge, skills, team performance, leadership, and communication. For this reason, the ACLS Course continues to incorporate this model in its design.

The AHA provides a range of experiences to engage different types of students with various learning styles, with a common goal of optimizing performance in real emergencies and saving lives.

To maximize student learning and retention, scenarios can be tailored to fit specific locations in certain sessions with certain groups.

Different course and program formats are available to accommodate the learning needs of individual students and offer flexibility for instructors:

- Instructor-led ACLS
- HeartCode ACLS
- RQI® (Resuscitation Quality Improvement®)
- Instructor-led ACLS for Experienced Providers

All formats use a different learning approach, with an emphasis on knowledge and skills integration. For more information on RQI programs, visit **rqipartners.com**. ACLS for Experienced Providers is an advanced ACLS Course for seasoned providers in emergency and critical care.

Instructor-Led Training

In instructor-led training, precourse preparation is required so that students are prepared for the course at a Training Center or other facility. The course is structured as follows:

- The Training Center may choose for students to complete online video lessons before coming to class, or may choose to conduct a traditional ACLS course, where all video lessons are conducted in class as interactive discussions with the students. Refer to the Sample Agenda for ACLS Traditional Course in Part 3.
- Core concepts are presented online through video lessons, instructor-led discussions, and case-based scenarios around a manikin.
- The instructor coaches students by using a feedback device as they practice CPR and ventilation skills.
- The instructor monitors as each student/team demonstrates skills proficiency as outlined in the skills testing checklist.
- Students take an exam to confirm their understanding of core concepts.

Blended Learning (HeartCode)

Blended learning combines the flexibility of online learning with on-site skills practice and testing.

Course Structure

A blended-learning course is structured as follows:

- Core concepts are presented in an online, adaptive, interactive format by using the HeartCode program. Engagement is enhanced by video and interactive learning activities. The online course is self-directed; the student controls the time, place, and pacing of the instruction.
- After successfully completing the online portion, students print a certificate of completion.
- Students will work with an AHA Instructor at a Training Center or other location or through a HeartCode-compatible manikin system for the hands-on session.
- The hands-on session with an AHA Instructor includes skills practice, which is the practical, hands-on portion of this blended-learning course. The hands-on session also includes skills testing—the same skills tests conducted in the full ACLS Course and the ACLS Update Course. For Megacode Testing (**required**), at least 3 students must be present for each case scenario.

Skills Practice and Testing

Students must demonstrate that they can successfully perform each skill as outlined in the skills testing checklists (eg, performing patient assessments, performing high-quality chest compressions, using a defibrillator, inserting an oropharyngeal airway [OPA], communicating effectively in a high-performance team, achieving a high CCF).

In HeartCode, skills practice and testing can be conducted by an AHA Instructor for that discipline or by a HeartCode-compatible manikin. The HeartCode-compatible manikin system is designed to allow students to practice and test without instructor assistance. An instructor can be present to assist with the HeartCode-compatible manikin, but one is not required.

Preparing to Teach Blended-Learning Courses

So that you are prepared to teach a blended-learning course, we recommend that you perform the precourse work online and/or take the online course for each discipline that you teach. This will help you understand what students learn and are being prepared to do. As with instructor-led courses, all online courses are developed by using educational principles and best practices. Course materials are presented in a way that helps students learn and retain the information. Students are required to complete all online course activities, which are designed to teach and test core concepts. The online instruction is also designed to help students transfer and apply their knowledge to skills performance.

Instructors should review all course materials, including the instructor manual, skills testing checklists, critical skills descriptors, and skills sections of the course videos.

For the HeartCode ACLS hands-on session, please use the following materials provided in this manual:

- Lesson Plans ACLS-HeartCode P1 and ACLS-HeartCode T1
- ACLS skills testing checklists in the Appendix

Understanding HeartCode

HeartCode is a Web-based, self-paced instructional program that uses adaptive technology to cover the following:

- Systems of Care
- Systematic Approach
- Adult BLS
- ACS
- Stroke
- Bradycardia
- Tachycardia
- High-Performance Teams
- Respiratory Arrest
- Cardiac Arrest and Post–Cardiac Arrest Care
- Megacode

Validation of Online Course Certificates

When a student has completed the online portion of any AHA course, a skills practice and testing session must be completed with an AHA Instructor or an approved HeartCode-compatible manikin.

As an ACLS Instructor, you may be asked to do a skills practice and testing session for HeartCode ACLS. You can confirm that the certificate that a student brings you is valid.

 To validate a student's online completion certificate, go to **www.elearning.heart.org/verify_certificate**.

Course Audience

Course Prerequisites

Providers who take the ACLS Course, ACLS Update Course, ACLS for Experienced Providers Course, or HeartCode ACLS must be proficient in the following:

- Performing high-quality BLS skills according to the current *AHA Guidelines for CPR and ECC*
- Reading and interpreting electrocardiograms (ECGs)
- Understanding ACLS pharmacology
- Providing bag-mask ventilation

Table 3 lists additional resources to help students fulfill each of these requirements. It is unlikely that students who are unable to complete the self-directed training modules listed will be able to pass the ACLS Course.

Table 3. Additional Resources for Meeting Course Prerequisites

Prerequisite	Measurements	Resources
BLS	Be able to perform high-quality CPR and demonstrate competency in adult CPR and AED use as well as bag-mask ventilation	• BLS Course • Current *AHA Guidelines for CPR and ECC* • *ACLS Provider Manual*
ECG rhythm interpretation	Be able to identify—on a monitor and paper tracing—rhythms associated with bradycardia, tachycardia with adequate perfusion, tachycardia with poor perfusion, and pulseless arrest. These rhythms include but are not limited to • Normal sinus rhythm • Sinus bradycardia • Type I second-degree atrioventricular (AV) block • Type II second-degree AV block • Third-degree AV block • Sinus tachycardia • Supraventricular tachycardias • Atrial fibrillation • Atrial flutter • Ventricular tachycardia (monomorphic and polymorphic) • Asystole • Ventricular fibrillation • Organized rhythm without a pulse	• Precourse self-assessment • *ACLS Provider Manual* • ACLS Supplementary Material
Pharmacology	Have a basic understanding of the essential drugs used in • Cardiac arrest • Bradycardia • Tachycardia with adequate perfusion • Tachycardia with poor perfusion • Post–cardiac arrest care • ACS • Stroke	• Precourse self-assessment • *ACLS Provider Manual*

BLS Provider Course Completion Card

The AHA has designed its advanced life support courses with BLS skills as the foundation. The ACLS Course does not test all the skills for BLS and does not include the BLS exam. If a BLS Provider card is to be issued, a BLS Instructor must be present to complete the infant CPR skills tests as well as the exam.

ACLS Instructors may choose to offer testing for BLS skills and to administer the BLS exam, but doing so will add time to the ACLS Course. Thus, renewal of BLS skills during an ACLS class should be a preplanned option, with registration for the BLS portion to allow for both the students and the instructor to prepare. To assist ACLS Instructors who are interested in pursuing this option, this manual includes a Sample Agenda for ACLS Course Plus BLS Card.

For more about exercising this option, including the specific requirements that must be met, refer to Students Obtaining BLS Cards in an ACLS Course later in this part.

ACLS Student Resources

ACLS Student Resources are accessed via **eLearning.heart.org**. These include the precourse self-assessment, precourse work (video lessons), and precourse resources (Table 4; see the Instructor Network for instructions on accessing ACLS Student Resources):

Table 4. ACLS Student Resources

Resource	Description	How to use
Mandatory precourse self-assessment	The precourse self-assessment evaluates a student's knowledge in 3 sections: rhythm recognition, pharmacology, and practical application.	Complete *before the course* to help evaluate your proficiency and determine the need for additional review and practice before the course. The passing score is 70%. There is no limit on how many times you can retake it to pass.
Video lessons (mandatory for Training Centers using the precourse work option)	Thirteen video lessons cover multiple medical subjects (eg, systematic approach, acute coronary syndromes) to prepare students for the course. Each lesson includes questions to engage students.	The video lessons must be completed before entering the instructor-led training course (except ACLS Traditional Course).
Precourse Preparation Checklist	Focuses student on how to prepare appropriately for the course.	Use as a checklist.
ACLS supplementary information	• Basic airway management • Advanced airway management • ACLS core rhythms • Defibrillation • Access for medications • ACS • Human, ethical, and legal dimensions of ECC and ACLS	This additional information supplements basic concepts presented in the ACLS Course. Some information is supplementary; other areas are for the interested student or advanced provider.

To ensure that students have prepared for the course, **they must pass the precourse self-assessment with a score of 70% or higher**. After taking the precourse self-assessment and completing the video lessons, students must print out a copy of their certificate indicating their score on the precourse self-assessment and completion of all video lessons and bring it to class. For Training

Centers following the traditional ACLS Course, students will not complete video lessons in advance of attending class but will need to bring their precourse self-assessment certificate with them to class. The time needed to complete the precourse self-assessment (approximately an hour) and precourse work (online video lessons; 2 to 3 hours) will vary among students. Depending on a student's particular needs, studying the *ACLS Provider Manual* and supplementary material will add to this time.

In addition, each student should complete the Precourse Preparation Checklist.

ACLS Course Flexibility

The AHA allows instructors to tailor the ACLS Course to meet audience-specific needs. You might choose to incorporate some local protocols related to CPR into both the **learning stations and the testing stations**. The use of different CPR protocols such as compression-only CPR in the first few minutes after arrest or continuous chest compressions with asynchronous ventilation once every 6 seconds with the use of a bag-mask device are a few examples of alternative approaches to the more traditional 30:2 ratio intended to optimize CCF with high-quality CPR. A default compression-to-ventilation ratio of 30:2 should be used by less-trained healthcare providers or if 30:2 is the established protocol. If you incorporate these or other local protocols, keep in mind that any protocols for CPR used in the learning and testing stations **should remain within the framework of 2-minute cycles (rhythm checks).**

Finally, an increased number of case scenarios for a more diverse audience, along with the option to build your own scenarios, further expand your flexibility to tailor the ACLS Course.

Any changes to the course are in addition to the basic course contents as outlined in this manual and will add to the length of the course. Instructors may not delete course lessons or course components. Any additions or alterations to the course must be specifically identified to students as *non-AHA material*. Please refer to the section titled Non-AHA Content in this instructor manual for further detail.

Creating Additional Case Scenarios

To expand course flexibility and meet audience-specific needs, experienced instructors can create additional scenarios. In developing your scenarios, follow the template provided here before advancing to the next section. These are things that you have to consider and do to create a realistic scenario:

- Choose a location.
- Choose the learning station that your case scenario applies to.
- Once your scenario is filled in, use the rating scale to rate the case scenario.
- The use of real cases is a preferred way to create a realistic scenario that will be physiologically sound.
- Make sure to match the scenario rating with providers' scope of practice.
  - For the full course, generally use a scenario rating of 1 or 2.
  - For the update course, generally use a scenario rating of 2 or 3.

Use current case scenarios as a guide (in the Appendix) to help fill in the appropriate information.

ACLS Case Scenario Template

Case number, location, and topic: (example)

Case 1: Out-of-Hospital Respiratory Arrest

Scenario Rating: 3

Lead-in: (example) You are a paramedic and you respond to a restaurant for a woman having an asthma attack.

Vital Signs
Heart rate:
Blood pressure:
Respiratory rate:
SpO$_2$:
Temperature:
Weight:
Age:

Initial Information   •   •   •   **What are your next actions?**
Additional Information   •   •   •   **What are your next actions?**
Additional Information (if needed)   •   •   •   **What are your next actions?**   **Instructor notes:** (example) The paramedic must decide whether to attempt an oral endotracheal intubation, which may worsen the airway swelling, or perform a needle cricothyrotomy. Oxygen should be initiated.
[Algorithm information, where applicable; not included for every case]   **Instructor notes:** (example) The team continues high-quality chest compressions, the patient has ROSC, and the team initiates the Adult Post–Cardiac Arrest Care Algorithm.

ACLS scenario difficulty rating is 1 through 3: 1 = easy, 2 = moderate, 3 = hard.

Students Obtaining BLS Cards in an ACLS Course

ACLS Instructors who wish to offer renewal of BLS skills during an ACLS Course must ensure that all of the following requirements are met:

- Students wishing to renew BLS skills must have a current BLS Provider card (printed or eCard) and either a *BLS Provider Manual* or a HeartCode BLS certificate of completion.
- An AHA BLS Instructor or ACLS Instructor (who can also teach the BLS Course) must conduct the BLS skills testing and administer the BLS exam.
- The course agenda must be based on one of the following:
  - Sample Agenda for ACLS Course Plus BLS Card (in this manual)
  - A comparable agenda created from the content listed in the Outline for ACLS Course or the Outline for ACLS Update Course (both in this manual)
  - The revised agenda must include the following BLS Course completion requirements:
    - Practice and testing of infant CPR skills (refer to the infant skills practice and infant skills testing lesson plans in the *BLS Instructor Manual*); skills testing must be documented on the BLS Infant CPR Skills Testing Checklist
    - Child choking (refer to the adult/child choking lesson plan in the *BLS Instructor Manual*)
    - Infant choking (refer to the infant choking lesson plan in the *BLS Instructor Manual*)
    - Infant bag-mask ventilation practice (refer to the infant bag-mask lesson plan in the *BLS Instructor Manual*)
    - BLS Provider Exam, unless the student can provide a HeartCode BLS certificate of completion
- The use of an instrumented feedback device or manikin is required for adult BLS skills practice and testing.
- During learning station cases and Megacode practice and testing, CCF will be measured and recorded on the station and testing checklists.
- Completion of a BLS Course Roster is required documentation for BLS skills renewal and issuance of a new BLS Provider card.
- If the student successfully fulfills all BLS Course completion requirements, a BLS Provider card will be issued regardless of the outcome of the ACLS Course and testing.

Instructor Requirements

Who Can Teach the Course

 AHA courses must be taught by AHA Instructors who have current instructor status in their specific disciplines. For detailed information about becoming an instructor, please go to **cpr.heart.org**, and select Instructors in the Resources tab.

Each AHA course must have a Course Director physically present throughout the course. The Course Director is responsible for course logistics and quality assurance and for ensuring that Instructors follow AHA guidelines in every course they teach.

An AHA Instructor in the appropriate discipline must also perform the formal assessment or testing of students.

Lead Instructor

If more than 1 instructor is teaching in an ACLS Course, a Lead Instructor needs to be designated. The Lead Instructor will oversee the communication among all instructors before and during class. The Lead Instructor will also be responsible for issuing and ensuring that students receive course completion cards from the instructor's Training Center and that all course paperwork (eg, roster, skills testing checklists, course evaluations) is supplied for the training.

The following guidelines apply to Lead Instructors for provider courses:

- Each ACLS Provider Course must have a Lead Instructor physically on-site throughout the class.
- The Lead Instructor can also fill the role of instructor in the course.
- The Lead Instructor is responsible for course logistics and quality assurance.
- The Lead Instructor is assigned by the Training Center Coordinator.

Faculty Requirements

Table 5 lists the roles and responsibilities of instructors teaching an ACLS Course. Note that one person may perform multiple roles. One instructor is needed for each of the learning stations as well as for the Megacode Testing Stations.

Table 5. ACLS Instructor Roles and Responsibilities

Role	Responsibilities
Course Director	• Oversees communication among instructors before and during class • Oversees the overall flow of the course • Ensures adherence to schedules • Oversees the quality of the program • Issues course completion cards from his or her Training Center
Course Instructor(s)	• Teaches the course • Facilitates case scenarios • Performs debriefing after each practice • Conducts all testing • Provides remediation as needed

Instructor-to-Student Ratio

The number of students allowed to participate in this course varies and usually depends on the facility, number of instructors, and available equipment.

The ACLS Course has been developed for 12 students: 2 stations of 6 students each and 1 instructor for each station. The preferred ratio is 6 students to 1 learning station with 1 instructor, and the station rotation schedules are designed for this ratio.

In some cases, a ratio of up to 8 students to 1 instructor to 1 learning station may be permitted. However, the class time will increase for each student over the ideal number of 6 per instructor. This is because each additional student must have practice time in each of the learning stations, additional cases need to be presented to accommodate the additional students, and additional time must be allotted for testing.

The ratio of students to instructors depends on the activity, as noted in Table 6.

Table 6. Student-to-Instructor Ratios

Activity	Recommended size or ratio
Large-group interactions	The size of the group is limited by the size of the room and the number of video monitors or projection screens.
Learning stations and Megacode testing	The student-to-instructor ratio should be 6:1 up to a maximum of 8:1 (with additional time).

Student-to-Manikin Ratio

For the Airway Management Practice and Testing Stations and the High-Quality BLS Practice and Testing Stations, there should be 1 manikin for every 3 students (or a ratio as low as 1:1 if the Training Center has the equipment).

For the Preventing Arrest: Bradycardia and Tachycardia Stations; High-Performance Teams: Cardiac Arrest and Post–Cardiac Arrest Care; High-Performance Teams: Megacode Practice; and High-Performance Teams: Megacode Testing Stations, the student-to-manikin ratio is 6:1 (with a maximum ratio of 8:1, minimum of 3:1).

Instructor Preparation

Preparing to Teach

An essential component of teaching the ACLS Course is instructor preparation. Before teaching the ACLS Course or the HeartCode ACLS hands-on skills session, please take the time to read and review in detail all of the following program components:

- The *ACLS Instructor Manual*
- All lesson plans (more information about the lesson plans is presented later in this manual)
- All video material
- The *ACLS Provider Manual* and Student Resources

As you view the videos and the lesson plans (Part 6), note how the course is organized and the expectations for you and the students. Make notes on your lesson plans as needed.

This important preparation will enable you to teach the course more effectively and anticipate what you will need to do as the course unfolds. This is especially true for those parts of the course that require you to organize the students for practice or testing; present the video to give information; facilitate discussions; distribute equipment; conduct prebriefs, case scenarios, and debriefs; and give exams or skills tests.

Without adequate preparation, you will not be successful teaching the ACLS Course.

Course Planning and Support Materials

Determining Course Specifics

Before you teach a course, determine the course specifics:

- Student background
- Number of students
- Special needs or equipment
- Special room reservations (eg, simulation lab)

You will teach both large-group and small-group sessions in this course. The small-group sessions are called *learning stations* and *testing stations*.

The following skills are tested in the testing stations:

- High-quality BLS
- Bag-mask ventilation with an OPA or a nasopharyngeal airway (NPA) insertion
- High-performance teams: Megacode

Please review the *ACLS Instructor Manual* and the *ACLS Provider Manual* as part of this process.

Templates

The *ACLS Instructor Manual* and Instructor Reference Material contain templates for letters, forms, and other materials to help you prepare to teach the course. You will need to customize some of these materials, including the precourse letter.

Sample Precourse Letter to Students (ACLS Course)

We recommend that you send a letter to students before class. The sample letter shown here can also be found in the Instructor Reference Materials (Instructor Network); please modify the letter to suit your needs or those of your Training Center.

(Date)

Dear ACLS Course Student:

Welcome to the Advanced Cardiovascular Life Support (ACLS) Provider Course.

When and Where the Class Will Be Given

Date:

Time:

Location:

Please plan to arrive on time, because it will be difficult for late students to catch up once we start. Students are expected to attend and participate in the entire course.

What We Sent You

We have enclosed the agenda and your copy of the *ACLS Provider Manual*. Use the following steps to access the Student Resources:

1. Visit **elearning.heart.org/courses**.
2. Find the course name (**instructor: insert the exact course name from the catalog here**).
3. Once you find your course, select Launch Course to begin.

Note: If you haven't already logged in, the system will ask you to do so. If you haven't visited the site before, you'll be prompted to set up an account.

How to Get Ready

The ACLS Course is designed to teach you the lifesaving skills required to be both a team member and a Team Leader in either an in-hospital or out-of-hospital setting. Because the ACLS Course covers extensive material in a short time, you will need to prepare for the course beforehand.

Precourse Requirements

You should **prepare for class** by doing the following:

1. Review and understand the information in your *ACLS Provider Manual*.
2. Review, understand, and **pass the mandatory precourse self-assessment**.
3. Review, understand, and **complete the mandatory precourse work (video lessons)**. You must pass the precourse self-assessment before gaining access to the video lessons. Once you have passed the ACLS Precourse Self-Assessment and completed the video lessons, print your certificate and score report, and bring them with you to class.

Ensure that your BLS skills and knowledge are current for the resuscitation scenarios. You will be tested on adult high-quality BLS skills using a feedback manikin at the beginning of the ACLS Course. You must know this in advance because you will not be taught how to do CPR or use an AED.

What to Bring and What to Wear

Bring your *ACLS Provider Manual* to each class. You will need it during each lesson in the course. You may wish to purchase the AHA's *Handbook of Emergency Cardiovascular Care for Healthcare Providers* (optional), which you may bring to class to use as a reference guide during some of the stations in the course.

Please wear loose, comfortable clothing to class. You will be practicing skills that require you to work on your hands and knees, and the course requires bending, standing, and lifting. If you have any physical condition that might prevent you from engaging in these activities, please tell an instructor. The instructor may be able to adjust the equipment if you have back, knee, or hip problems.

We look forward to welcoming you on (day and date of class). If you have any questions about the course, please call (name) at (telephone number).

Sincerely,

(Name), Lead Instructor

Sample Precourse Letter to Students (ACLS Traditional Course)

We recommend that you send a letter to students before class. The sample letter included here is also in the Instructor Reference Materials (Instructor Network); please modify the letter to suit your needs or those of your Training Center.

(Date)

Dear ACLS Course Student:

Welcome to the Advanced Cardiovascular Life Support (ACLS) Provider Course.

When and Where the Class Will Be Given
Date:

Time:

Location:

Please plan to arrive on time, because it will be difficult for late students to catch up once we start. Students are expected to attend and participate in the entire course.

What We Sent You
We have enclosed the agenda and your copy of the *ACLS Provider Manual*.

Use the following steps to access the Student Resources:

1. Visit **elearning.heart.org/courses**.
2. Find the course name (**instructor: insert the exact course name from the catalog here**).
3. Once you find your course, select Launch Course to begin.

Note: If you haven't already logged in, the system will ask you to do so. If you haven't visited the site before, you'll be prompted to set up an account.

How to Get Ready
The ACLS Course will teach you the lifesaving skills required to be both a team member and a Team Leader in either an in-hospital or out-of-hospital setting. Because the ACLS Course covers extensive material in a short time, you will need to prepare for the course beforehand.

Precourse Requirements
You should **prepare for class** by doing the following:

1. Review and understand the information in your *ACLS Provider Manual*.
2. Review, understand, and **pass the mandatory precourse self-assessment**. Print your certificate and score report and bring them with you to class.
3. Ensure that your BLS skills and knowledge are current for the resuscitation scenarios. At the beginning of the ACLS Course, you will be tested on adult high-quality BLS skills, using a feedback manikin. You must know these skills in advance because the ACLS Course will not teach you how to do CPR or use an AED.

What to Bring and What to Wear
Bring your *ACLS Provider Manual* to class. You will need it during each lesson in the course. You may wish to purchase the AHA's *Handbook of Emergency Cardiovascular Care for Healthcare Providers* (optional), which you may bring to class to use as a reference guide during some of the learning stations.

Please wear loose, comfortable clothing to class. You will be practicing skills that require working on your hands and knees, bending, standing, and lifting. If you have any physical condition that might prevent you from engaging in these activities, please tell an instructor. The instructor may be able to adjust the equipment if you have back, knee, or hip problems.

We look forward to welcoming you on (day and date of class). If you have any questions about the course, please call (name) at (telephone number).

Sincerely,

(Name), Lead Instructor

Sample Precourse Letter to Students (HeartCode ACLS)

The letter provided here is a sample that you may modify and send to students enrolled in HeartCode ACLS.

(Date)

Dear ACLS Course Student:

Welcome to the HeartCode® ACLS Course. This course has 2 components: an online portion and an instructor-led classroom portion. You must complete the online portion first.

You can access the online portion of the course by using this unique URL: [student's license URL].

Important: You must print the certificate of completion at the end of the online portion. You will need to give this to your instructor when you attend the classroom portion. It is necessary to show that you completed the online portion. If you do not have your certificate of completion, you will not be able to complete the skills practice and testing portion of the course.

The classroom portion is scheduled for

Date:

Time:

Location:

Please wear loose, comfortable clothing. You will be practicing skills that require working on your hands and knees, bending, standing, and lifting. If you have physical conditions that might prevent you from participating in the course, please tell one of the instructors when you arrive for class. The instructor will work to accommodate your needs within the stated course completion requirements. In the event that you are ill, please notify your instructor to reschedule your training.

We look forward to welcoming you on (day and date of class). If you have any questions about the course, please call (name) at (telephone number).

Sincerely,

(Name), Lead Instructor

Room Requirements

You can teach a typical course—for example, with 12 students and 2 instructors—in 1 large room and 2 small rooms. The large room should comfortably hold at least 20 people. The smaller rooms must hold up to 8 students plus 1 instructor and the required manikins and equipment.

Both large and small rooms should have:

- Good acoustics
- Bright lighting that can be adjusted for video presentations
- An instructor-controlled video player or computer and a monitor large enough to be viewed by all the students (although a TV may be acceptable for small classes with only a few students, larger classes may require a large-screen TV or a computer and LCD projector)
- A chair for each student
- A table for completing the ACLS exam (if not taking online)

Core Curriculum

Each AHA course must follow the guidelines and core curriculum in the most current editions of the *ACLS Provider Manual* and *ACLS Instructor Manual*. Current editions of AHA course materials must serve as the primary training resources during the course.

The instructor tools include extensive materials to help you teach the ACLS Course, as described in this section.

ACLS Instructor Manual and Instructor Reference Material

The Instructor Reference Material (which includes content formerly found on the Instructor CD) contains copies of many of the important materials included in the *ACLS Instructor Manual*, for example, lesson plans, case scenarios, and electronic versions of the learning stations checklists, Megacode Testing Checklists, and High-Quality BLS and Airway Management Testing Checklists. Having the material available in 2 formats gives instructors and course coordinators flexibility in retrieving the information.

Lesson Plans

Located in Part 6, these lesson plans are full-color, 2-sided, 3-hole–punched information cards used to guide the instructor through each lesson. The lesson plans will guide you in teaching each lesson in the course. The **lesson plans are very important to use because they ensure that the instructional design is preserved and all content is covered.** The AHA recommends that instructors use the lesson plans **every time** they teach an ACLS class.

Posters (Optional)

Ten 4-color, 22 × 34-inch wall posters:

- Adult Cardiac Arrest Algorithm
- Acute Coronary Syndromes Algorithm
- Adult Suspected Stroke Algorithm
- Adult Tachycardia With a Pulse Algorithm
- Adult Bradycardia Algorithm
- Adult Cardiac Arrest Circular Algorithm
- Relationship of 12-Lead ECG to Coronary Artery Anatomy
- Adult Post–Cardiac Arrest Care Algorithm
- Cardiac Arrest in Pregnancy In-Hospital ACLS Algorithm
- Adult Ventricular Assist Device Algorithm

Place the posters in a prominent location, or have students use other AHA materials that contain the AHA algorithms in each of the learning stations in the course to guide and reinforce skills practice. Also place such materials in common areas of the workplace or organization (eg, emergency department resuscitation rooms and break room, crash carts, intensive care unit break room) to remind employees and staff of steps to take in an emergency.

High-Performance Teams: Megacode Testing Checklist Masters

Use the High-Performance Teams: Megacode Testing Checklist (in the Appendix) to evaluate Team Leaders and team members during the Megacode Test.

Learning Station Checklists

- Preventing Arrest: Bradycardia Learning Station Checklist
- Preventing Arrest: Tachycardia (Stable and Unstable) Learning Station Checklist
- High-Performance Teams: Cardiac Arrest and Post–Cardiac Arrest Care Learning Station Checklist
- High-Performance Teams: Megacode Practice Learning Station Checklist

Use the learning station checklists (in the Appendix) to evaluate Team Leaders and team members during the Bradycardia, Tachycardia, High-Performance Teams: Cardiac Arrest and Post–Cardiac Arrest Care, and High-Performance Teams: Megacode Practice Learning Stations.

Handbook of ECC (Optional)

The *Handbook of Emergency Cardiovascular Care for Healthcare Providers* (Handbook of ECC) may be purchased (optional) through the AHA website at **ShopCPR.Heart.org**. Students may use the Handbook of ECC during all learning stations and exams, as well as during the Megacode test, with the following restrictions:

- A student may use the Handbook of ECC to check a drug dose during the learning and testing stations.
- The students should be able to complete the Megacode Test without looking up a majority of the questions. However, it is OK for a student to occasionally look things up during the Megacode Test.

ACLS Provider Manual

The *ACLS Provider Manual* is designed to be both a stand-alone publication and a complement to the ACLS Course. We strongly recommend that both instructors and students review the appropriate sections before each course session. Students should keep their manuals with them during all course activities.

The provider manual should be used to enhance the student's learning process throughout the ACLS Course. **To achieve this, lesson plans will call out when students should refer to specific sections of the provider manual. Instructors should refer to the provider manual often during each class session.**

The ACLS Student Resources contains the following content:

- Precourse self-assessment (a passing score is 70%)
- 13 interactive video lessons (precourse work except for students in the ACLS Traditional Course; see sample agendas)
- Precourse Preparation Checklist
- Additional supplementary ACLS information
- Two optional videos (IO and Coping With Death)
- Each student must have the current *ACLS Provider Manual* readily available for use before, during, and after class.

The *ACLS Provider Manual* is designed for individual use and is an integral part of the student's education. Students may reuse their manuals for future courses until new science guidelines are published.

ACLS Course Videos

The course videos (DVD or streaming option) included with the instructor package or purchased separately cover these major topics:

- High-Performance Teams: In-Hospital
- High-Performance Teams: Out-of-Hospital

Optional section (students see most of these videos in their precourse work unless they are taking the ACLS Traditional Course):

- Systems of Care
- Science of Resuscitation
- Systematic Approach
- CPR Coach
- High-Quality BLS
- Airway Management (short version)
- Airway Management (long version)
- Recognition: Signs of Clinical Deterioration
- Acute Coronary Syndromes
- Stroke
- Algorithms (4)
  - Cardiac Arrest
  - Bradycardia
  - Tachycardia
  - Post–Cardiac Arrest Care
- Intraosseous Access
- Coping With Death

The following videos become mandatory for the classroom if the traditional agenda is followed (see Sample Agenda for ACLS Traditional Course):

- Systems of Care
- Science of Resuscitation
- Systematic Approach
- CPR Coach
- High-Quality BLS
- Airway Management (short version)
- Recognition: Signs of Clinical Deterioration
- Acute Coronary Syndromes
- Stroke
- Algorithms (4)
  - Cardiac Arrest
  - Bradycardia
  - Tachycardia
  - Post–Cardiac Arrest Care

Precourse Preparation

Student preparation is essential for participating in and completing the ACLS Course. Passing the precourse self-assessment and completing the online interactive video lessons (if the precourse work option is selected) is required for entrance into the course. The precourse self-assessment allows the student to understand any gaps in the knowledge needed to participate in and successfully complete the course. A student who enters the ACLS Course without basic arrhythmia, pharmacology, high-quality BLS, and bag-mask ventilation knowledge and skills will not be able to function in the learning and testing stations and is unlikely to successfully complete the ACLS Course. The video lessons provide further core cognitive knowledge to participate in the course and allow more hands-on time in person.

Students should prepare for the ACLS Course by doing the following:

1. View the Precourse Preparation Checklist found in the ACLS Student Resources.
2. Review the course agenda.
3. Review and understand the information in their *ACLS Provider Manual*.
4. Review, understand, and pass the precourse self-assessment in the Student Resources.
5. Review, understand, and complete the precourse work video lessons in the Student Resources (except for traditional courses; see Sample Agenda for ACLS Traditional Course).
6. Ensure that their BLS skills and knowledge are current for the resuscitation scenarios. Students will be tested on adult compressions and AED skills as well as on bag-mask ventilation skills at the beginning of the ACLS Course.

Course Equipment

All AHA ECC courses require that manikins and equipment allow demonstration of the core skills of the course being taught (eg, airway management, correct hand placement, compression depth, chest recoil).

Equipment List

Equipment required for each class held is listed in the table in this section. All equipment used must be clean and in proper working order and good repair.

Table 7 lists the equipment and supplies needed to optimally conduct this course. This includes a code cart for in-hospital providers and a jump kit and defibrillator unit for prehospital providers.

Table 7. Classroom Equipment and Supplies

Equipment and supplies	Quantity needed	Learning/testing station where equipment needed
Paperwork		
Course roster	1/class	Beginning of course
Listing of student groups	1/class	All
Name tags	1/student and instructor	All
Course agenda	1/student and instructor	All
Course completion card	1/student	End of course
ACLS Provider Manual	1/student and instructor	All
Handbook of ECC (optional)	1/student and instructor	All
ACLS posters	1 set/class	All
Precourse letter	1/student	Precourse
Airway Management Skills Testing Checklist	1/student	Airway Management

(continued)

Equipment and supplies	Quantity needed	Learning/testing station where equipment needed
Adult High-Quality BLS Skills Testing Checklist	1/student	High-Quality BLS
High-Performance Teams: Megacode Testing Checklist	1/student	Megacode Testing
ACLS Provider Course exam (if not taking online)	1/student	Exam
Blank exam answer sheet (if not taking online)	1/student	Exam
Exam answer key (if not taking online)	1/class	Exam
ACLS Instructor Manual (including case scenarios) and ACLS Lesson Plans	1/instructor	All
Learning station checklists	1/student	High-Quality BLS; Airway Management; Preventing Arrest: Bradycardia; Preventing Arrest: Tachycardia (Stable and Unstable); High-Performance Teams: Cardiac Arrest and Post–Cardiac Arrest Care and High-Performance Teams: Megacode Practice
Audiovisual Equipment		
Course video: TV with DVD player or computer with internet access/streaming capability and projection screen	1/station	High-Performance Teams: Megacode; all other videos are optional if completed in the precourse work
CPR and AED Equipment		
Adult CPR manikin with shirt	1/every 3 students	High-Quality BLS
Adult airway manikin	1/every 3 students	Airway Management
Adult manikin (airway, CPR, and defibrillation capable)	1/every 6 students	Technology Review; Preventing Arrest: Bradycardia; Preventing Arrest: Tachycardia (Stable and Unstable); High-Performance Teams: Cardiac Arrest and Post–Cardiac Arrest Care; High-Performance Teams: Megacode Practice; and High-Performance Teams: Megacode Testing
CPR/short board	1/station	High-Quality BLS; High-Performance Teams: Cardiac Arrest and Post–Cardiac Arrest Care; High-Performance Teams: Megacode Practice; and High-Performance Teams: Megacode Testing
Code cart or jump kit	1/station	Technology Review; Bradycardia; Tachycardia; High-Performance Teams: Cardiac Arrest and Post–Cardiac Arrest Care; High-Performance Teams: Megacode Practice; and High-Performance Teams: Megacode Testing

(continued)

Equipment and supplies	Quantity needed	Learning/testing station where equipment needed
Stopwatch/timing device (ventilation timing or CCF)	1/instructor	Airway Management; High-Performance Teams: Cardiac Arrest and Post–Cardiac Arrest Care; High-Performance Teams: Megacode Practice; and High-Performance Teams: Megacode Testing
Countdown timer	1/instructor	All
Feedback device (required)	1/station	High-Quality BLS; Airway Management; High-Performance Teams: Cardiac Arrest and Post–Cardiac Arrest Care; High-Performance Teams: Megacode Practice; and High-Performance Teams: Megacode Testing
AED trainer with adult AED training pads	1/every 3 students	High-Quality BLS
Step stools to stand on for CPR	1/every 3 students	High-Quality BLS; High-Performance Teams: Cardiac Arrest and Post–Cardiac Arrest Care; High-Performance Teams: Megacode Practice; and High-Performance Teams: Megacode Testing
Ultrasound (optional)	1 every 6 students	High-Performance Teams: Cardiac Arrest and Post–Cardiac Arrest Care; High-Performance Teams: Megacode Practice; and High-Performance Teams: Megacode Testing
Airway and Ventilation		
Bag-mask device, reservoir, and tubing	1/every 3 students	All but High-Quality BLS; Preventing Arrest: Bradycardia; and Preventing Arrest: Tachycardia (Stable and Unstable)
Oral and nasal airways	1 set/station	All but High-Quality BLS; Preventing Arrest: Bradycardia; and Preventing Arrest: Tachycardia (Stable and Unstable)
Water-soluble lubricant	1/station	All but High-Quality BLS; Preventing Arrest: Bradycardia; and Preventing Arrest: Tachycardia (Stable and Unstable)
Nonrebreathing mask	1/every 3 students	All but High-Quality BLS
Waveform capnography	1/station	Airway Management; High-Performance Teams: Cardiac Arrest and Post–Cardiac Arrest Care; High-Performance Teams: Megacode Practice; and High-Performance Teams: Megacode Testing
Rhythm Recognition and Electrical Therapy		
ECG simulator/rhythm generator	1/station	All but High-Quality BLS and Airway Management

(continued)

Equipment and supplies	Quantity needed	Learning/testing station where equipment needed
Electrodes	1/station	All but High-Quality BLS and Airway Management
Monitor capable of defibrillation/ synchronized cardioversion, transcutaneous pacing	1/station	All but High-Quality BLS and Airway Management
Pacing pads, defibrillator pads, or defibrillator gel (if pads are not used)	1/station	All but High-Quality BLS and Airway Management
Spare batteries or power cord	1/station	All but High-Quality BLS and Airway Management
Spare ECG paper	1/station	All but High-Quality BLS and Airway Management
Recommended Drugs, Drug Packages, or Drug Cards (Appendix)		
Epinephrine	1/station	Preventing Arrest: Bradycardia; High-Performance Teams: Cardiac Arrest and Post–Cardiac Arrest Care; High-Performance Teams: Megacode Practice; and High-Performance Teams: Megacode Testing
Atropine sulfate	1/station	Preventing Arrest: Bradycardia; High-Performance Teams: Cardiac Arrest and Post–Cardiac Arrest Care; High-Performance Teams: Megacode Practice; and High-Performance Teams: Megacode Testing
Amiodarone and/or lidocaine	1/station	Preventing Arrest: Bradycardia; Preventing Arrest: Tachycardia (Stable and Unstable); High-Performance Teams: Cardiac Arrest and Post–Cardiac Arrest Care; High-Performance Teams: Megacode Practice; and High-Performance Teams: Megacode Testing
Adenosine	1/station	Preventing Arrest: Tachycardia (Stable and Unstable); High-Performance Teams: Megacode Practice; and High-Performance Teams: Megacode Testing
Dopamine	1/station	Preventing Arrest: Bradycardia; High-Performance Teams: Cardiac Arrest and Post–Cardiac Arrest Care; High-Performance Teams: Megacode Practice; and High-Performance Teams: Megacode Testing
Saline fluid bags/bottles	1/station	All but ACS, Stroke, Airway Management, and High-Quality BLS
IV pole	1/station	All but High-Quality BLS and Airway Management
Safety		
Sharps container (if using real needles)	1/station	All but High-Quality BLS and Airway Management

(continued)

Equipment and supplies	Quantity needed	Learning/testing station where equipment needed
Advanced Airways (must choose endotracheal tube and at least 1 supraglottic device)		
Endotracheal tube and all equipment and supplies necessary for correct insertion	1/station	Airway Management; High-Performance Teams: Cardiac Arrest and Post–Cardiac Arrest Care; High-Performance Teams: Megacode Practice; and High-Performance Teams: Megacode Testing
Laryngeal tube and supplies necessary for correct insertion	1/station	Airway Management; High-Performance Teams: Cardiac Arrest and Post–Cardiac Arrest Care; High-Performance Teams: Megacode Practice; and High-Performance Teams: Megacode Testing
Laryngeal mask airway and supplies necessary for correct insertion	1/station	Airway Management, High-Performance Teams: Cardiac Arrest and Post–Cardiac Arrest Care, High-Performance Teams: Megacode Practice, and High-Performance Teams: Megacode Testing
Regionally available supraglottic airway and all equipment and supplies necessary for correct insertion	1/station	Airway Management; High-Performance Teams: Cardiac Arrest and Post–Cardiac Arrest Care; High-Performance Teams: Megacode Practice; and High-Performance Teams: Megacode Testing
Cleaning Supplies for Use Between Student Practice and After Every Class		
Manikin cleaning supplies	Varies	All

Note: Consider an emergency department or intensive care unit bed and/or stretcher to place manikins on for a more realistic case-based scenario during appropriate learning stations.

Teaching the Course

Interacting With Students

Greeting Students

Be sure to greet each student as they arrive so that everyone feels welcome and comfortable with you as the instructor.

During the Course

Throughout the course, try to get to know each student, observe each person's strengths and weaknesses, and work with each individual to ensure that learning is taking place. As the course progresses, share information about each student with other instructors so that every student has an opportunity for coaching, feedback, and encouragement from all instructors.

Learning Stations and Skills Practice

Introduction

During the learning stations, you will review specific skills and case scenarios with the students. There are several case scenarios for each of the learning and testing stations; both out-of-hospital and in-hospital scenarios are provided in the Appendix.

Required: An audiovisual feedback device for compression rate and depth must be present to provide real-time feedback during **all learning and testing stations** requiring CPR. In addition, CCF must be measured for the High-Performance Teams: Cardiac Arrest and Post–Cardiac Arrest Care; High-Performance Teams: Megacode Practice; and High-Performance Teams: Megacode Testing Stations.

Chest recoil can also be measured if your audiovisual feedback device provides that measure. Manual ventilation timing should be done for the Airway Management Learning and Testing Station unless an audiovisual feedback device is present (rate and volume).

Timing and real-time feedback on skills is a key focus of the course, allowing for objective measures in the pursuit of competence.

All learning and testing stations case scenarios should be conducted as if they were real emergency situations.

It is critical that every student has a role in each case and that every student has an opportunity to be the Team Leader at least 3 times in the full course and at least 1 time in the update course. Assigned student roles may vary depending on the number of students in the station. Additional students may be given roles as additional compressors, additional recorders, or as a second person managing the airway. Instructors are not required to present cases in any specific sequence, but assigned student roles should not be changed. Case order in subsequent learning stations rotates students so that no one student always goes first in the station.

Instructors should include prebriefing before each case and structured and supported debriefing after each case in the learning stations as a technique to facilitate learning, particularly when covering high-performance team concepts. Debrief students on what happened, how issues were addressed, and outcomes. **Every student must take the role of Team Leader at least 3 times during the full ACLS Course:**

- Preventing Arrest: Bradycardia or Tachycardia
- High-Performance Teams: Cardiac Arrest and Post–Cardiac Arrest Care
- High-Performance Teams: Megacode Practice
- High-Performance Teams: Megacode Testing

Every student must take the role of Team Leader at least 1 time during the ACLS Update Course:

- High-Performance Teams: Megacode Practice
- High-Performance Teams: Megacode Testing

Preparing for Learning Stations

Facilitate the learning stations:

- High-Quality BLS
- Airway Management
- Technology Review
- Preventing Arrest: Bradycardia
- Preventing Arrest: Tachycardia (Stable and Unstable)
- High-Performance Teams: Cardiac Arrest and Post–Cardiac Arrest Care
- High-Performance Teams: Megacode Practice
- High-Performance Teams: Megacode Testing

The sample agendas provided can be modified based on the needs of the Training Center. The first 3 lessons should be done in numerical order because they are the foundation of the course: Course Overview, High-Quality BLS, and Airway Management.

To prepare for the learning stations, carefully review all the material for each station in the lesson plans (Part 6) in this manual and in the *ACLS Provider Manual*. Preparation includes practicing components of a learning station. For the first few times, it may be helpful for you and other instructors to rehearse with each other. The practice sessions will make you familiar with the materials and which instructor can best cover particular sections of the content.

Additional preparation includes the following:

- Set up your learning station—make sure you have all the necessary equipment and supplies.
- Confirm that you can properly operate the simulators and manikins.
- Review the lesson plans.
- Review the Handbook of ECC (optional) and the current *AHA Guidelines for CPR and ECC*.

Conducting Learning Stations

When conducting the learning stations, introduce yourself (if necessary) as students enter the room. Describe the objectives of the learning stations. Remember that time for hands-on practice by students is essential in the learning stations.

Your responsibility is to coach the students as they perform skills, not to lecture them about specific skills. Rather than explaining everything the students should know and do ahead of each learning station, instructors will provide a brief explanation of the case called a *prebrief*. During the prebrief, you will set the stage for learning by letting the students know the purpose of that learning station and what they should be able to do by the end. Tell students that you are there to help them learn and that they should also help each other as team members. Finally, have the group members set goals that they hope to achieve as a team in the station. Facilitate skills practice in the station, and demonstrate only when indicated on the lesson plans for the station. ECC prebriefing should cover

- **Psychological safety**, ensuring a safe learning environment (it's OK to make mistakes and learn from them)
- Setting **expectations,** including discussing realism for the case
- Explaining the **rules** for the case
- Conducting the case with **mutual respect**
- Helping the team **set goals** (eg, CCF of 82%) for the case (these goals will be evaluated in the structured debriefing)

Instructors should spend more time in the beginning of the course instructing, facilitating, and guiding students in the case-based learning stations and then gradually spend less time as students acclimate to the roles and their responsibilities during each case. Encourage students to work together to help each other, making sure that key points are not missed or misunderstood. Remember that your goal as an ACLS Instructor is for your students to be ready and able to save someone's life, not just to pass the course. It is important for learning purposes that students lead and actually perform skills required in that station in real time, with real equipment. The learning stations are also designed to encourage teamwork. When the students get acclimated to their roles and responsibilities and all of these aspects come together, the team functions much better as a whole than any individual team member could function alone. As an instructor, emphasize to students the importance and advantage of teamwork, which ultimately leads to more lives being saved.

Conduct a prebriefing before the case and a structured and supported debriefing after the case (Figure 2). During the debriefing, evaluating the goals set in the prebrief will allow the team to evaluate, discuss, and determine how they performed and what they can do differently in the next case to perform better. Provide quantitative performance data, including time to key interventions, number and length of unnecessary pauses, quality of chest compressions, and CCF from the feedback manikin or with the use of timers. This gives the students clear targets for improvement.

Figure 2. Flow for High-Performance Teams: Cardiac Arrest and Post–Cardiac Arrest Care and High-Performance Teams: Megacode Practice Stations.

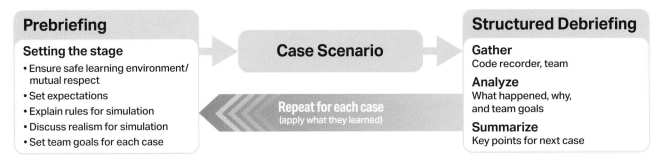

If the station includes a case-based scenario, give the Team Leader and other team members information about the case. The Team Leader will primarily manage the case with the help of the team and, as needed, with some coaching by the instructor. (Refer to Figure 3 for suggested locations for the Team Leader and team members during the case scenario.)

Be prepared to provide key information about the case as it unfolds. If the group strays from the learning station objectives, guide them back to the objectives. You can give hints or advice, but let the students work through the algorithms and the BLS, Primary, and Secondary Assessments under the direction of the student playing the role of Team Leader.

If you are a new instructor or are teaching for the first time, you may want to watch and work with an experienced ACLS Instructor before conducting a learning station on your own.

Figure 3. Suggested locations for the Team Leader and team members during case simulations and real emergencies.

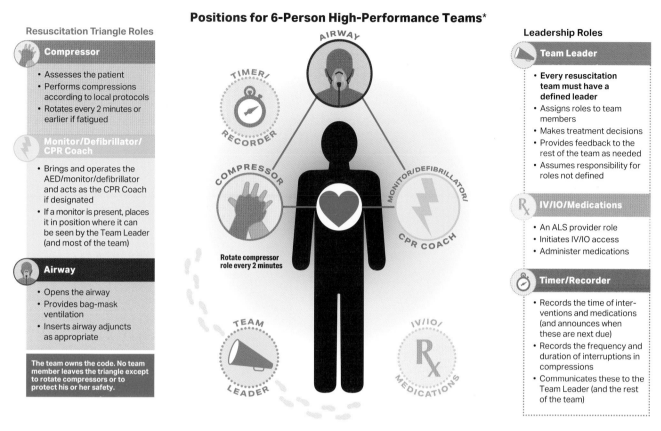

Positions for 6-Person High-Performance Teams*

Resuscitation Triangle Roles

Compressor
- Assesses the patient
- Performs compressions according to local protocols
- Rotates every 2 minutes or earlier if fatigued

Monitor/Defibrillator/ CPR Coach
- Brings and operates the AED/monitor/defibrillator and acts as the CPR Coach if designated
- If a monitor is present, places it in position where it can be seen by the Team Leader (and most of the team)

Airway
- Opens the airway
- Provides bag-mask ventilation
- Inserts airway adjuncts as appropriate

The team owns the code. No team member leaves the triangle except to rotate compressors or to protect his or her safety.

Rotate compressor role every 2 minutes

Leadership Roles

Team Leader
- **Every resuscitation team must have a defined leader**
- Assigns roles to team members
- Makes treatment decisions
- Provides feedback to the rest of the team as needed
- Assumes responsibility for roles not defined

IV/IO/Medications
- An ALS provider role
- Initiates IV/IO access
- Administer medications

Timer/Recorder
- Records the time of interventions and medications (and announces when these are next due)
- Records the frequency and duration of interruptions in compressions
- Communicates these to the Team Leader (and the rest of the team)

*This is a suggested team formation. Roles may be adapted to local protocol.

Be sure to provide adequate time for prebriefing and debriefing. It is not necessary to resolve each case clinically during the case practice; rather, end the case in a timely way to provide sufficient opportunity for discussion.

Students can wear gloves during learning station simulations just as they would in a real emergency. Donning gloves should not delay the initiation of chest compressions.

Learning Stations

CPR Coach

CPR Coaches provide peer coaching in the High-Quality BLS and Airway Management stations and in the High-Performance Teams Learning and Testing Stations (Monitor/ Defibrillator position)—as well as in real-life emergencies. During class, the CPR Coach (a student) should encourage the other students to make compression and ventilation adjustments on the basis of the audiovisual feedback and data from the timing devices. The CPR Coach should also assist the Team Leader in keeping pauses in compressions to a minimum (high CCF).

High-Quality BLS

During the High-Quality BLS Learning and Testing Stations, allow time for all students to practice compressions. Students should conduct peer coaching (CPR Coach) during the compressions practice, using feedback devices. This will influence coaching in real emergencies. The instructor can coach both the CPR Coach and the student performing the compressions (Figure 4). Test each student. Give students the feedback generated by the device in real time so that they can self-correct if possible. The goal is to develop motor memory so that the student will automatically perform compressions at the correct rate and depth without leaning on the chest. The more they do it correctly during practice, the more likely they will do it correctly in a real emergency. If the feedback device gives chest recoil feedback as well, it should be used to adjust the student.

Figure 4. Positions for High-Quality BLS Learning Station with a CPR Coach.

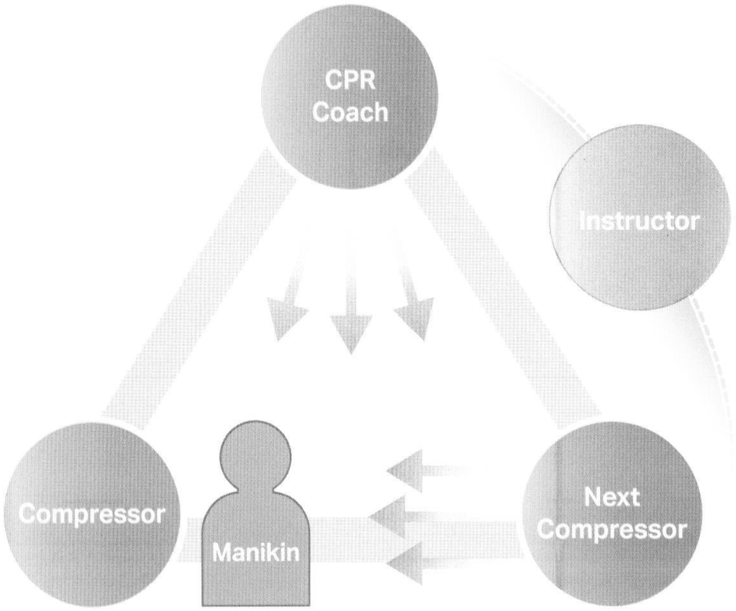

Airway Management

During the Airway Management Learning and Testing Station, allow time for all students to practice placing an OPA and an NPA, hooking up oxygen, suctioning, and ventilating with a bag-mask device for 1 minute (use a timer to monitor ventilation rates or a feedback device for rate and volume). Students should conduct peer coaching (CPR Coach) during the bag-mask ventilation practice with the use of a timer or feedback device. This will influence coaching in real emergencies. The instructor can coach both the CPR Coach and the student providing ventilation (Figure 5). Test each student. **Make sure students allow adequate pauses between breaths, because rapid ventilation is a common finding in real emergencies.** Remind students to attach the $ETCO_2$ monitor and to use it during actual resuscitation attempts, both as a signal that there is air exchange during ventilation and as an indirect measure of cardiac output during chest compressions. This includes use with a bag-mask device.

Figure 5. Positions for Airway Management Learning and Testing Station with a CPR Coach.

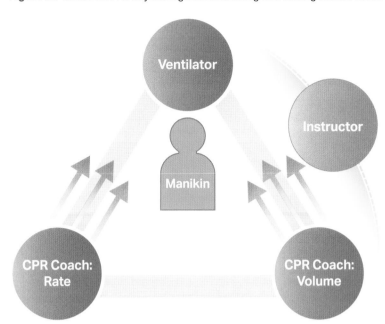

Technology and Equipment Review

Before conducting the learning stations, be sure each student is familiar with all equipment and is able to operate the monitor/defibrillator and any other necessary equipment. It is important that students get hands-on experience with the equipment they will be responsible for using during the learning stations and testing stations. Ideally, equipment would be the same as would be used in a real emergency. Demonstrate, review, and have the students practice the following:

- Monitor/defibrillator functions, buttons, and connections (features of your equipment may vary)
  - Power button
  - Transcutaneous pacing
  - Synchronized cardioversion
  - Blood pressure
  - PETCO$_2$
  - Pulse oximetry
  - Pad connections
  - ECG connections and lead placement (3-lead, 4-lead, 5-lead)
  - Optional 12-lead placement and right-sided 12-lead placement
- Review crash cart/jump kit supply locations (eg, airways, drugs)
- Explain the use of **feedback devices** (audiovisual) during the **learning and testing stations** involving CPR and ventilation. Also, explain how **timing** and objective measures are critical components of the learning and testing stations.

Be sure each student is familiar with the proper use of an AED and the transition to a manual defibrillator. Emphasize

- Remedies for pads-connector incompatibility (use an adapter, or switch pads as quickly as possible) for EMS-to–emergency department transfers
- The importance of continuous, uninterrupted chest compressions

Preventing Arrest: Bradycardia and Tachycardia

During the Bradycardia and Tachycardia Learning Stations, review the monitor/defibrillator technology if needed and review bradycardia and tachycardia rhythms with the use of a rhythm generator or static ECGs. Once these activities are completed, conduct learning station case scenarios (3 per station), assigning roles for each case. Facilitate a structured and supported debriefing after each case (refer to the Appendix).

High-Performance Teams: Cardiac Arrest and Post–Cardiac Arrest Care

During the High-Performance Teams: Cardiac Arrest and Post–Cardiac Arrest Care Learning Station, review the monitor/defibrillator technology if needed. Conduct prebriefing before each learning station case scenario (1 per student), assigning roles for each case. Facilitate a structured and supported debriefing after each case (refer to the Appendix). Students should apply what they learned from the previous case to subsequent cases. **A feedback device is required for this station, and CCF must be calculated.**

High-Performance Teams: Megacode Practice

The High-Performance Teams: Megacode Learning and Testing Station incorporates multiple algorithms in a large, case-based scenario. By the time students are ready to practice Megacode scenarios, they should have a good understanding of the component parts, so the focus here is on smooth transitions between one algorithm to another as a patient's status changes, as well as on working as a team to make sure the key actions are collaboratively and exquisitely completed.

Lead the first prebriefing, case scenario, and debriefing as the Team Leader in the demonstration case. Conduct learning station case scenarios (1 per student), assigning roles for each case. Perform prebriefing before each case and a structured and supported debriefing after each case. The team should identify and focus on areas for improvement so that every repetition is better than the last. This process should reinforce the practice of reviewing and debriefing every real resuscitation attempt, a practice that has been shown to improve subsequent resuscitation attempts (refer to the Appendix).

Case Scenarios for the Learning Stations

Learning stations can be customized for your students. The case objectives become key concepts with discussion points detailed in the instructor notes.

To vary the learning station scenarios, there are several case presentations in 3 settings: out-of-hospital, emergency department, and in-hospital. Each case contains a rating from 1 (easy) to 3 (hard). A rating of 1 or 2 should generally be used for new or returning students during the full ACLS Course. A rating of 2 or 3 should generally be used for students in the update course. A rating of 1 to 3 can be used for students during the HeartCode ACLS hands-on session. Choose the scenario that fits best for each student. Select 1 of the case scenarios in the Appendix for each student:

Respiratory Arrest

- Case 1: Respiratory Arrest—Out-of-Hospital
- Case 2: Respiratory Arrest—Out-of-Hospital
- Case 3: Respiratory Arrest—Out-of-Hospital
- Case 4: Respiratory Arrest—Out-of-Hospital
- Case 5: Respiratory Arrest—Emergency Department
- Case 6: Respiratory Arrest—Emergency Department
- Case 7: Respiratory Arrest—Emergency Department
- Case 8: Respiratory Arrest—Emergency Department
- Case 9: Respiratory Arrest—Emergency Department
- Case 10: Respiratory Arrest—In-Hospital
- Case 11: Respiratory Arrest—In-Hospital
- Case 12: Respiratory Arrest—In-Hospital
- Case 13: Respiratory Arrest—In-Hospital

Preventing Arrest: Bradycardia

- Case 14: Sinus Bradycardia—Out-of-Hospital
- Case 15: Sinus Bradycardia—Out-of-Hospital
- Case 16: Sinus Bradycardia—Out-of-Hospital
- Case 17: Sinus Bradycardia—Out-of-Hospital
- Case 18: Sinus Bradycardia—Emergency Department
- Case 19: Sinus Bradycardia—Emergency Department
- Case 20: Sinus Bradycardia—Emergency Department
- Case 21: Sinus Bradycardia—In-Hospital
- Case 22: Sinus Bradycardia—In-Hospital
- Case 23: Sinus Bradycardia—In-Hospital

Preventing Arrest: Tachycardia (Stable and Unstable)

- Case 24: Tachycardia—Out-of-Hospital
- Case 25: Tachycardia—Out-of-Hospital
- Case 26: Tachycardia—Out-of-Hospital
- Case 27: Tachycardia—Emergency Department
- Case 28: Tachycardia—Emergency Department
- Case 29: Tachycardia—Emergency Department
- Case 30: Tachycardia—In-Hospital
- Case 31: Tachycardia—In-Hospital
- Case 32: Tachycardia—In-Hospital

High-Performance Teams: Cardiac Arrest and Post–Cardiac Arrest Care

- Case 33: Cardiac Arrest—Out-of-Hospital
- Case 34: Cardiac Arrest—Out-of-Hospital
- Case 35: Cardiac Arrest—Out-of-Hospital
- Case 36: Cardiac Arrest—Out-of-Hospital
- Case 37: Cardiac Arrest—Emergency Department
- Case 38: Cardiac Arrest—Emergency Department
- Case 39: Cardiac Arrest—Emergency Department
- Case 40: Cardiac Arrest—In-Hospital
- Case 41: Cardiac Arrest—In-Hospital
- Case 42: Cardiac Arrest—In-Hospital
- Case 43: Cardiac Arrest—In-Hospital
- Case 44: Cardiac Arrest—In-Hospital
- Case 45: Cardiac Arrest—In-Hospital
- Case 46: Cardiac Arrest—In-Hospital
- Case 47: Cardiac Arrest—In-Hospital

High-Performance Teams: Megacode Practice

- Case 48: Megacode Practice—Out-of-Hospital
- Case 49: Megacode Practice—Out-of-Hospital
- Case 50: Megacode Practice—Out-of-Hospital
- Case 51: Megacode Practice—Out-of-Hospital
- Case 52: Megacode Practice—Out-of-Hospital
- Case 53: Megacode Practice—Out-of-Hospital
- Case 54: Megacode Practice—Out-of-Hospital
- Case 55: Megacode Practice—Out-of-Hospital
- Case 56: Megacode Practice—Emergency Department
- Case 57: Megacode Practice—Emergency Department
- Case 58: Megacode Practice—Emergency Department
- Case 59: Megacode Practice—Emergency Department
- Case 60: Megacode Practice—In-Hospital
- Case 61: Megacode Practice—In-Hospital
- Case 62: Megacode Practice—In-Hospital

Each case scenario has instructor notes to guide you through the scenario sequence. For your convenience, the Appendix in this manual includes a debriefing tool for each case scenario in which debriefing should be performed.

Complete the learning station checklist for each student depending on the station (in the Appendix or in the Instructor Reference Material).

Instructor Teaching Materials

Understanding Icons

The icons used in the lesson plans as well as in the course videos are there to remind you of what specific action needs to be taken at that point in the course. The icons used throughout the course are included in Table 8.

Table 8. Lesson Plan Icons

Icon	Definition
▶	Play the video
⏸	Pause the video
💬	Interactive discussion
🏃	Students practice
🔄	Students rotate
☑	Exam or skills test

Understanding Lesson Plans

All AHA ECC instructor manuals include lesson plans. The purposes of lesson plans are to

- Help you as an instructor to facilitate your courses
- Ensure consistency from course to course
- Keep you focused on the main objectives for each lesson
- Explain your responsibilities during the course

Lesson plans are meant to be used only by you as the instructor. They are your tools to guide you, so make notations on them and make them your own. Figure 6 depicts a sample lesson plan.

Figure 6. Sample Lesson Plan.

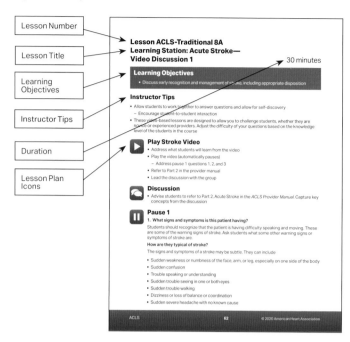

Using Lesson Plans

Your lesson plans were created to be used before and during class and during skills practice and testing sessions, as noted in Table 9.

Table 9. When and How to Use Lesson Plans

When	How to use
Before class	Review your lesson plans to understand • Objectives for each lesson • Your role for each lesson plan • Resources that you need for each lesson Make notes of things you want to remember or add.
During class	• Follow each lesson plan as you conduct the course. • Remind students what each video segment covers. • Make sure you have all the resources, equipment, and supplies ready for each lesson. • Help the students achieve the objectives identified for each lesson.
During practice before a skills test	A student may have a question about a certain part of skills they will be tested on. The lesson plans serve as a resource for you when answering those questions.

Course Outlines and Agendas

The ACLS Provider Course is made up of 9 lessons plus the Megacode and exam. The course was designed with a ratio of 6 students to 1 instructor to 1 manikin or station. The High-Quality BLS and Airway Management stations require 1 instructor and 2 manikins for 6 students per station.

The ratio of students to instructors in an AHA ACLS Provider Course may not exceed 8 students to 1 instructor. Adding a seventh or eighth student will cause the total course time to increase by approximately 80 minutes per student.

This section provides sample agendas and outlines for the ACLS Course, the ACLS Traditional Course, and the ACLS Traditional Update Course. Please note that times given in the charts are approximate and may vary from class to class. In addition, the Course Director will need to factor in transition times between activities and rooms.

Sample Agenda for ACLS Course

12 Students, 2 ACLS Instructors; approximately 12 to 13 hours with breaks

Day 1		
8:30 **Lesson START:** Welcome, Introductions, and Course Administration 8:45 **Lesson 1:** ACLS Course Overview and Organization		
Divide class into 2 groups	**Lesson 2** Learning/Testing Station: High-Quality BLS	**Lesson 2** Learning/Testing Station: High-Quality BLS
8:55	Group 1	Group 2
Divide class into 2 groups	**Lesson 3** Learning/Testing Station: Airway Management	**Lesson 3** Learning/Testing Station: Airway Management
9:40	Group 2	Group 1
10:25 **Break**		
One large group (or 2 small groups) 10:40 **Lesson 4:** Technology Review		
Divide class into 2 groups	**Lesson 5** Learning Station: Preventing Arrest: Bradycardia	**Lesson 6** Learning Station: Preventing Arrest: Tachycardia (Stable and Unstable)
10:55	Group 1	Group 2
11:55 **Lunch**		
12:50	Group 2	Group 1
One large group (or 2 small groups) 1:50 **Lesson 7:** High-Performance Teams 2:20 **Break**		
Divide class into 2 groups	**Lesson 8** Learning Station: High-Performance Teams: Cardiac Arrest and Post–Cardiac Arrest Care	**Lesson 8** Learning Station: High-Performance Teams: Cardiac Arrest and Post–Cardiac Arrest Care
2:35	Group 1	Group 2
5:05 **End of Day 1**		

Day 2		
Divide class into 2 groups	**Lesson 9** Learning Station: High-Performance Teams: Megacode Practice	**Lesson 9** Learning Station: High-Performance Teams: Megacode Practice
8:30	Group 2	Group 1
10:50 **Break**		
Divide class into 2 groups	High-Performance Teams: Megacode Testing and Megacode Testing Details **Lessons T2-T4**	High-Performance Teams: Megacode Testing and Megacode Testing Details **Lessons T2-T4**
11:00	Group 1	Group 2
One large group (as students finish the Megacode Test) 12:15 Exam (T5-T6) 1:00 Remediation/Class Ends		

Sample Agenda for ACLS Update Course

12 Students, 2 ACLS Instructors; approximately 7.25 to 8.25 hours with breaks

Single day		
8:30 **Lesson START:** Welcome, Introductions, and Course Administration		
8:45 **Lesson 1:** ACLS Course Overview and Organization		
Divide class into 2 groups	**Lesson 2** Learning/Testing Station: High-Quality BLS	**Lesson 2** Learning/Testing Station: High-Quality BLS
8:55	Group 1	Group 2
Divide class into 2 groups	**Lesson 3** Learning/Testing Station: Airway Management	**Lesson 3** Learning/Testing Station: Airway Management
9:40	Group 2	Group 1
10:25 **Break**		
One large group (or 2 small groups)		
10:40 **Lesson 4:** Technology Review		
10:55 **Lesson 5:** High-Performance Teams **(Lesson 7 in ACLS Lesson Plans)**		
11:25 **Lunch**		
Divide class into 2 groups	**Lesson 6** Learning Station: High-Performance Teams: Megacode Practice **(Lesson 9 in ACLS Lesson Plans)**	**Lesson 6** Learning Station: High-Performance Teams: Megacode Practice **(Lesson 9 in ACLS Lesson Plans)**
12:15	Group 2	Group 1
2:35 **Break**		
Divide class into 2 groups	High-Performance Teams: Megacode Testing and Megacode Testing Details **Lessons T2-T4**	High-Performance Teams: Megacode Testing and Megacode Testing Details **Lessons T2-T4**
2:50	Group 1	Group 2
One large group (as students finish the Megacode Test)		
4:05 Exam (T5-T6)		
4:50 Remediation/Class Ends		

Sample Agenda for ACLS Traditional Course

12 Students, 2 ACLS Instructors; approximately 15 to 16 hours with breaks

Day 1		
8:30 **Lesson START:** Welcome, Introductions, and Course Administration		
8:45 **Lesson 1:** ACLS Course Overview and Organization		
8:55 **Lesson ACLS-Traditional 2:** Systems of Care		
9:05 **Lesson ACLS-Traditional 3:** The Science of Resuscitation		
9:20 **Lesson ACLS-Traditional 4:** Systematic Approach		
9:35 **Lesson ACLS-Traditional 5:** CPR Coach		
Divide class into 2 groups	**Lesson 6** Learning/Testing Station: High-Quality BLS **(Lesson 2 in ACLS Lesson Plans)**	**Lesson 6** Learning/Testing Station: High-Quality BLS **(Lesson 2 in ACLS Lesson Plans)**
9:45	Group 1	Group 2
10:30 **Break**		
Divide class into 2 groups	**Lesson 7** Learning/Testing Station: Airway Management **(Lesson 3 in ACLS Lesson Plans)**	**Lesson 7** Learning/Testing Station: Airway Management **(Lesson 3 in ACLS Lesson Plans)**
10:40	Group 2	Group 1
One large group (or 2 small groups) 11:25 **Lesson 8:** Technology Review **(Lesson 4 in ACLS Lesson Plans)** 11:40 **Lesson 9:** Recognition: Signs of Clinical Deterioration **(Lesson ACLS-Traditional 6)**		
Divide class into 2 groups	**Lesson 10** Learning Station: Acute Coronary Syndromes **(Lesson ACLS-Traditional 7)**	**Lesson 11** Learning Station: Acute Stroke **(Lesson ACLS-Traditional 8)**
11:50	Group 1	Group 2
12:20	Group 2	Group 1
12:50 **Lunch**		
One large group (or 2 small groups) 1:35 **Lesson 12:** High-Performance Teams **(Lesson 7 in ACLS Lesson Plans)**		
2:05 **Break**		
Divide class into 2 groups	**Lessons 13** Learning Station: High-Performance Teams: Cardiac Arrest and Post–Cardiac Arrest Care **(Lesson 8 in ACLS Lesson Plans)**	**Lesson 13** Learning Station: High-Performance Teams: Cardiac Arrest and Post–Cardiac Arrest Care **(Lesson 8 in ACLS Lesson Plans)**
2:20	Group 1	Group 2
4:50 **End of Day 1**		

Day 2		
Divide class into 2 groups	**Lesson 14** Learning Station: Preventing Arrest: Bradycardia **(Lesson 5 in ACLS Lesson Plans)**	**Lesson 15** Learning Station: Preventing Arrest: Tachycardia (Stable and Unstable) **(Lesson 6 in ACLS Lesson Plans)**
8:30	Group 2	Group 1
9:30	Group 1	Group 2
10:30 **Break**		
Divide class into 2 groups	**Lesson 16** Learning Station: High-Performance Teams: Megacode Practice **(Lesson 9 in ACLS Lesson Plans)**	**Lesson 16** Learning Station: High-Performance Teams: Megacode Practice **(Lesson 9 in ACLS Lesson Plans)**
10:45	Group 2	Group 1
1:05 **Lunch**		
Divide class into 2 groups	High-Performance Teams: Megacode Testing and Megacode Testing Details **(Lessons T2-T4 in ACLS Lesson Plans)**	High-Performance Teams: Megacode Testing and Megacode Testing Details **(Lessons T2-T4 in ACLS Lesson Plans)**
2:00	Group 1	Group 2
3:15 **Break**		
One large group (as students finish Megacode Test) 3:25 Exam (T5-T6) 4:10 Remediation/Class Ends		

Sample Agenda for ACLS Traditional Update Course

12 Students, 2 ACLS Instructors; approximately 8 to 9 hours with breaks

8:30	**Lesson START:** Welcome, Introductions, and Course Administration
8:45	**Lesson 1:** ACLS Course Overview and Organization
8:55	**Lesson ACLS-Traditional 2:** Systems of Care
9:05	**Lesson ACLS-Traditional 3:** The Science of Resuscitation
9:20	**Lesson ACLS-Traditional 4:** Systematic Approach
9:35	**Lesson ACLS-Traditional 5:** CPR Coach

Divide class into 2 groups	**Lesson 6** Testing Station: High-Quality BLS **(Lesson 2 in ACLS Lesson Plans)**	**Lesson 7** Testing Station: Airway Management **(Lesson 3 in ACLS Lesson Plans)**
9:45	Group 1	Group 2
10:30 **Break**		
10:40	Group 2	Group 1

One large group (or 2 small groups)

11:25	**Lesson 8:** Technology Review **(Lesson 4 in ACLS Lesson Plans)**
11:40	**Lesson 9:** High-Performance Teams **(Lesson 7 in ACLS Lesson Plans)**
12:10	**Lunch**

Divide class into 2 groups	**Lesson 10** Learning Station: High-Performance Teams: Megacode Practice **(Lesson 9 in ACLS Lesson Plans)**	**Lesson 10** Learning Station: High-Performance Teams: Megacode Practice **(Lesson 9 in ACLS Lesson Plans)**
1:05	Group 1	Group 2
3:25 **Break**		
Divide class into 2 groups	High-Performance Teams: Megacode Testing and Megacode Testing Details **(Lessons T2-T4 in ACLS Lesson Plans)**	High-Performance Teams: Megacode Testing and Megacode Testing Details **(Lessons T2-T4 in ACLS Lesson Plans)**
3:35	Group 1	Group 2

One large group (as students finish Megacode Test)

4:45	Exam (T5-T6)
5:30	Remediation/Class Ends **Optional: ACS and Stroke Lessons (Lessons ACLS-Traditional 7 and ACLS-Traditional 8)**

Outline for ACLS Course

Approximate course duration: 10.25 to 11.25 hours (without breaks); student-to-instructor ratio for learning stations is 6:1

Lesson number	Course event	Duration (minutes)	Type of lesson
ACLS START	Welcome, Introductions, and Course Administration	15	
ACLS 1	ACLS Course Overview and Organization	10	
ACLS 2	Learning/Testing Station: High-Quality BLS	45	
ACLS 3	Learning/Testing Station: Airway Management	45	
ACLS 4	Technology Review	15	
ACLS 5	Learning Station: Preventing Arrest: Bradycardia	60	
ACLS 6	Learning Station: Preventing Arrest: Tachycardia (Stable and Unstable)	60	
ACLS 7	High-Performance Teams	30	
ACLS 8	Learning Station: High-Performance Teams: Cardiac Arrest and Post–Cardiac Arrest Care	148	
ACLS 9	Learning Station: High-Performance Teams: Megacode Practice	138	
ACLS T2-T4	High-Performance Teams: Megacode Testing and Megacode Testing Details	12–75	
ACLS T5, T6	Exam and Exam Details	45	

(continued)

Lesson number	Course event	Duration (minutes)	Type of lesson
ACLS REM	Remediation	Variable	
ACLS VAS	Learning Station: Vascular Access (Optional)*	Variable	
ACLS COP	Learning Station: Coping With Death (Optional)*	Variable	

Optional lessons may be facilitated at any portion of the agenda.

Outline for ACLS Update Course

Approximate course duration: 6 to 7 hours (without breaks);
student-to-instructor ratio for learning stations is 6:1

Lesson number	Course event	Duration (minutes)	Type of lesson
ACLS START	Welcome, Introductions, and Course Administration	15	
ACLS 1	ACLS Course Overview and Organization	10	
ACLS 2	Learning/Testing Station: High-Quality BLS	45	
ACLS 3	Learning/Testing Station: Airway Management	45	
ACLS 4	Technology Review	15	
ACLS 5	High-Performance Teams **(Lesson 7 in ACLS Lesson Plans)**	30	
ACLS 6	Learning Station: High-Performance Teams: Megacode Practice **(Lesson 9 in ACLS Lesson Plans)**	138	
ACLS T2-T4	High-Performance Teams: Megacode Testing and Megacode Testing Details	12–75	
ACLS T5, T6	Exam and Exam Details	45	
ACLS REM	Remediation	Variable	
ACLS VAS	Learning Station: Vascular Access (Optional)*	Variable	
ACLS COP	Learning Station: Coping With Death (Optional)*	Variable	

*Optional lessons may be facilitated at any portion of the agenda.

Outline for HeartCode ACLS Hands-on Skills (Option 1)

Approximate course duration: 4.75 to 5.75 hours (without breaks); student-to-instructor ratio for learning stations is 6:1

Lesson number	Course event	Duration (minutes)	Type of lesson
ACLS START	Welcome, Introductions, and Course Administration	15	
ACLS 1	ACLS Course Overview and Organization	10	
ACLS 2	Learning Station: High-Quality BLS Practice (**Lesson 2A in ACLS Lesson Plans**)	30	
ACLS 3	Learning Station: Airway Management Practice (**Lesson 3A in ACLS Lesson Plans**)	30	
ACLS 4	Technology Review	15	
ACLS 5	Learning Station: High-Performance Teams: Megacode Practice (**Lesson 9 in ACLS Lesson Plans**)	138	
ACLS T	High-Quality BLS Testing—Testing Details (**Lesson 2B in ACLS Lesson Plans**)	15	
ACLS T	Airway Management Testing— Testing Details (**Lesson 3B in ACLS Lesson Plans**)	15	
ACLS T2-T4	High-Performance Teams: Megacode Testing and Megacode Testing Details	12–75	
ACLS REM	Remediation	Variable	

Outline for HeartCode ACLS Hands-on Skills (Option 2)

Approximate course duration: 4.75 to 5.75 hours (without breaks);
student-to-instructor ratio for learning stations is 6:1

Lesson number	Course event	Duration (minutes)	Type of lesson
ACLS START	Welcome, Introductions, and Course Administration	15	
ACLS 1	ACLS Course Overview and Organization	10	
ACLS 2	Learning/Testing Station: High-Quality BLS	45	
ACLS 3	Learning/Testing Station: Airway Management	45	
ACLS 4	Technology Review	15	
ACLS 5	Learning Station: High-Performance Teams: Megacode Practice **(Lesson 9 in ACLS Lesson Plans)**	138	
ACLS T2-T4	High-Performance Teams: Megacode Testing and Megacode Testing Details	12–75	
ACLS REM	Remediation	Variable	

Outline for ACLS Traditional Course

Approximate course duration: 12.25 to 13.25 hours (without breaks); student-to-instructor ratio for learning stations is 6:1

Lesson number	Course event	Duration (minutes)	Type of lesson
ACLS START	Welcome, Introductions, and Course Administration	15	
ACLS 1	ACLS Course Overview and Organization	10	
ACLS-Traditional 2	Systems of Care	10	
ACLS-Traditional 3	The Science of Resuscitation	15	
ACLS-Traditional 4	Systematic Approach	15	
ACLS-Traditional 5	CPR Coach	10	
ACLS 6	Learning/Testing Station: High-Quality BLS Practice (**Lesson 2 in ACLS Lesson Plans**)	45	
ACLS 7	Learning/Testing Station: Airway Management (**Lesson 3 in ACLS Lesson Plans**)	45	
ACLS 8	Technology Review (**Lesson 4 in ACLS Lesson Plans**)	15	
ACLS 9	Recognition: Signs of Clinical Deterioration (**Lesson ACLS-Traditional 6**)	10	
ACLS 10	Learning Station: Acute Coronary Syndromes (**Lesson ACLS-Traditional 7**)	30	
ACLS 11	Learning Station: Acute Stroke (**Lesson ACLS-Traditional 8**)	30	

(continued)

Lesson number	Course event	Duration (minutes)	Type of lesson
ACLS 12	High-Performance Teams (**Lesson 7 in ACLS Lesson Plans**)	30	▶ 💬
ACLS 13	Learning Station: High-Performance Teams: Cardiac Arrest and Post–Cardiac Arrest Care (**Lesson 8 in ACLS Lesson Plans**)	148	▶ 💬 🧑 🔄
ACLS 14	Learning Station: Preventing Arrest: Bradycardia (**Lesson 5 in ACLS Lesson Plans**)	60	▶ 💬 🧑 🔄
ACLS 15	Learning Station: Preventing Arrest: Tachycardia (Stable and Unstable) (**Lesson 6 in ACLS Lesson Plans**)	60	▶ 💬 🧑 🔄
ACLS 16	Learning Station: High-Performance Teams: Megacode Practice (**Lesson 9 in ACLS Lesson Plans**)	138	💬 🧑 🔄
ACLS T	High-Performance Teams: Megacode Testing and Megacode Testing Details (**Lessons T2-T4 in ACLS Lesson Plans**)	12–75	☑
ACLS T	Exam (**Lessons T5-T6 in ACLS Lesson Plans**)	45	☑
ACLS REM	Remediation	Variable	☑
ACLS VAS	Learning Station: Vascular Access	Optional	▶ 🧑
ACLS COP	Learning Station: Coping With Death	Optional	▶ 💬

Outline for ACLS Traditional Update Course

Approximate course duration: 6.75 to 7.75 hours (without breaks); student-instructor ratio for learning stations is 6:1

Lesson plan number	Course event	Duration (minutes)	Type of lesson
ACLS START	Welcome, Introductions, and Course Administration	15	
ACLS 1	ACLS Update Course Overview and Organization	10	
ACLS-Traditional 2	Systems of Care	10	
ACLS-Traditional 3	The Science of Resuscitation	15	
ACLS-Traditional 4	Systematic Approach	15	
ACLS-Traditional 5	CPR Coach	10	
ACLS 6	Learning/Testing Station: High-Quality BLS (**Lesson 2 in ACLS Lesson Plans**)	45	
ACLS 7	Learning/Testing Station: Airway Management (**Lesson 3 in ACLS Lesson Plans**)	45	
ACLS 8	Technology Review (**Lesson 4 in ACLS Lesson Plans**)	15	
ACLS 9	High-Performance Teams (**Lesson 7 in ACLS Lesson Plans**)	30	
ACLS 10	Learning Station: High-Performance Teams: Megacode Practice (**Lesson 9 in ACLS Lesson Plans**)	138	

(continued)

Lesson plan number	Course event	Duration (minutes)	Type of lesson
ACLS T	High-Performance Teams: Megacode Testing and Megacode Testing Details (**Lessons T2-T4 in ACLS Lesson Plans**)	12–75	☑
ACLS T	Exam (**Lessons T5-T6 in ACLS Lesson Plans**)	45	☑
ACLS REM	Remediation	Variable	☑

Sample Agenda for ACLS Course Plus BLS Card*

12 Students, 2 ACLS Instructors; approximately 13 to 14 hours with breaks

Day 1		
8:30 **Lesson START:** Welcome, Introductions, and Course Administration		
8:45 **Lesson 1**: ACLS Course Overview and Organization		
8:55 **Lesson 1A**: Infant CPR and Bag-Mask Ventilation Practice*		
9:10 **Lesson 1B**: Infant CPR Testing*		
9:30 **Lesson 1C**: Adult/Child Choking*		
9:35 **Lesson 1D**: Infant Choking*		
9:40 **Lesson 1E**: BLS Exam		
Divide class into 2 groups	**Lesson 2** Learning/Testing Station: High-Quality BLS	**Lesson 2** Learning/Testing Station: High-Quality BLS
10:10	Group 1	Group 2
10:55 **Break**		
Divide class into 2 groups	**Lesson 3** Learning/Testing Station: Airway Management	**Lesson 3** Learning/Testing Station: Airway Management
11:10	Group 2	Group 1
One large group (or 2 small groups)		
11:55 **Lunch**		
12:50 **Lesson 4**: Technology Review		
Divide class into 2 groups	**Lesson 5** Learning Station: Preventing Arrest: Bradycardia	**Lesson 6** Learning Station: Preventing Arrest: Tachycardia (Stable and Unstable)
1:05	Group 1	Group 2
2:05	Group 2	Group 1
One large group (or 2 small groups)		
3:05 **Break**		
3:20 **Lesson 7**: High-Performance Teams		
Divide class into 2 groups	**Lesson 8** Learning Station: High-Performance Teams: Cardiac Arrest and Post–Cardiac Arrest Care	**Lesson 8** Learning Station: High-Performance Teams: Cardiac Arrest and Post–Cardiac Arrest Care
3:50	Group 1	Group 2
6:10 **End of Day 1**		
Day 2		
Divide class into 2 groups	**Lesson 9** Learning Station: High-Performance Teams: Megacode Practice	**Lesson 9** Learning Station: High-Performance Teams: Megacode Practice
8:30	Group 2	Group 1
10:50 **Break**		

(continued)

Day 2		
Divide class into 2 groups	High-Performance Teams: Megacode Testing and Megacode Testing Details **Lessons T2-T4**	High-Performance Teams: Megacode Testing and Megacode Testing Details **Lessons T2-T4**
11:00	Group 1	Group 2
One large group (as students finish the Megacode Test)		
12:15	Exam (T5-T6)	
1:00	Remediation/Class Ends	

*See BLS Lesson Plans in the *BLS Instructor Manual.*

Sample Agenda for ACLS Update Course Plus BLS Card*

12 Students, 2 ACLS Instructors; approximately 8.5 to 9.5 hours with breaks

Single day		
8:30 **Welcome, Introductions, and Course Administration**		
8:45 **Lesson 1**: ACLS Course Overview and Organization		
8:55 **Lesson 1A**: Infant CPR and Bag-Mask Ventilation Practice*		
9:10 **Lesson 1B**: Infant CPR Testing*		
9:30 **Lesson 1C**: Adult/Child Choking*		
9:35 **Lesson 1D**: Infant Choking*		
9:40 **Lesson 1E**: BLS Exam		
Divide class into 2 groups	**Lesson 2** Learning/Testing Station: High-Quality BLS	**Lesson 2** Learning/Testing Station: High-Quality BLS
10:10	Group 1	Group 2
10:55 **Break**		
Divide class into 2 groups	**Lesson 3** Learning/Testing Station: Airway Management	**Lesson 3** Learning/Testing Station: Airway Management
11:10	Group 2	Group 1
One large group (or 2 small groups) 11:55 **Lunch** 12:45 **Lesson 4**: Technology Review 1:00 **Lesson 5**: High-Performance Teams		
Divide class into 2 groups	**Lesson 6** Learning Station: High-Performance Teams: Megacode Practice **(Lesson 9 in ACLS Lesson Plans)**	**Lesson 6** Learning Station: High-Performance Teams: Megacode Practice **(Lesson 9 in ACLS Lesson Plans)**
1:30	Group 2	Group 1
3:50 **Break**		
Divide class into 2 groups	High-Performance Teams: Megacode Testing and Megacode Testing Details **Lessons T2-T4**	High-Performance Teams: Megacode Testing and Megacode Testing Details **Lessons T2-T4**
4:00	Group 1	Group 2
One large group (as students finish the Megacode Test) 5:15 Exam (T5-T6) 6:00 Remediation/Class Ends		

*See BLS Lesson Plans in the *BLS Instructor Manual.*

Part 4

Testing

Testing for Course Completion

The AHA requires successful completion of skills tests, as well as an exam in instructor-led courses or successful completion of the online portion of HeartCode, for a student to receive an ACLS Provider course completion card. Additional information about testing and criteria for completion is presented throughout this part.

The prompt and accurate delivery of ACLS skills and knowledge by high-performance teams is critically important for patient survival. Accurate, objective, and uniform testing reinforces these lifesaving skills and knowledge and is critical for the consistent delivery of the ACLS Provider Course content by all instructors. Ensuring competent, well-trained, high-performance teams is the goal.

All ACLS Instructors are expected to maintain high standards of performance for all ACLS skills tests, as discussed in the next section.

Course Completion Requirements

To receive a course completion card, students taking the full course or the update course must attend and participate in all lessons of the respective course, pass all skills tests, and pass the exam.

The recommended update or renewal interval for all AHA courses is 2 years. **Due to natural decay of skills, institutions should conduct practice codes every 3 to 6 months or as necessary to help their providers stay sharp on high-performance team skills.** Providers who intend to take an update course must show a valid provider card to enroll in an update (or renewal) course. At the discretion of the Training Center Coordinator, Course Director, or Lead Instructor, exceptions may be allowed. The Training Center Coordinator has the final authority and responsibility for allowing a student to take an update course if he or she does not have a current AHA Provider card. Students who present an expired provider card or who do not possess a provider card may be allowed to take an update course but will not be given the option of remediation. These students will need to complete the entire provider course if they cannot successfully meet the course completion requirements when tested. If the student fails any skills test, he or she should retake the full ACLS Course.

In addition, HeartCode ACLS students must participate in a hands-on session, which includes skills practice and skills testing. Students must pass the skills tests with an AHA Instructor or HeartCode-compatible manikin system after completing the online portion.

Explain clearly to the students which actions, if not performed correctly, will result in a "no pass" and require remediation (eg, failure to confirm airway placement, shocking a perfusing rhythm).

It will be the student's responsibility to be familiar with the latest *AHA Guidelines for CPR and ECC*.

Students who meet all course prerequisites and are eligible to receive a course completion card must do the following (Table 10):

Table 10. Skills Testing and Exam Requirements

Skills testing requirements	Exam requirements
Students must successfully pass these skills tests: • High-Quality BLS Skills Test • Airway Management Skills Test with OPA/NPA insertion • Learning station competencies • High-Performance Teams: Megacode Test	Students must score at least 84% on the exam (does not apply to HeartCode students)

Skills Testing

Students must demonstrate competency in all required skills. Refer to the skills testing checklists in the Appendix for a description of requirements.

Instructors of the appropriate discipline will evaluate each student's didactic knowledge and proficiency in all core psychomotor skills of the course.

Students may use the *Handbook of ECC* and ECC algorithms for the Megacode Test.

No AHA course completion card is issued without hands-on manikin skills testing by either an AHA Instructor for that discipline or an AHA-approved computerized manikin in an AHA eLearning course.

Students in advanced life support courses are not required by the AHA to have a current BLS Provider card, but they are expected to be proficient in appropriate BLS skills. Training Centers have the option to require a current BLS Provider card.

High-Quality BLS Skills Testing

All ACLS Course students must pass the High-Quality BLS Skills Test regardless of the method of preparation or prior CPR training. All CPR testing should be done with an audiovisual feedback device (required). Table 11 describes how to use the Adult High-Quality BLS Skills Testing Checklist.

Please refer to the Remediation section in Part 1 for additional information.

High-Quality BLS Test Scenario

The High-Quality BLS Skills Testing scenario for all ACLS students is an in-hospital or out-of-hospital scenario at the top of the skills testing checklist.

Airway Management Skills Testing

All ACLS Course students must pass the Airway Management Skills Test that includes bag-mask ventilation with OPA/NPA insertion, regardless of the method of preparation or prior airway training. Ventilation should be timed to meet objective testing criteria.

Please refer to the Remediation section in Part 1 for additional information.

Mandatory Audiovisual Feedback Device

All CPR practice and testing must be performed with an audio and/or visual feedback device (required). In addition, all CPR performed in real life should be done with an audiovisual feedback device for optimal quality and timing.

Skills Testing of Blended-Learning Students

Instructors may need to conduct the hands-on session of a blended-learning course. Specific content from the ACLS Course has been incorporated into the hands-on session for a blended-learning solution. The hands-on session includes skills practice and skills testing (refer to the HeartCode Lesson Plans). The skills testing portion of the hands-on session should be conducted the same as in an instructor-led course. A minimum of 3 students should be present to conduct the required Megacode Test.

Table 11. How to Use the Adult High-Quality BLS Skills Testing Checklist

Section	How to use
Assessment and Activation	The steps in this box do not have to be completed in a specific order; the student only needs to complete all of the steps before beginning compressions. For educational purposes, it is best that students complete the steps in order, so they commit them to memory. Pulse and breathing checks can be done simultaneously. **Script** Once the student shouts for help, the instructor should say, "Here's the barrier device. I am going to get the AED."
Adult Compressions	During this section, the student should perform 2 minutes of continuous compressions before the second rescuer (student) arrives with the AED. Evaluate the student's ability to perform high-quality chest compressions. High-fidelity manikins are optimal feedback devices and are highly recommended to objectively evaluate chest compressions. If a high-fidelity manikin is not available, **feedback devices are required** to objectively evaluate chest compressions. Compressions should be initiated within 10 seconds after recognition of cardiac arrest. **Hand Placement** Evaluate the student to ensure that hand placement is in the center of the chest, on the lower half of the sternum, and that the heel of the hand is used. When the student uses 2 hands, the second hand is placed on top of or grasping the wrist of the first hand. **Rate** Compression rate should be evaluated by a feedback device to achieve a rate of 100 to 120 compressions per minute. Focusing on a midrange rate of 110 is recommended. **Depth and Recoil** Compression depth and recoil should be at least 2 inches (5 cm). Use feedback devices to monitor depth and, if possible, chest recoil. *Note:* **All CPR practice and testing should be performed with an audiovisual feedback device (required). In addition, all CPR performed in real life should be done with an audiovisual feedback device for optimal quality and timing**. *Tip*: To help students achieve adequate compression depth and to minimize fatigue, instruct them to perform chest compressions with their elbows locked and their shoulders (fulcrum) directly over the patient.

(continued)

Section	How to use
AED	The second student or instructor can arrive with an AED and hand it to the first student after completing 2 minutes of compressions. The second student or the instructor can take over compressions immediately after handing the AED to the first student and instruct the student to use the AED. The instructor can tell the student that another rescuer is providing chest compressions. In a 2-rescuer scenario, it is important that students understand that the use of an AED should not interrupt chest compressions. The student should turn the AED on as required for his or her specific device; this may require the student to push the power button on the AED, or the AED may turn on automatically when the case is opened. Students should attach the AED pads to the manikin by following the pictures on the pads. Students should follow the prompts of the AED they are using.
	Instructors should be aware that some of the AED steps outlined on the skills testing checklist might not be completely applicable to all devices. Some AEDs require the patient to be cleared during the analysis and charging cycle, and some AEDs allow compressions to be continued while the device is charging. Once the AED is ready to deliver a shock, the student should clear the patient both verbally and visually. Once everyone is clear, the student should press the shock button. The student should resume compressions immediately.
Resumes Compressions	The student being evaluated moves to the head of the manikin and prepares to use the bag-mask device while the other student or instructor resumes compressions immediately after the shock is delivered. Evaluate the student's ability to direct the other student or instructor to resume compressions immediately after the shock is delivered. When the student directs the other student or instructor to resume compressions immediately after the shock delivery, stop the test.
Test Results	If the student successfully performs all of the skills, circle "Pass" on the student's skills testing checklist. If the student does not successfully perform all of the skills, circle "NR" for needs remediation. The instructor should use a new skills testing checklist to retest (reevaluate) the student on the skills that were not performed correctly. If remediation is needed, both the skills testing checklist that indicated the need for remediation and the new skills testing checklist indicating that the student passed should be stored with the course records. Provide your initials, your instructor ID, and the date in the box at the end of the checklist.

Using the Skills Testing Checklist and Critical Skills Descriptors

Use the skills testing checklists to document the student's performance during the skills testing portion of the course. The skills testing checklist should be filled out while the student is performing the skills. Use the skills testing critical skills descriptors to determine if a student has demonstrated each step of the skill correctly.

- If the student successfully completes a step, place a check (✓) in the box to the right of the step on the skills testing checklist.
- If the student is unsuccessful, leave the box next to the step blank on the skills testing checklist. Circle the step under the critical skills descriptor that the student did not complete successfully.

If a student demonstrates each step of the skills test successfully, mark the student as passing that skills test on the skills testing checklist. If a student does not receive checks in all boxes, refer the student to the remediation lesson at the end of the course for further testing in that skill. Also, discuss with the student the areas that you circled on the critical skills descriptors and how to correctly perform each of those skills.

You should be very familiar with all of the critical skills descriptors to be able to test BLS skills correctly.

Skills Testing Checklist Rules

When using the skills testing checklist, remember the rules listed in Table 12.

Table 12. Skills Testing Checklist Rules and Reminders

Rule	Reminders
Check only the steps that the student performs correctly.	• On the Adult High-Quality BLS Skills Testing Checklist, put a check in the box next to a specific step if the student performs that step correctly based on the critical skills descriptor. • If the student does not perform that step correctly, do not mark the checklist for that step. • Once the student has correctly performed all steps, the student has passed the skills test.

Do not give hints during the test.	• Do not tell the student any specific information about the assessment steps. For example, do not say "no breathing" as the student checks for breathing.
	• Do not comment on the skills performance of the student during the test. This ensures that
	    – The student relies on his or her own assessments of the victim, makes decisions about what to do, and performs CPR *independent of the instructor*
	    – The test more accurately reflects a real-life CPR situation; *this is an important criterion to determine skills competency in CPR*

Refer to the critical skills descriptors for detailed information about what to observe.	• Do not interpret or read into the critical skills descriptors or evaluate anything not specifically identified in the skills descriptions for each skill.
	• Determine whether the student has performed a step exactly as the description indicates.
	    – If yes, place a "correct" check on the checklist for that step.
	    – If no, leave the checklist blank for that step.

Stop the test when the Adult High-Quality BLS Skills Testing Checklist indicates to do so.	• Mark the student as "Pass" or "NR" (needs remediation).
	• For those with a mark of NR:
	    – Check the steps that need more practice on the student's practice sheet
	    – Tell the student to practice those steps before retesting later in the course
	    – Conduct additional practice and retesting as part of the remediation lesson later in the course

Do not retest the student at this time.	• If the student stops the test before the stop point indicated on the checklist,
	    – Mark the student as "NR"
	    – Refer the student for more practice

Retest the entire skill.	When retesting a student during the remediation lesson, you must test the entire skill.

Advanced Cardiovascular Life Support
Adult High-Quality BLS
Skills Testing Checklist

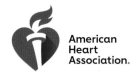

American Heart Association.

Student Name _____   Date of Test _____

Hospital Scenario: "You are working in a hospital or clinic, and you see a person who has suddenly collapsed in the hallway. You check that the scene is safe and then approach the patient. Demonstrate what you would do next."

Prehospital Scenario: "You arrive on the scene for a suspected cardiac arrest. No bystander CPR has been provided. You approach the scene and ensure that it is safe. Demonstrate what you would do next."

Assessment and Activation

☐ Checks responsiveness   ☐ Shouts for help/Activates emergency response system/Sends for AED

☐ Checks breathing   ☐ Checks pulse

Once student shouts for help, instructor says, "I am going to get the AED."

Compressions   *Audio/visual feedback device required for accuracy*

☐ Hand placement on lower half of sternum

☐ Perform continuous compressions for 2 minutes (100-120/min)

☐ Compresses at least 2 inches (5 cm)

☐ Complete chest recoil. (Optional, check if using a feedback device that measures chest recoil)

Rescuer 2 says, "Here is the AED. I'll take over compressions, and you use the AED."

AED (follows prompts of AED)

☐ Powers on AED   ☐ Correctly attaches pads   ☐ Clears for analysis   ☐ Clears to safely deliver a shock

☐ Safely delivers a shock   ☐ Shocks within 45 seconds of AED arrival

---

Resumes Compressions

☐ Ensures compressions are resumed immediately after shock delivery

• Student directs instructor to resume compressions *or*

• Second student resumes compressions

STOP TEST

Instructor Notes
• Place a check in the box next to each step the student completes successfully.
• If the student does not complete all steps successfully (as indicated by at least 1 blank check box), the student must receive remediation. Make a note here of which skills require remediation (refer to instructor manual for information about remediation).

Test Results	Circle **PASS** or **NR** to indicate pass or needs remediation:	**PASS**	**NR**

Instructor Initials _____   Instructor Number _____   Date _____

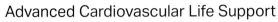

Advanced Cardiovascular Life Support
Adult High-Quality BLS
Skills Testing Critical Skills Descriptors

1. **Assesses patient and activates emergency response system (this *must* precede starting compressions) within a maximum of 30 seconds. After determining that the scene is safe:**
   - Checks for responsiveness by tapping and shouting
   - Shouts for help or directs someone to call for help and get an AED/defibrillator
   - Checks for absent or abnormal breathing (no breathing or only gasping)
     - Scans from the head to the chest looking for rise and fall for a minimum of 5 seconds and no more than 10 seconds
   - Checks carotid pulse
     - Can be done simultaneously with check for breathing
     - Checks for a minimum of 5 seconds and no more than 10 seconds
2. **Performs high-quality chest compressions (initiates compressions immediately after recognition of cardiac arrest) for 2 minutes**
   - Demonstrates correct hand placement
     - Center of the chest on the lower half of the sternum
     - 2-handed (second hand on top of the first or grasping the wrist of the first hand)
   - Achieves compression rate of 100 to 120/min
   - Performs compressions for 2 minutes (at a rate of 100/120 min)
   - Achieves correct compression depth and recoil
     - Depth: at least 2 inches (5 cm)*
     - Complete chest recoil after each compression
   - Minimizes interruptions in compressions
     - Compressions not interrupted until AED analyzes rhythm
     - Compressions resumed immediately after shock/no shock indicated
3. **AED use**
   - Powers on the AED
     - Turns the AED on by pushing the button or lifting the lid as soon as it arrives
   - Correctly attaches pads
     - Places proper-sized (adult) pads for the patient's age in the correct locations
   - Clears for analysis
     - Clears providers from the victim to allow the AED to analyze the heart rhythm (pushes the analyze button if required by the device)
     - Communicates clearly to all other providers to stop touching the victim
   - Clears to safely deliver shock
     - Communicates clearly to all other providers to stop touching the victim
   - Delivers a shock
     - Resumes chest compressions immediately after shock delivery
     - Does *not* turn off the AED during CPR
4. **Ensures that compressions are resumed immediately after shock delivery**
   - Performs the same steps for compressions

*If you have a CPR quality feedback device that allows adjustment of depth, it is optimal to target your compression depth from 2 to 2.4 inches (5 to 6 cm). This is a narrow target, so the student should not fail the test simply for compressing to a depth of more than 2.4 inches but for compressing to a shallow depth of less than 2 inches on average.

Retesting Students

If time permits in the High-Quality BLS Testing Station, you may retest a student 1 additional time if the student did not pass. All additional retesting is done at the end of the course during the remediation lesson. (Refer to the Remediation section in Part 1 and the lesson plans in Part 6.)

In every retesting case, test the student on the entire skill.

In some cases, you may defer retesting to a later time after class. For example, if remediation is not successful, you might develop a plan of improvement and schedule retesting once the student completes the plan. If a student needs substantial additional remediation, you may recommend that the student repeat the BLS or ACLS Course. The exam measures the mastery of cognitive skills and is an open-resource exam.

In some self-directed learning courses, the exam is included in the software program according to the policy for that individual course. Students can print a certificate upon successful completion of the online part of the course.

Instructors may read the exam to a student who has a learning disability or language barrier.

Each student must score at least 84% on the exam.

High-Performance Teams: Megacode

Assessment and Testing Guidelines

The ACLS Provider Course includes High-Performance Teams: Megacode Testing. Students will rotate through the Megacode Test Station. Each Megacode station is designed to test the student in the ventricular fibrillation (VF)/pulseless ventricular tachycardia (pVT) rhythm and 3 other rhythms. The Megacode Testing Checklists are included in the Appendix and in the Instructor Reference Material. You will randomly select the testing checklist to be used.

To vary the testing scenarios, there are several case presentations. Select 1 of the case scenarios from the Appendix or the Instructor Reference Material for each student:

ACLS High-Performance Teams: Megacode

- Case 1: Megacode—Out-of-Hospital
- Case 2: Megacode—Out-of-Hospital
- Case 3: Megacode—Out-of-Hospital
- Case 4: Megacode—Out-of-Hospital
- Case 5: Megacode—Emergency Department
- Case 6: Megacode—In-Hospital
- Case 7: Megacode—In-Hospital
- Case 8: Megacode—In-Hospital
- Case 9: Megacode—In-Hospital
- Case 10: Megacode—In-Hospital
- Case 11: Megacode—In-Hospital
- Case 12: Megacode—In-Hospital

Each case scenario has instructor notes to guide you through the scenario sequence. The notes will help you achieve uniform testing of students. An instructor can use the High-Performance Teams: Megacode Practice scenarios for testing to increase the selection of cases for testing. It is best practice to use the case scenarios that the students have not seen and used for practice.

Complete the testing checklist for each student (in the Appendix or in the Instructor Reference Material).

Passing the Megacode Test

At the end of the course, students will participate in a Megacode Testing Station to validate their achievement of the course objectives. A simulated case scenario will evaluate the following:

- CPR quality and timing (meeting objective goals by using a feedback device/timer)
- Achieving a CCF of greater than 80% (objective measure)
- Team communication
- Knowledge of core case material and skills
- Knowledge of algorithms
- Arrhythmia interpretation
- Use of appropriate basic ACLS drug therapy
- Performance as an effective member of a high-performance team (within the team member's scope of practice)
- Performance of the team working together to achieve prebriefing goals

During the Megacode Testing Station, the instructor or the team can decide who will be the Team Leader (within scope of practice, if possible) and assign all other roles on the basis of scope of practice (if possible). The team will be tested (ie, evaluating the team's overall performance) using objective (eg, CCF) and subjective measures (eg, team communication). If the team passes the first Megacode case, it's done. If not, it will continue with additional

Megacode cases until the team passes. The team members can keep the same roles, if they choose, or switch roles. Megacode testing is about the team members performing well together, including the Team Leader as a key member of the team. If a student is having trouble mastering skills, the instructor should address this well before the student moves all the way through the course to the Megacode Test. Students will take the role of Team Leader and all team member roles multiple times in the practice scenarios during class. If a group (team) consists of 6 students, that group should participate in 3 bradycardia and 3 tachycardia cases, 6 cardiac arrest/post–cardiac arrest cases, and 6 Megacode cases (18 cases total) before entering the Megacode Test. As previously stated, there is ample opportunity for an instructor to evaluate and decide if a student should continue the class. Megacode Testing should take place with at least 3 students (during the full ACLS Course, ACLS Update Course, and HeartCode ACLS hands-on session). *Note:* For Megacode Testing, all healthcare providers who would normally be Team Leaders (eg, emergency department physicians, paramedics) during a real cardiac arrest should be tested as Team Leader (ie, may need more than one passing Megacode test with the whole team).

Objective and Uniform Testing of Students

Each student, related to the team, must be able to demonstrate competency as a Team Leader or as a team member during the case scenario to pass the Megacode Test. It will take the whole team working together to achieve the objective and subjective requirements on the skills testing checklist.

Competency in the Megacode means that the team, in the roles of Team Leader and team members, successfully managed a resuscitation team's completion of all skills steps on the critical performance checklist, including objective measure (eg, CCF). The team's actions and communication should result in a satisfactory application of appropriate ACLS guidelines and principles in the Megacode as well as objective measures.

To ensure that the Megacode Test is objective and uniform, you must accomplish all of the following:

- Follow the testing checklist. The basic criteria for each step of the testing checklist are the content, principles, and actions that are taught in the ACLS Provider Course. Students should avoid performing steps or skills that are not part of this course.
- To pass, the team must successfully perform all skills steps on the testing checklist, including objectives measures.
- Do not coach, guide, or lead the team through the Megacode Test.
- Do not answer questions or give hints about what the team should do or not do during the Megacode Test.
- Permit the team members to rely on each other for help, but do not permit students to rely too heavily on the high-performance team to manage most or all of the case. Do not pass students who consistently hesitate or who ask the high-performance team for significant guidance throughout the test. A student may use the Handbook of ECC during the Megacode Test to check a drug dose. A student may not spend a significant amount of time looking up details of case management in the Handbook of ECC.
- Make sure that all students play their roles realistically during the test (eg, compressions should be done and not simulated). *Ensure that all students understand this requirement before the test begins.*
- Observe carefully and check off as correct only those skills that you see the student demonstrate through appropriate verbal directions to or appropriate actions with the high-performance team.
- Do not allow the Megacode Test to degenerate into a conversation about what is being done or should be done. Make the test a realistic scenario with hands-on skills being demonstrated or simulated in real time.
- Do not pause the test. If the student pauses, remind the student that real-life ACLS does not permit a pause in the actions required to resuscitate a patient.

- Record the team's performance on the testing checklist during the test, not afterward. *Do not rely on your memory to determine what the learner did or did not do during the test.*

- Do not allow a team to progress through a part of the test and then start over. If a student is not doing well, stop the test, give private feedback about performance deficiencies, and refer the student for remediation.

- Stop the test when the team demonstrates performance of all critical steps on the checklist, or when it is evident that the team needs remediation. For testing purposes, it is not necessary to bring each case scenario to a realistic ending. Many case scenarios end in ROSC for education and teaching purposes. This does not reflect the actual survival percentages in real life.

- Avoid deliberate misdirection of the students. Do not subvert the team's performance. If someone is doing very well, allow the case to continue to a reasonable end point without trying to see how much more the team members know or whether they can handle more difficult aspects of the case.

- Allow students to direct actions that are appropriate to the scope of practice of the high-performance team and team members. For example, insertion of an advanced airway is not required to pass the Megacode Test, but if it is ordered by the Team Leader and within the scope of practice of the person managing the airway, it may be done (consistent with ACLS guidelines for interruption of resuscitation).

- Give feedback to the team after the conclusion of the Megacode Test. Continue with the team members until they pass the test (or show signs that they should retake the course).

- Be fair, consistent, and as objective as possible when testing. Pass those teams who correctly manage the case as identified on the testing checklist; fail those who do not. Avoid passing those who should not pass or failing those who should pass.

- Remember, the consistency and quality of an ACLS Provider Course is often measured by the fairness and objectivity of testing.

ACLS Megacode Cases: General Information

Instructor Guide: Select and read the appropriate case scenario from the Appendix.

Students will rotate through this Megacode station and be tested in the sequence of bradycardia/tachycardia, VF/pVT, asystole/pulseless electrical activity (PEA), and ROSC.

- **Bradycardia/Tachycardia:** The student will manage the patient according to the Bradycardia/Tachycardia Algorithm.

- **VF/pVT:** The patient then develops VF/pVT that is unresponsive to an initial shock.

- **Asystole/PEA:** After administration of a second and third shock, epinephrine, and amiodarone/lidocaine, the patient testing scenario moves into asystole/PEA with delivery of a vasopressor.

- **Post–Cardiac Arrest Care:** The high-performance team continues high-quality chest compressions, the patient has ROSC, and the Team Leader initiates the Adult Post–Cardiac Arrest Care Algorithm.

The following items are tested in the case scenarios:

- **The team:** First, the Team Leader should assign the high-performance team members to specific roles.

- **High-quality CPR monitored by the CPR Coach:** When cardiac arrest occurs, the team members initiate BLS, Primary, and Secondary Assessments and interventions. The Team Leader must ensure that the high-performance team provides effective CPR at all times with minimal interruption of chest compressions.

- **CCF measured and calculated at the end of the test:** Students must pass with a score of at least 81% (greater than 80%).

- **Bradycardia or Tachycardia, Cardiac Arrest (VF/pVT, asystole, PEA), and Post–Cardiac Arrest Care Algorithms:** Then the instructor tests the critical actions on the checklist of the Bradycardia, Tachycardia, Cardiac Arrest (VF/pVT/Asystole/PEA), and Post–Cardiac Arrest Algorithms.

During each of these scenarios, the instructor should observe the student for effective leadership skills.

Part 5

Appendixes

Learning Station Scenarios, Megacode Scenarios, and Debriefing Tool

ACLS Case Scenarios

For all cases, instructors have the flexibility to withhold or add information based on the students' skills and experience levels.

For the *respiratory arrest cases,* instructors need to use only the lead-in and initial information to lead the student through the bag-mask ventilation and OPA/NPA skills testing. Instructors may use the entire respiratory scenario to go deeper into respiratory distress, respiratory failure, and respiratory arrest. To accommodate this approach, the instructor or the Course Coordinator will need to schedule extra time for the airway management station.

Instructor's Note: At the start of every case, inform students that "the scene is safe."

Airway Management Skills Testing Checklist

Student Name _____ Date of Test _____

Critical Performance Steps	Check if done correctly
BLS Assessment and Interventions	
Checks for responsiveness • Taps and shouts, "Are you OK?"	
Activates the emergency response system • Shouts for nearby help/Activates the emergency response system and gets the AED *or* • Directs second rescuer to activate the emergency response system and get the AED	
Checks breathing • Scans chest for movement (5-10 seconds)	
Checks pulse (5-10 seconds) **Breathing and pulse check can be done simultaneously**	
Notes that pulse is present and does not initiate chest compressions or attach AED	
Inserts oropharyngeal or nasopharyngeal airway	
Administers oxygen	
Performs effective bag-mask ventilation for 1 minute • Gives proper ventilation rate (once every 6 seconds) • Gives proper ventilation speed (over 1 second) • Gives proper ventilation volume (about half a bag)	

STOP TEST

Instructor Notes
- Place a check in the box next to each step the student completes successfully.
- If the student does not complete all steps successfully (as indicated by at least 1 blank check box), the student must receive remediation. Make a note here of which skills require remediation (refer to Instructor Manual for information about remediation).

Test Results
Circle **PASS** or **NR** to indicate pass or needs remediation:

PASS	NR

Instructor Initials _____

Instructor Number _____ Date _____

Case 1: Out-of-Hospital Respiratory Arrest

Scenario Rating: 3

Lead-in: You are a paramedic and respond to a call for a woman having an asthma attack at a restaurant.

Vital Signs
Heart rate: 120/min
Blood pressure: 60/38 mm Hg
Respiratory rate:
SpO₂: <50% on room air
Temperature:
Weight:
Age:

Initial Information
- The patient is unconscious on the floor, with agonal respirations.

What are your initial actions?

Additional Information
- She reported difficulty breathing while eating.
- She began gasping for air and had a decrease in mental status.
- Her pulse is weak and regular.
- She has only moderate chest rise and no improvement with bag-mask ventilation.
- One friend says that the woman is allergic to peanuts.

What are your next actions?

Additional Information (if needed)
- You gave the following treatments without improvement:
  – Epinephrine 0.3 mg (1:1000) IM
  – Diphenhydramine 50 mg IV
  – Albuterol 2.5 mg via the bag-mask device

What are your next actions?

Instructor notes: The paramedic must decide whether to attempt an oral endotracheal intubation, which may worsen the airway swelling, or perform a needle cricothyrotomy. Oxygen should be initiated.

Case 2: Out-of-Hospital Respiratory Arrest

Scenario Rating: 1

Lead-in: You are in the lounge, and your partner enters, holding her throat with both hands.

Vital Signs
Heart rate: 64/min
Blood pressure: 110/70 mm Hg
Respiratory rate:
SpO$_2$: 62%
Temperature:
Weight:
Age:

Initial Information
- Your partner cannot speak or cough.
- **What are your actions?**

Additional Information
- You perform abdominal thrusts several times without dislodging the obstruction.
- Your partner becomes unresponsive.
- **What are your actions?**

Additional Information (if needed)
- You activate the emergency response system, lower your partner to the ground, and start CPR.
- Every time you open the airway to give breaths, you look for an object and try to remove it.
- Assistance arrives and your partner is placed on a cardiac monitor.
- Pulse oximeter and airway equipment are available as you retrieve a food bolus from your partner's mouth.
- You can now ventilate, but your partner is unresponsive and not breathing.
- **What are your next actions?**

Airway Management Skills Testing Checklist

Student Name _____   Date of Test _____

Critical Performance Steps	Check if done correctly
BLS Assessment and Interventions	
Checks for responsiveness • Taps and shouts, "Are you OK?"	
Activates the emergency response system • Shouts for nearby help/Activates the emergency response system and gets the AED _or_ • Directs second rescuer to activate the emergency response system and get the AED	
Checks breathing • Scans chest for movement (5-10 seconds)	
Checks pulse (5-10 seconds) **Breathing and pulse check can be done simultaneously** Notes that pulse is present and does not initiate chest compressions or attach AED	
Inserts oropharyngeal or nasopharyngeal airway	
Administers oxygen	
Performs effective bag-mask ventilation for 1 minute • Gives proper ventilation rate (once every 6 seconds) • Gives proper ventilation speed (over 1 second) • Gives proper ventilation volume (about half a bag)	

STOP TEST

Instructor Notes
- Place a check in the box next to each step the student completes successfully.
- If the student does not complete all steps successfully (as indicated by at least 1 blank check box), the student must receive remediation. Make a note here of which skills require remediation (refer to Instructor Manual for information about remediation).

Test Results
Circle **PASS** or **NR** to indicate pass or needs remediation:

	PASS	NR

Instructor Initials _____
Instructor Number _____   Date _____

Case 3: Out-of-Hospital Respiratory Arrest

Scenario Rating: 2

Lead-in: You are a paramedic and respond to a call for breathing difficulty.

Vital Signs
Heart rate:
Blood pressure:
Respiratory rate:
SpO$_2$:
Temperature:
Weight:
Age:

Initial Information
- The patient is lying in bed, unresponsive and with severe difficulty breathing.

What are your actions?

Additional Information
- You attach a cardiac monitor/defibrillator.
- A rhythm check shows sinus tachycardia.

Instructor notes: Show ECG strip.

What are your actions?

Additional Information (if needed)
- The patient's wife says her husband did not feel well yesterday and had a very restless night.

Instructor notes: If the paramedic begins assisting ventilation quickly, the heart rate remains the same. If not, bradycardia develops and quickly progresses to asystole.

What are your next actions?

Airway Management Skills Testing Checklist

Student Name _____   Date of Test _____

Critical Performance Steps	Check if done correctly
BLS Assessment and Interventions	
Checks for responsiveness • Taps and shouts, "Are you OK?"	
Activates the emergency response system • Shouts for nearby help/Activates the emergency response system and gets the AED *or* • Directs second rescuer to activate the emergency response system and get the AED	
Checks breathing • Scans chest for movement (5-10 seconds)	
Checks pulse (5-10 seconds) **Breathing and pulse check can be done simultaneously**	
Notes that pulse is present and does not initiate chest compressions or attach AED	
Inserts oropharyngeal or nasopharyngeal airway	
Administers oxygen	
Performs effective bag-mask ventilation for 1 minute • Gives proper ventilation rate (once every 6 seconds) • Gives proper ventilation speed (over 1 second) • Gives proper ventilation volume (about half a bag)	

STOP TEST

Instructor Notes
- Place a check in the box next to each step the student completes successfully.
- If the student does not complete all steps successfully (as indicated by at least 1 blank check box), the student must receive remediation. Make a note here of which skills require remediation (refer to Instructor Manual for information about remediation).

Test Results Circle **PASS** or **NR** to indicate pass or needs remediation:	PASS	NR

Instructor Initials _____
Instructor Number _____   Date _____

Case 4: Out-of-Hospital Respiratory Arrest

Scenario Rating: 2

Lead-in: You are a paramedic responding to a call for shortness of breath in an obese man with a severe asthma attack.

Vital Signs
Heart rate: 120/min
Blood pressure: 184/100 mm Hg
Respiratory rate: 28/min
SpO_2: 85% on room air
Temperature:
Weight:
Age: 32 years

Initial Information
- The patient is in a chair in the tripod position.
- He is in severe respiratory distress, cyanotic, and diaphoretic.
- His wife says he has been using his asthma inhaler "all day" and became worse over the past 20 minutes.

What are your initial actions?

Additional Information
- Your assessment reveals silent breath sounds with minimal air movement.
- He is tachycardic.

What are your actions?

Additional Information (if needed)
- You obtain IV access, but the patient becomes increasingly agitated and restless.
- He removes his nonrebreathing mask and nebulizer.
- His SpO_2 decreases immediately after this.

Airway Management Skills Testing Checklist

Student Name _____ Date of Test _____

Critical Performance Steps	Check if done correctly
BLS Assessment and Interventions	
Checks for responsiveness • Taps and shouts, "Are you OK?"	
Activates the emergency response system • Shouts for nearby help/Activates the emergency response system and gets the AED *or* • Directs second rescuer to activate the emergency response system and get the AED	
Checks breathing • Scans chest for movement (5-10 seconds)	
Checks pulse (5-10 seconds)	
Breathing and pulse check can be done simultaneously	
Notes that pulse is present and does not initiate chest compressions or attach AED	
Inserts oropharyngeal or nasopharyngeal airway	
Administers oxygen	
Performs effective bag-mask ventilation for 1 minute • Gives proper ventilation rate (once every 6 seconds) • Gives proper ventilation speed (over 1 second) • Gives proper ventilation volume (about half a bag)	
STOP TEST	

Instructor Notes
- Place a check in the box next to each step the student completes successfully.
- If the student does not complete all steps successfully (as indicated by at least 1 blank check box), the student must receive remediation. Make a note here of which skills require remediation (refer to Instructor Manual for information about remediation).

Test Results
Circle **PASS** or **NR** to indicate pass or needs remediation:

	PASS
	NR

Instructor Initials _____
Instructor Number _____ Date _____

Airway Management Skills Testing Checklist

Student Name _____ Date of Test _____

Critical Performance Steps	Check if done correctly
BLS Assessment and Interventions	
Checks for responsiveness • Taps and shouts, "Are you OK?"	
Activates the emergency response system • Shouts for nearby help/Activates the emergency response system and gets the AED *or* • Directs second rescuer to activate the emergency response system and get the AED	
Checks breathing • Scans chest for movement (5–10 seconds)	
Checks pulse (5–10 seconds)	
Breathing and pulse check can be done simultaneously	
Notes that pulse is present and does not initiate chest compressions or attach AED	
Inserts oropharyngeal or nasopharyngeal airway	
Administers oxygen	
Performs effective bag-mask ventilation for 1 minute • Gives proper ventilation rate (once every 6 seconds) • Gives proper ventilation speed (over 1 second) • Gives proper ventilation volume (about half a bag)	
STOP TEST	

Instructor Notes
• Place a check in the box next to each step the student completes successfully.
• If the student does not complete all steps successfully (as indicated by at least 1 blank check box), the student must receive remediation. Make a note here of which skills require remediation (refer to Instructor Manual for information about remediation).

Test Results
Circle **PASS** or **NR** to indicate pass or needs remediation:

Instructor Initials _____

Instructor Number _____ Date _____

PASS	NR

Case 5: Emergency Department Respiratory Arrest

Scenario Rating: 3

Lead-in: You are an emergency department care provider. You are asked by the charge nurse to see a patient in your resuscitation bay. A storekeeper called 9-1-1 after finding an unconscious man in his 30s in an alley. On arrival, EMTs found the man unconscious and not breathing, and they noticed drug paraphernalia on the scene and an empty syringe.

Vital Signs
Heart rate: 120/min
Blood pressure: 100/55 mm Hg
Respiratory rate: 0/min
SpO₂: 75%
Temperature: 36.7°C
Weight:
Age:

Initial Information
• The patient appears disheveled and unconscious, with mildly cyanotic lips.
• EMTs perform the BLS Assessment and try to ventilate him with a bag-mask device.

What are your actions?

Additional Information
• You attach a cardiac monitor/defibrillator.
• The patient has a strong pulse but no spontaneous respirations.
• A rhythm check finds a **narrow-complex rapid tachycardia.**
• Numerous track marks are on the patient's arms.
• He has a Glasgow Coma Scale score of 3; his pupils are dilated bilaterally at 7 mm.

Instructor notes: Show ECG strip.

What are your actions?

Additional Information (if needed)
• EMTs were having difficulty achieving adequate ventilation with the bag-mask device.

What are some actions you can take to improve bag-mask ventilation?

Instructor notes: Actions to improve ventilation include positioning the airway, ensuring a good seal, using the 2-rescuer technique, and inserting an oral or nasopharyngeal airway.

• After you use some of these techniques, ventilation and oxygen saturation improve.
 – SpO₂ is now 100% oxygen by bag-mask device.
• The patient remains unconscious and apneic.
 – Heart rate is now 100/min with a normal sinus rhythm; blood pressure is unchanged.

What are your next actions?

Instructor notes: Options include trial of naloxone, starting with small, escalating doses.

Case 6: Emergency Department Respiratory Arrest

Scenario Rating: 2

Lead-in: You are a nurse practitioner in a double-coverage emergency department (a physician is the other provider) when a patient arrives via EMS, reporting shortness of breath. Paramedics report a history of heart failure and medical noncompliance. The patient arrives on continuous positive airway pressure (CPAP).

Vital Signs
Heart rate: 145/min
Blood pressure: 210/115 mm Hg
Respiratory rate:
SpO₂: 82% on 100% oxygen
Temperature:
Weight:
Age:

Initial Information
- The patient is transferred onto an emergency department stretcher.
- He looks tired and cannot speak in complete sentences.

What are your new actions?

Additional Information
- The patient is placed on a monitor.
- He is transitioned to bilevel positive airway pressure.
- After 10 minutes, he slumps over and becomes apneic.

What are your actions now?

Additional Information (if needed)
- The family arrives and states that the patient has been noncompliant with his medications.
- He has progressively become short of breath, with swollen lower extremities.
- This happened a few times in the past, often requiring hospitalization.

Instructor notes: A definitive airway should be obtained.
Treatment for heart failure should be initiated after the patient is placed on bilevel positive airway pressure. ECG, chest x-ray, and laboratory analysis should help confirm the diagnosis. A patient who becomes apneic should be removed from bilevel positive airway pressure (BiPAP) or CPAP and be intubated.

Airway Management Skills Testing Checklist

Student Name _____ Date of Test _____

Critical Performance Steps	Check if done correctly
BLS Assessment and Interventions	
Checks for responsiveness • Taps and shouts, "Are you OK?"	
Activates the emergency response system • Shouts for nearby help/Activates the emergency response system and gets the AED *or* • Directs second rescuer to activate the emergency response system and get the AED	
Checks breathing • Scans chest for movement (5-10 seconds)	
Checks pulse (5-10 seconds)	
Breathing and pulse check can be done simultaneously	
Notes that pulse is present and does not initiate chest compressions or attach AED	
Inserts oropharyngeal or nasopharyngeal airway	
Administers oxygen	
Performs effective bag-mask ventilation for 1 minute • Gives proper ventilation rate (once every 6 seconds) • Gives proper ventilation speed (over 1 second) • Gives proper ventilation volume (about half a bag)	
STOP TEST	

Instructor Notes
- Place a check in the box next to each step the student completes successfully.
- If the student does not complete all steps successfully (as indicated by at least 1 blank check box), the student must receive remediation. Make a note here of which skills require remediation (refer to Instructor Manual for information about remediation).

Test Results
Circle **PASS** or **NR** to indicate pass or needs remediation:

PASS	NR

Instructor Initials _____

Instructor Number _____ Date _____

Airway Management Skills Testing Checklist

Student Name _____ Date of Test _____

Critical Performance Steps	Check if done correctly
BLS Assessment and Interventions	
Checks for responsiveness • Taps and shouts, "Are you OK?"	
Activates the emergency response system • Shouts for nearby help/Activates the emergency response system and gets the AED *or* • Directs second rescuer to activate the emergency response system and get the AED	
Checks breathing • Scans chest for movement (5-10 seconds)	
Checks pulse (5-10 seconds) **Breathing and pulse check can be done simultaneously** Notes that pulse is present and does not initiate chest compressions or attach AED	
Inserts oropharyngeal or nasopharyngeal airway	
Administers oxygen	
Performs effective bag-mask ventilation for 1 minute • Gives proper ventilation rate (once every 6 seconds) • Gives proper ventilation speed (over 1 second) • Gives proper ventilation volume (about half a bag)	

STOP TEST

Instructor Notes
- Place a check in the box next to each step the student completes successfully.
- If the student does not complete all steps successfully (as indicated by at least 1 blank check box), the student must receive remediation. Make a note here of which skills require remediation (refer to Instructor Manual for information about remediation).

Test Results
Circle **PASS** or **NR** to indicate pass or needs remediation:

	PASS	NR

Instructor Initials _____

Instructor Number _____ Date _____

Case 7: Emergency Department Respiratory Arrest (Smoke Inhalation)

Scenario Rating: 2

Lead-in: You are a nurse/respiratory therapist/physician/paramedic covering the emergency department when a man is transported for evaluation of injuries related to a house fire.

Vital Signs
Heart rate: 125/min
Blood pressure: 180/94 mm Hg
Respiratory rate:
SpO₂: 100% on room air
Temperature:
Weight:
Age: 23

Initial Information
- The patient is tachypneic and says that he has shortness of breath and chest pain.

What are your initial actions?

Additional Information
- The patient has singed nasal hair, and second-degree burns are noted on his face, neck, and upper chest.
- Arterial blood gases are obtained, and analysis by hemoximetry reveals the following:
  - pH: 7.50
  - PCO₂: 29
  - PO₂: 45
  - HCO₃: 22
  - SaO₂: 80%
  - BE: 1
- Lab values:
  - Hgb: 12 g/100 mL
  - WBC: 8000

After blood gases are obtained, the patient shows a decrease in mental status as well as decreased chest rise and fall, with no improvement with bag-mask ventilation.

What are your next actions?

Additional Information (if needed)
You have used the following treatments without improvement:
- 100% oxygen
- Bag-mask device
- Albuterol 2.5 mg via bag-mask device

What are your next actions?

Instructor notes: The healthcare provider must decide whether to attempt an oral endotracheal intubation, which may be very difficult due to potential inhalation injury and associated swelling. Additionally, this patient may have elevated carboxyhemoglobin level that is impairing oxygen delivery. Hyperbaric oxygen therapy may be required. Other considerations are cyanide and mechanical trauma.

103

Case 8: Emergency Department Respiratory Arrest (Stroke)

Scenario Rating: 1

Lead-in: You are a nurse/respiratory therapist/physician/paramedic covering the emergency department when a male patient with chronic obstructive pulmonary disease (COPD) presents at the emergency department after his daughter found him slumped over in a chair at home. The patient is approximately 6 feet tall. He was receiving home oxygen at 2 L/min by nasal cannula. The patient arrives in the emergency department with his home prescription. The patient is exhibiting unilateral facial weakness.

Vital Signs
Heart rate: 94/min
Blood pressure: 165/95 mm Hg
Respiratory rate:
SpO_2: 89% on 2 L/min on home therapy
Temperature:
Weight: 155
Age: 58

Initial Information
- The patient has stertorous breathing. Snoring sounds are audible on inspiration.
- The patient is unconscious and unresponsive to painful stimuli.

What are your actions?

Additional Information
- Respiratory rate of 16/min has been slowing since admission.
- Pupils respond slowly and unequally to light.
- Breath sounds are clear but diminished bibasilarly.

What are your next actions?

Additional Information (if needed)
You have used the following treatments without improvement:
- Repositioned the patient's head and opened his airway
- Increased the nasal cannula to 4 L/min

What are your next actions?

Instructor notes: The healthcare provider must suspect a cerebral vascular accident and begin the stroke protocol. The patient is unable to protect his airway, so intubation is required. Noninvasive ventilation places the patient at risk for aspiration. Reasonable initial ventilator settings would include the following:
- Set heart rate: 12-16/min
- Tidal volume: 6-8 mL/kg
- FiO_2: 0.4-0.5
- PEEP: 5-6 cm H_2O
- $PaCO_2$ target: normal of 35-45 mm Hg; or $ETCO_2$ target: normal of 30-40 mm Hg

---

Airway Management Skills Testing Checklist

Student Name _____ Date of Test _____

Critical Performance Steps	Check if done correctly
BLS Assessment and Interventions	
Checks for responsiveness • Taps and shouts, "Are you OK?"	
Activates the emergency response system • Shouts for nearby help/Activates the emergency response system and gets the AED *or* • Directs second rescuer to activate the emergency response system and get the AED	
Checks breathing • Scans chest for movement (5-10 seconds)	
Checks pulse (5-10 seconds) **Breathing and pulse check can be done simultaneously** Notes that pulse is present and does not initiate chest compressions or attach AED	
Inserts oropharyngeal or nasopharyngeal airway	
Administers oxygen	
Performs effective bag-mask ventilation for 1 minute • Gives proper ventilation rate (once every 6 seconds) • Gives proper ventilation speed (over 1 second) • Gives proper ventilation volume (about half a bag)	

STOP TEST

Instructor Notes
- Place a check in the box next to each step the student completes successfully.
- If the student does not complete all steps successfully (as indicated by at least 1 blank check box), the student must receive remediation. Make a note here of which skills require remediation (refer to Instructor Manual for information about remediation).

Test Results
Circle **PASS** or **NR** to indicate pass or needs remediation:

PASS	NR

Instructor Initials _____
Instructor Number _____ Date _____

Case 9: Emergency Department Respiratory Arrest (TBI With Pneumonia)

Scenario Rating: 2

Lead-in: You are a nurse/respiratory therapist/physician/paramedic covering the emergency department when you are called to evaluate a female patient who sustained a traumatic brain injury 3 years ago. The patient resides in a long-term care facility and does not have a DNAR order. She has been unresponsive.

Vital Signs
Heart rate: 120/min
Blood pressure: 90/40 mm Hg
Respiratory rate: 24/min
SpO$_2$: 88% on room air
Temperature: 38.9°C (102°F)
Weight:
Age: 55

Initial Information
- The patient is tachypneic, exhibits intercostal retractions, and is warm and clammy to the touch.

What are your initial actions?

Additional Information
- Heart rate: 130/min, an increase since admission
- Skin: warm and clammy
- Capillary refill: 3 seconds
- Breath sounds: decreased aeration bilaterally in the bases. Course rhonchi scattered throughout lung fields. A spontaneous, moist, productive cough is present.
- As you watch, respiration starts to slow, and the SpO$_2$ drops to 78%.

What are your next actions?

Additional Information (if needed)
You have used the following treatments, with some improvement:
- You opened the patient's airway, and bag-mask ventilation has helped improve her SpO$_2$ to 92% on 100% oxygen.
- You gave a fluid bolus.

What are your next actions?

Instructor notes: The healthcare provider must suspect an overwhelming pneumonia and possible sepsis. Although the bag-mask ventilation helped, the patient is unresponsive and the pneumonia is not likely to resolve in a few hours, so the patient is not an ideal candidate for noninvasive airway management and, therefore, should be intubated for long-term management.

Airway Management Skills Testing Checklist

Student Name _____   Date of Test _____

Critical Performance Steps	Check if done correctly
BLS Assessment and Interventions	
Checks for responsiveness • Taps and shouts, "Are you OK?"	
Activates the emergency response system • Shouts for nearby help/Activates the emergency response system and gets the AED *or* • Directs second rescuer to activate the emergency response system and get the AED	
Checks breathing • Scans chest for movement (5–10 seconds)	
Checks pulse (5–10 seconds) **Breathing and pulse check can be done simultaneously** Notes that pulse is present and does not initiate chest compressions or attach AED	
Inserts oropharyngeal or nasopharyngeal airway	
Administers oxygen	
Performs effective bag-mask ventilation for 1 minute • Gives proper ventilation rate (once every 6 seconds) • Gives proper ventilation speed (over 1 second) • Gives proper ventilation volume (about half a bag)	

STOP TEST

Instructor Notes
- Place a check in the box next to each step the student completes successfully.
- If the student does not complete all steps successfully (as indicated by at least 1 blank check box), the student must receive remediation. Make a note here of which skills require remediation (refer to Instructor Manual for information about remediation).

Test Results
Circle **PASS** or **NR** to indicate pass or needs remediation:

	PASS	NR

Instructor Initials _____
Instructor Number _____   Date _____

Case 10: In-Hospital—Medical-Surgical Unit Respiratory Arrest

Scenario Rating: 1

Lead-in: You are a healthcare provider caring for a patient who just returned from a surgical procedure.

Vital Signs

Heart rate: 112/min
Blood pressure: 122/64 mm Hg
Respiratory rate: 10 to 12/min (assisted)
SpO₂:
Temperature:
Weight:
Age: 32 years

Initial Information

- The patient is a woman returning for recovery from an appendectomy.
- The postanesthesia care unit was experiencing overflow, so she was returned to the surgical unit for postsurgical care.
- Before surgery, she was a healthy, active mother.
- Her husband runs out to the nurses' station, screaming that his wife is not breathing.
- When entering her room, you note that she is unresponsive.

What are your initial actions?

- You perform the BLS Assessment and discover that she is unconscious and is not making any respiratory effort.

What are your actions?

Additional Information

- Upon initial assessment, the Team Leader discovers that the patient has a strong radial pulse.
- Simultaneous ventilation with 100% oxygen is given via bag-mask device and OPA, and a rhythm check of the cardiac monitor/defibrillator shows a **narrow-complex tachycardia.**

Additional Information (if needed)

- The patient was symptom free the previous day.
- On the basis of the diagnostics, the patient was rushed to surgery for an emergency appendectomy.
- Her weight was estimated because of the urgent nature of the procedure.
- Her husband notes that she has no health problems that he knows of and has never had surgery.

What additional information would you like to know?
What additional actions would you perform?

Airway Management Skills Testing Checklist

Student Name _____ Date of Test _____

Critical Performance Steps	Check if done correctly
BLS Assessment and Interventions	
Checks for responsiveness • Taps and shouts, "Are you OK?"	
Activates the emergency response system • Shouts for nearby help/Activates the emergency response system and gets the AED *or* • Directs second rescuer to activate the emergency response system and get the AED	
Checks breathing • Scans chest for movement (5-10 seconds)	
Checks pulse (5-10 seconds) **Breathing and pulse check can be done simultaneously** Notes that pulse is present and does not initiate chest compressions or attach AED	
Inserts oropharyngeal or nasopharyngeal airway	
Administers oxygen	
Performs effective bag-mask ventilation for 1 minute • Gives proper ventilation rate (once every 6 seconds) • Gives proper ventilation speed (over 1 second) • Gives proper ventilation volume (about half a bag)	

STOP TEST

Instructor Notes

- Place a check in the box next to each step the student completes successfully.
- If the student does not complete all steps successfully (as indicated by at least 1 blank check box), the student must receive remediation. Make a note here of which skills require remediation (refer to Instructor Manual for information about remediation).

Test Results
Circle **PASS** or **NR** to indicate pass or needs remediation:

	PASS	NR

Instructor Initials _____
Instructor Number _____ Date _____

Case 11: In-Hospital Respiratory Arrest

Scenario Rating: 2

Lead-in: You are the medical resident on call in a large urban teaching hospital. The nurse calls you about a patient who has lip swelling and itching while receiving an IV medication.

Vital Signs
Heart rate: 130/min
Blood pressure: 170/82 mm Hg
Respiratory rate: 35/min
SpO₂: 87%
Temperature:
Weight:
Age: 73 years

Initial Information
- The patient has swollen lips and tongue and noticeable stridor.
- She appears anxious.
- **What are your initial actions?**

Additional Information
- You attach a cardiac monitor/defibrillator.
- You discover that the patient has new IV antibiotic infusing for lower extremity cellulitis.
- Hives are apparent on the neck and upper chest.
- **What are your actions?**

Additional Information (if needed)
- Your initial impression is anaphylaxis.
- You give the patient IM epinephrine, IV H₂/H₁ blockers, and steroids.
- The condition is unchanged, except the tongue is now more swollen.
- The stridor is worsening.
- Her husband says she is allergic to penicillin.
- **What are your next actions?**
  Options to consider:
  - A rapid sequence intubation
  - Double setup with surgical airway
- **Instructor notes:** Consider a double setup in case an emergency cricothyrotomy is needed.
- The patient is transferred to the ICU.

Airway Management Skills Testing Checklist

Student Name _____   Date of Test _____

Critical Performance Steps	Check if done correctly
BLS Assessment and Interventions	
Checks for responsiveness • Taps and shouts, "Are you OK?"	
Activates the emergency response system • Shouts for nearby help/Activates the emergency response system and gets the AED *or* • Directs second rescuer to activate the emergency response system and get the AED	
Checks breathing • Scans chest for movement (5–10 seconds)	
Checks pulse (5–10 seconds) **Breathing and pulse check can be done simultaneously**	
Notes that pulse is present and does not initiate chest compressions or attach AED	
Inserts oropharyngeal or nasopharyngeal airway	
Administers oxygen	
Performs effective bag-mask ventilation for 1 minute • Gives proper ventilation rate (once every 6 seconds) • Gives proper ventilation speed (over 1 second) • Gives proper ventilation volume (about half a bag)	
STOP TEST	

Instructor Notes
- Place a check in the box next to each step the student completes successfully.
- If the student does not complete all steps successfully (as indicated by at least 1 blank check box), the student must receive remediation. Make a note here of which skills require remediation (refer to Instructor Manual for information about remediation).

Test Results
Circle **PASS** or **NR** to indicate pass or needs remediation:

	PASS	NR

Instructor Initials _____
Instructor Number _____   Date _____

Case 12: In-Hospital Respiratory Arrest

Scenario Rating: 2

Lead-in: A woman who is postoperative day 1 from a cholecystectomy is found to be unresponsive with poor respirations.

Vital Signs
Heart rate:
Blood pressure:
Respiratory rate:
SpO₂:
Temperature:
Weight:
Age: 70 years

Initial Information

- A Code Blue is called.
- You enter the room to assist with the patient.

What are your initial actions?

Additional Information

- You find the patient to be apneic, but she has a strong carotid pulse.
- You initiate bag-mask ventilation.

What are your actions?

Instructor notes: The student should recognize respiratory arrest without cardiac arrest. Bag-mask ventilation should be initiated, ideally with supplementary use of an NPA or OPA. Use this to test appropriate techniques and both 1- and 2-person bag-mask ventilation. The patient is completely unresponsive and will tolerate either but, over time with ventilation, becomes more responsive and unable to tolerate the oral airway.

Additional Information (if needed)

- Bag-mask ventilation with airway adjuncts continues.
- On further questioning, you learn that the patient is receiving morphine continuously through a pump for postoperative pain management.
- With naloxone, the patient becomes responsive and the airway is maintained.

Instructor notes: The origin of the respiratory failure is overdose of morphine. This should be recognized during the event and naloxone provided. The dose of naloxone should be discussed. The scenario ends when naloxone is administered.

Airway Management Skills Testing Checklist

Student Name _____ Date of Test _____

Critical Performance Steps	Check if done correctly
BLS Assessment and Interventions	
Checks for responsiveness • Taps and shouts, "Are you OK?"	
Activates the emergency response system • Shouts for nearby help/Activates the emergency response system and gets the AED *or* • Directs second rescuer to activate the emergency response system and get the AED	
Checks breathing • Scans chest for movement (5–10 seconds)	
Checks pulse (5–10 seconds)	
Breathing and pulse check can be done simultaneously	
Notes that pulse is present and does not initiate chest compressions or attach AED	
Inserts oropharyngeal or nasopharyngeal airway	
Administers oxygen	
Performs effective bag-mask ventilation for 1 minute • Gives proper ventilation rate (once every 6 seconds) • Gives proper ventilation speed (over 1 second) • Gives proper ventilation volume (about half a bag)	

STOP TEST

Instructor Notes
- Place a check in the box next to each step the student completes successfully.
- If the student does not complete all steps successfully (as indicated by at least 1 blank check box), the student must receive remediation. Make a note here of which skills require remediation (refer to Instructor Manual for information about remediation).

Test Results Circle **PASS** or **NR** to indicate pass or needs remediation:	PASS	NR

Instructor Initials _____
Instructor Number _____   Date _____

Case 13: In-Hospital Respiratory Failure (Asthma)

Scenario Rating: 3

Lead-in: You are a nurse/respiratory therapist/physician/paramedic covering the intermediate care unit when you are called to evaluate a female patient with a history of diabetes, coronary artery disease, asthma, and congestive heart failure. The patient is well known to the cardiology and pulmonary staff and is noncompliant with her numerous medications for asthma and heart failure. She has been intubated before for asthma exacerbations.

Vital Signs
Heart rate: 80/min
Blood pressure: 132/88 mm Hg
Respiratory rate: 26/min
SpO$_2$: 82% on CPAP with 100% oxygen
Temperature: 37.2°C (99°F)
Weight:
Age: 62 years

Initial Information
- You find the patient on CPAP of 10 as part of her treatment for congestive heart failure. She is short of breath and wanting to take the mask off.

What are your initial actions?

Additional Information
- Heart rate of 80/min hasn't really changed despite her increase in anxiety.
- Respiratory rate is regular, but the patient says that she "can't do this much longer."
- Skin: cool to the touch
- Capillary refill: 3 seconds
- Breath sounds: diminished, wheezing, prolonged expiratory phase with crackles
- She refuses to continue wearing the CPAP mask and takes it off in front of you.

What are your next actions?

Additional Information (if needed)
You have given the following treatments, with no improvement:
- Albuterol 2.5 mg
- Sedation for anxiety
- Placed the patient back on CPAP

What are your next actions?

Instructor notes: The healthcare provider must consider intubation for respiratory failure. You can try BiPAP to see whether that helps with her work of breathing, but she should probably be moved to a higher level of care. It's best to determine whether this is an asthma exacerbation or heart failure or both. β-Blockers appear to pose the greatest risk to patients with asthma or COPD. With this patient's lack of heart rate response, it appears that she is on a β-blocker. This may be why bronchodilators like albuterol are not effective.

Airway Management Skills Testing Checklist

Student Name _____ Date of Test _____

Critical Performance Steps	Check if done correctly
BLS Assessment and Interventions	
Checks for responsiveness • Taps and shouts, "Are you OK?"	
Activates the emergency response system • Shouts for nearby help/Activates the emergency response system and gets the AED *or* • Directs second rescuer to activate the emergency response system and get the AED	
Checks breathing • Scans chest for movement (5-10 seconds)	
Checks pulse (5-10 seconds) **Breathing and pulse check can be done simultaneously** Notes that pulse is present and does not initiate chest compressions or attach AED	
Inserts oropharyngeal or nasopharyngeal airway	
Administers oxygen	
Performs effective bag-mask ventilation for 1 minute • Gives proper ventilation rate (once every 6 seconds) • Gives proper ventilation speed (over 1 second) • Gives proper ventilation volume (about half a bag)	
STOP TEST	

Instructor Notes
- Place a check in the box next to each step the student completes successfully.
- If the student does not complete all steps successfully (as indicated by at least 1 blank check box), the student must receive remediation. Make a note here of which skills require remediation (refer to Instructor Manual for information about remediation).

Test Results
Circle **PASS** or **NR** to indicate pass or needs remediation:

	PASS	NR

Instructor Initials _____
Instructor Number _____ Date _____

Case 14: Out-of-Hospital Unstable Bradycardia

Scenario Rating: 2

Lead-in: You are a paramedic and respond to a call for a patient with an altered mental status.

Vital Signs
Heart rate:
Blood pressure:
Respiratory rate:
SpO₂:
Temperature:
Weight:
Age: 59 years

Initial Information
- The patient is sitting upright on a couch.
- He is disoriented, pale, and diaphoretic.

What are your actions?

Additional Information
- You attach a cardiac monitor/defibrillator.
- A rhythm check finds a **third-degree heart block**.

Instructor notes: Show ECG strip.

What are your actions?

Additional Information (if needed)
- The patient's wife says the condition came on quickly, and the patient had chest pain just before he became unresponsive.

Instructor notes: If the paramedic correctly initiates the transcutaneous pacing procedure, the patient's condition improves. If not, the patient quickly deteriorates to pulseless.

What are your next actions?

Adult Bradycardia Learning Station Checklist

Adult Bradycardia Algorithm

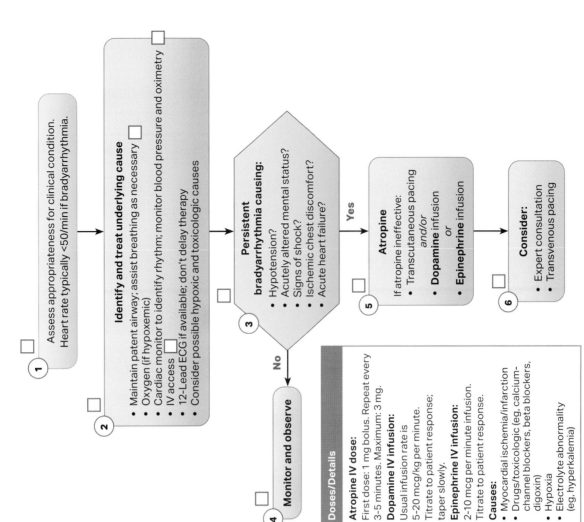

1 ☐ Assess appropriateness for clinical condition. Heart rate typically <50/min if bradyarrhythmia.

2 ☐ **Identify and treat underlying cause**
- Maintain patent airway; assist breathing as necessary ☐
- Oxygen (if hypoxemic)
- Cardiac monitor to identify rhythm; monitor blood pressure and oximetry ☐
- IV access
- 12-Lead ECG if available; don't delay therapy
- Consider possible hypoxic and toxicologic causes

3 ☐ **Persistent bradyarrhythmia causing:**
- Hypotension?
- Acutely altered mental status?
- Signs of shock?
- Ischemic chest discomfort?
- Acute heart failure?

No →

4 ☐ **Monitor and observe**

Yes →

5 ☐ **Atropine**
If atropine ineffective:
- Transcutaneous pacing
  and/or
- **Dopamine** infusion
  or
- **Epinephrine** infusion

6 ☐ **Consider:**
- Expert consultation
- Transvenous pacing

Doses/Details

Atropine IV dose:
First dose: 1 mg bolus. Repeat every 3-5 minutes. Maximum: 3 mg.

Dopamine IV infusion:
Usual infusion rate is 5-20 mcg/kg per minute. Titrate to patient response; taper slowly.

Epinephrine IV infusion:
2-10 mcg per minute infusion. Titrate to patient response.

Causes:
- Myocardial ischemia/infarction
- Drugs/toxicologic (eg, calcium-channel blockers, beta blockers, digoxin)
- Hypoxia
- Electrolyte abnormality (eg, hyperkalemia)

Debriefing Tool

ACLS Sample Scenario: Bradycardia

Learning Objectives

- Apply the BLS, Primary, and Secondary Assessments sequence for a systematic evaluation of adult patients
- Recognize bradyarrhythmias that may result in cardiac arrest or complicate resuscitation outcome
- Perform early management of bradyarrhythmias that may result in cardiac arrest or complicate resuscitation outcome
- Model effective communication as a member or leader of a high-performance team
- Recognize the impact of team dynamics on overall team performance

General Debriefing Principles

- Use the table on the right to guide your debriefing.
- Debriefings are 4 to 6 minutes long (unless more time is needed).
- Address all objectives.
- Summarize take-home messages at the end of the debriefing.
- **Encourage** students to self-reflect, and engage all participants.
- **Avoid** mini-lectures, and prevent closed-ended questions from dominating the discussion.

Action	Gather	Analyze	Summarize
- Assigns team roles and directs the team (effective team dynamics) - Directs the systematic approach - Directs team to apply monitor leads - Directs IV or IO access - Directs appropriate drug treatment or transcutaneous pacing - Directs reassessment of patient in response to treatments - Summarizes specific treatments - Verbalizes indications for advanced airway if needed	**Student Observations** (primary is Team Leader and Timer/Recorder) - Can you describe the events from your perspective? - How did you think your treatments went? - Can you review the events of the scenario? *(directed to the Timer/Recorder)* - What could you have improved? - What did the team do well?	**Done Well** - How were you able to *[insert action here]*? - Why do you think you were able to *[insert action here]*? - Tell me a little more about how you *[insert action here]*.	**Student-Led Summary** - What are the main things you learned? - Can someone summarize the key points made? - What are the main take-home messages?
	Instructor Observations - I noticed that *[insert action here]*. - I observed that *[insert action here]*. - I saw that *[insert action here]*.	**Needs Improvement** - Why do you think *[insert action here]* occurred? - How do you think *[insert action here]* could have been improved? - What was your thinking while *[insert action here]*? - What prevented you from *[insert action here]*?	**Instructor-Led Summary** - Let's summarize what we learned… - Here is what I think we learned… - The main take-home messages are…

Case 15: Out-of-Hospital Unstable Bradycardia

Scenario Rating: 2

Lead-in: You are called to the scene for a man who says he is weak and light-headed.

Vital Signs

Heart rate: 48/min, irregular
Blood pressure: 78/40 mm Hg
Respiratory rate: 20/min
SpO₂: 96%
Temperature:
Weight:
Age:

Initial Information

- The patient is sitting in a chair, ashen and diaphoretic.
- He reports indigestion and weakness.

What are your actions?

Additional Information

- You assess your patient while your partner obtains vital signs and attaches a cardiac monitor and pulse oximeter.

Now, what would you do?

- The rhythm is **second-degree type II AV block.**

Additional Information (if needed)

- Atropine is unsuccessful, and the transcutaneous pacemaker fails to capture.

What are your next actions?

- Rapid transport to the hospital

Adult Bradycardia Learning Station Checklist

Adult Bradycardia Algorithm

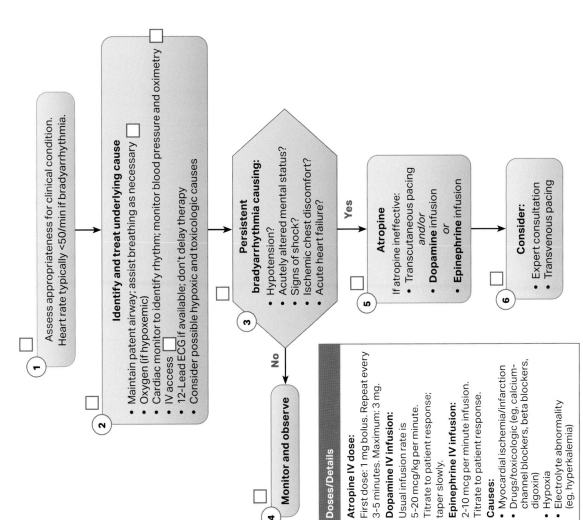

1
Assess appropriateness for clinical condition.
Heart rate typically <50/min if bradyarrhythmia.

2
Identify and treat underlying cause
- Maintain patent airway; assist breathing as necessary
- Oxygen (if hypoxemic)
- Cardiac monitor to identify rhythm; monitor blood pressure and oximetry
- IV access
- 12-Lead ECG if available; don't delay therapy
- Consider possible hypoxic and toxicologic causes

3
Persistent bradyarrhythmia causing:
- Hypotension?
- Acutely altered mental status?
- Signs of shock?
- Ischemic chest discomfort?
- Acute heart failure?

No → **4** **Monitor and observe**

Yes →

5
Atropine
If atropine ineffective:
- Transcutaneous pacing
  and/or
- **Dopamine** infusion
  or
- **Epinephrine** infusion

6
Consider:
- Expert consultation
- Transvenous pacing

Doses/Details

Atropine IV dose:
First dose: 1 mg bolus. Repeat every 3-5 minutes. Maximum: 3 mg.
Dopamine IV infusion:
Usual infusion rate is 5-20 mcg/kg per minute.
Titrate to patient response; taper slowly.
Epinephrine IV infusion:
2-10 mcg per minute infusion.
Titrate to patient response.
Causes:
- Myocardial ischemia/infarction
- Drugs/toxicologic (eg, calcium-channel blockers, beta blockers, digoxin)
- Hypoxia
- Electrolyte abnormality (eg, hyperkalemia)

Debriefing Tool

ACLS Sample Scenario: Bradycardia

Action	Gather	Analyze	Summarize
	Student Observations (primary is Team Leader and Timer/Recorder)	**Done Well**	**Student-Led Summary**
• Assigns team roles and directs the team (effective team dynamics)	• Can you describe the events from your perspective?	• How were you able to [insert action here]?	• What are the main things you learned?
• Directs the systematic approach	• How did you think your treatments went?	• Why do you think you were able to [insert action here]?	• Can someone summarize the key points made?
• Directs team to apply monitor leads	• Can you review the events of the scenario? (directed to the Timer/ Recorder)	• Tell me a little more about how you [insert action here].	• What are the main take-home messages?
• Directs IV or IO access	• What could you have improved?		
• Directs appropriate drug treatment or transcutaneous pacing	• What did the team do well?		
• Directs reassessment of patient in response to treatments			
• Summarizes specific treatments	**Instructor Observations**	**Needs Improvement**	**Instructor-Led Summary**
• Verbalizes indications for advanced airway if needed	• I noticed that [insert action here].	• Why do you think [insert action here] occurred?	• Let's summarize what we learned...
	• I observed that [insert action here].	• How do you think [insert action here] could have been improved?	• Here is what I think we learned...
	• I saw that [insert action here].	• What was your thinking while [insert action here]?	• The main take-home messages are...
		• What prevented you from [insert action here]?	

Learning Objectives

- Apply the BLS, Primary, and Secondary Assessments sequence for a systematic evaluation of adult patients
- Recognize bradyarrhythmias that may result in cardiac arrest or complicate resuscitation outcome
- Perform early management of bradyarrhythmias that may result in cardiac arrest or complicate resuscitation outcome
- Model effective communication as a member or leader of a high-performance team
- Recognize the impact of team dynamics on overall team performance

General Debriefing Principles

- Use the table on the right to guide your debriefing.
- Debriefings are 4 to 6 minutes long (unless more time is needed).
- Address all objectives.
- Summarize take-home messages at the end of the debriefing.
- *Encourage* students to self-reflect, and engage all participants.
- *Avoid* mini-lectures, and prevent closed-ended questions from dominating the discussion.

Case 16: Out-of-Hospital Unstable Bradycardia

Scenario Rating: 1

Lead-in: You are a paramedic and respond to a home for a patient who has reportedly had a syncopal episode.

Vital Signs

Heart rate: 40/min, weak and regular
Blood pressure: 54/36 mm Hg
Respiratory rate:
SpO₂: 70% on room air
Temperature:
Weight:
Age:

Initial Information

- The patient is lying on the floor with an altered level of consciousness.
- She is breathing and appears extremely pale.

What are your initial actions?

Additional Information

- Her husband tells you that she has a history of high blood pressure.
- She began feeling light-headed after taking her medication.
- Cardiac monitor shows **sinus bradycardia.**

What are your next actions?

Instructor notes: The patient just changed medication from lisinopril to atenolol. She never took atenolol before.

Additional Information (if needed)

- You have started an IV and pushed a bolus of normal saline, but there is no significant improvement in perfusion.

What are your next actions?

Adult Bradycardia Learning Station Checklist

Adult Bradycardia Algorithm

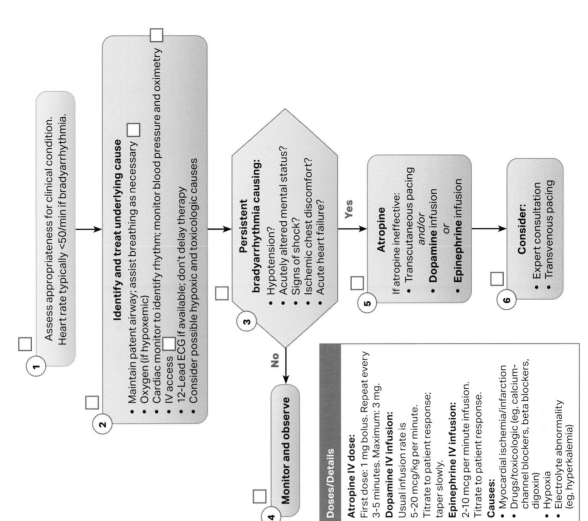

1
Assess appropriateness for clinical condition.
Heart rate typically <50/min if bradyarrhythmia.

2 Identify and treat underlying cause
- Maintain patent airway; assist breathing as necessary
- Oxygen (if hypoxemic)
- Cardiac monitor to identify rhythm; monitor blood pressure and oximetry
- IV access
- 12-Lead ECG if available; don't delay therapy
- Consider possible hypoxic and toxicologic causes

3 Persistent bradyarrhythmia causing:
- Hypotension?
- Acutely altered mental status?
- Signs of shock?
- Ischemic chest discomfort?
- Acute heart failure?

No → **4 Monitor and observe**

Yes →

5 Atropine
If atropine ineffective:
- Transcutaneous pacing
  and/or
- **Dopamine** infusion
  or
- **Epinephrine** infusion

6 Consider:
- Expert consultation
- Transvenous pacing

Doses/Details

Atropine IV dose:
First dose: 1 mg bolus. Repeat every 3-5 minutes. Maximum: 3 mg.
Dopamine IV infusion:
Usual infusion rate is 5-20 mcg/kg per minute.
Titrate to patient response; taper slowly.
Epinephrine IV infusion:
2-10 mcg per minute infusion.
Titrate to patient response.
Causes:
- Myocardial ischemia/infarction
- Drugs/toxicologic (eg, calcium-channel blockers, beta blockers, digoxin)
- Hypoxia
- Electrolyte abnormality (eg, hyperkalemia)

Debriefing Tool

ACLS Sample Scenario: Bradycardia

Learning Objectives

- Apply the BLS, Primary, and Secondary Assessments sequence for a systematic evaluation of adult patients
- Recognize bradyarrhythmias that may result in cardiac arrest or complicate resuscitation outcome
- Perform early management of bradyarrhythmias that may result in cardiac arrest or complicate resuscitation outcome
- Model effective communication as a member or leader of a high-performance team
- Recognize the impact of team dynamics on overall team performance

General Debriefing Principles

- Use the table on the right to guide your debriefing.
- Debriefings are 4 to 6 minutes long (unless more time is needed).
- Address all objectives.
- Summarize take-home messages at the end of the debriefing.
- **Encourage** students to self-reflect, and engage all participants.
- **Avoid** mini-lectures, and prevent closed-ended questions from dominating the discussion.

Action	Gather	Analyze	Summarize
- Assigns team roles and directs the team (effective team dynamics) - Directs the systematic approach - Directs team to apply monitor leads - Directs IV or IO access - Directs appropriate drug treatment or transcutaneous pacing - Directs reassessment of patient in response to treatments - Summarizes specific treatments - Verbalizes indications for advanced airway if needed	**Student Observations** (primary is Team Leader and Timer/Recorder) - Can you describe the events from your perspective? - How did you think your treatments went? - Can you review the events of the scenario? *(directed to the Timer/Recorder)* - What could you have improved? - What did the team do well?	**Done Well** - How were you able to *[insert action here]*? - Why do you think you were able to *[insert action here]*? - Tell me a little more about how you *[insert action here]*.	**Student-Led Summary** - What are the main things you learned? - Can someone summarize the key points made? - What are the main take-home messages?
	Instructor Observations - I noticed that *[insert action here]*. - I observed that *[insert action here]*. - I saw that *[insert action here]*.	**Needs Improvement** - Why do you think *[insert action here]* occurred? - How do you think *[insert action here]* could have been improved? - What was your thinking while *[insert action here]*? - What prevented you from *[insert action here]*?	**Instructor-Led Summary** - Let's summarize what we learned… - Here is what I think we learned… - The main take-home messages are…

Case 17: Out-of-Hospital Unstable Bradycardia

Scenario Rating: 2

Lead-in: You are the paramedic dispatched to help a woman who reports epigastric abdominal pain and vomiting.

Vital Signs
Heart rate: 46/min
Blood pressure: 76/30 mm Hg
Respiratory rate: 18/min
SpO₂: 98% on room air
Temperature:
Weight:
Age: 76 years

Initial Information

- The patient is a thin, elderly woman who is diaphoretic, pale, and in obvious discomfort, holding her epigastrium.
- She states that she feels very weak.
- She denies any chest pain but feels short of breath.

What are your initial actions?

Additional Information

- You place her on oxygen.

What do you do, and what are your priorities?

- A 12-lead ECG shows an **acute inferior wall STEMI** with a **wide-complex third-degree AV block.**

Instructor notes: The student should recognize the STEMI and contact the receiving hospital so that a cardiac STEMI alert can be activated.

Additional Information (if needed)

Instructor notes: The student should verbalize to try either dopamine 2 to 20 mcg/kg per minute, titrating to patient's response, or transcutaneous pacing. If atropine is considered, discuss the precautions of using it in the presence of myocardial ischemia; in addition, atropine may not be effective given the cardiac rhythm.

It is appropriate for the paramedic to also administer aspirin and an analgesic to this patient.

The patient should be transported to the emergency department with anticipation of rapidly going to the cath lab.

Adult Bradycardia Learning Station Checklist

Adult Bradycardia Algorithm

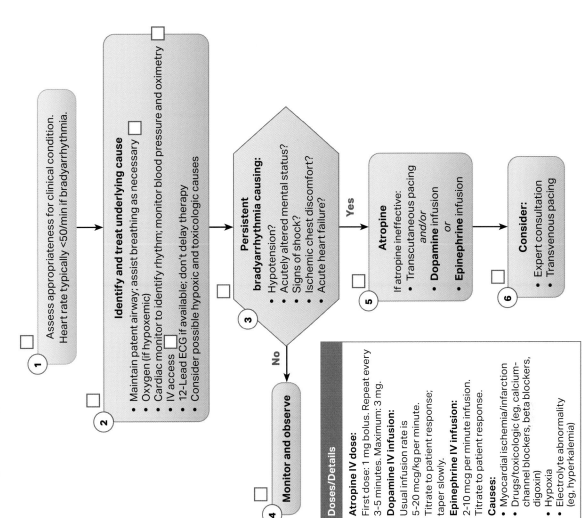

1
Assess appropriateness for clinical condition.
Heart rate typically <50/min if bradyarrhythmia.

2
Identify and treat underlying cause
- Maintain patent airway; assist breathing as necessary
- Oxygen (if hypoxemic)
- Cardiac monitor to identify rhythm; monitor blood pressure and oximetry
- IV access
- 12-Lead ECG if available; don't delay therapy
- Consider possible hypoxic and toxicologic causes

3
Persistent bradyarrhythmia causing:
- Hypotension?
- Acutely altered mental status?
- Signs of shock?
- Ischemic chest discomfort?
- Acute heart failure?

No → **4** **Monitor and observe**

Yes

5
Atropine
If atropine ineffective:
- Transcutaneous pacing
and/or
- **Dopamine** infusion
or
- **Epinephrine** infusion

6
Consider:
- Expert consultation
- Transvenous pacing

Doses/Details

Atropine IV dose:
First dose: 1 mg bolus. Repeat every 3-5 minutes. Maximum: 3 mg.
Dopamine IV infusion:
Usual infusion rate is 5-20 mcg/kg per minute. Titrate to patient response; taper slowly.
Epinephrine IV infusion:
2-10 mcg per minute infusion. Titrate to patient response.
Causes:
- Myocardial ischemia/infarction
- Drugs/toxicologic (eg, calcium-channel blockers, beta blockers, digoxin)
- Hypoxia
- Electrolyte abnormality (eg, hyperkalemia)

Debriefing Tool

ACLS Sample Scenario: Bradycardia

Learning Objectives

- Apply the BLS, Primary, and Secondary Assessments sequence for a systematic evaluation of adult patients
- Recognize bradyarrhythmias that may result in cardiac arrest or complicate resuscitation outcome
- Perform early management of bradyarrhythmias that may result in cardiac arrest or complicate resuscitation outcome
- Model effective communication as a member or leader of a high-performance team
- Recognize the impact of team dynamics on overall team performance

General Debriefing Principles

- Use the table on the right to guide your debriefing.
- Debriefings are 4 to 6 minutes long (unless more time is needed).
- Address all objectives.
- Summarize take-home messages at the end of the debriefing.
- *Encourage* students to self-reflect, and engage all participants.
- *Avoid* mini-lectures, and prevent closed-ended questions from dominating the discussion.

Action	Gather	Analyze	Summarize
	Student Observations (primary is Team Leader and Timer/Recorder)	**Done Well**	**Student-Led Summary**
• Assigns team roles and directs the team (effective team dynamics)	• Can you describe the events from your perspective?	• How were you able to *[insert action here]*?	• What are the main things you learned?
• Directs the systematic approach	• How did you think your treatments went?	• Why do you think you were able to *[insert action here]*?	• Can someone summarize the key points made?
• Directs team to apply monitor leads	• Can you review the events of the scenario? *(directed to the Timer/Recorder)*	• Tell me a little more about how you *[insert action here]*.	• What are the main take-home messages?
• Directs IV or IO access	• What could you have improved?		
• Directs appropriate drug treatment or transcutaneous pacing	• What did the team do well?		
• Directs reassessment of patient in response to treatments			
• Summarizes specific treatments	**Instructor Observations**	**Needs Improvement**	**Instructor-Led Summary**
• Verbalizes indications for advanced airway if needed	• I noticed that *[insert action here]*.	• Why do you think *[insert action here]* occurred?	• Let's summarize what we learned...
	• I observed that *[insert action here]*.	• How do you think *[insert action here]* could have been improved?	• Here is what I think we learned...
	• I saw that *[insert action here]*.	• What was your thinking while *[insert action here]*?	• The main take-home messages are...
		• What prevented you from *[insert action here]*?	

Case 18: Emergency Department Unstable Bradycardia

Scenario Rating: 2

Lead-in: You are working in a community emergency department. In one room is a patient who reports generalized weakness. She tells the triage nurse that she had difficulty getting off the toilet.

Vital Signs

Heart rate: 32/min
Blood pressure: 72/45 mm Hg
Respiratory rate:
SpO₂: 92% on room air
Temperature:
Weight:
Age: 74 years

Initial Information

- The patient is in no distress, but she looks tired and pale.
- She is not on the monitor.

What are your actions?

Additional Information

- The patient is afebrile.
- She is placed on a monitor.
- She takes "hypertension medication" every day.
- The ECG reads **second-degree type I AV block.**

What are your actions now?

Instructor notes: The patient is given IV atropine without response and then IV dopamine (epinephrine may be used also) and glucagon for presumptive β-blocker overdose.

Additional Information (if needed)

- The family arrives and notes that the patient has been reporting nausea and vague heartburn and has been more tired recently.
- She sometimes becomes confused and takes too many of her medications.

Adult Bradycardia Learning Station Checklist

Adult Bradycardia Algorithm

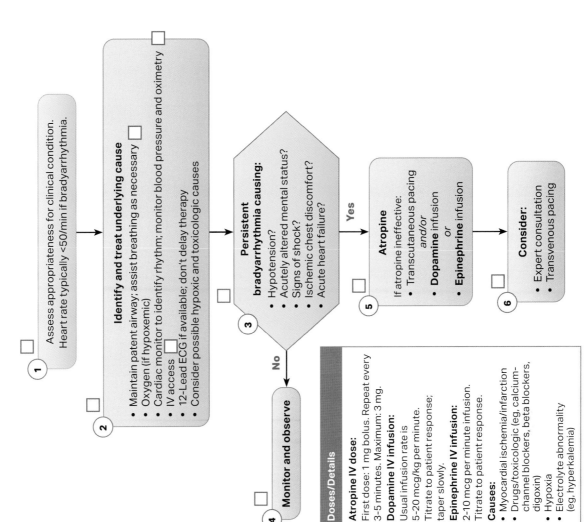

1

Assess appropriateness for clinical condition.
Heart rate typically <50/min if bradyarrhythmia.

2

Identify and treat underlying cause

- Maintain patent airway; assist breathing as necessary
- Oxygen (if hypoxemic)
- Cardiac monitor to identify rhythm; monitor blood pressure and oximetry
- IV access
- 12-Lead ECG if available; don't delay therapy
- Consider possible hypoxic and toxicologic causes

3

Persistent bradyarrhythmia causing:

- Hypotension?
- Acutely altered mental status?
- Signs of shock?
- Ischemic chest discomfort?
- Acute heart failure?

No

4 **Monitor and observe**

Yes

5 **Atropine**

If atropine ineffective:

- Transcutaneous pacing
and/or
- **Dopamine** infusion
or
- **Epinephrine** infusion

6 **Consider:**

- Expert consultation
- Transvenous pacing

Doses/Details

Atropine IV dose:
First dose: 1 mg bolus. Repeat every 3-5 minutes. Maximum: 3 mg.
Dopamine IV infusion:
Usual infusion rate is
5-20 mcg/kg per minute.
Titrate to patient response; taper slowly.
Epinephrine IV infusion:
2-10 mcg per minute infusion. Titrate to patient response.

Causes:

- Myocardial ischemia/infarction
- Drugs/toxicologic (eg, calcium-channel blockers, beta blockers, digoxin)
- Hypoxia
- Electrolyte abnormality (eg, hyperkalemia)

Debriefing Tool

ACLS Sample Scenario: Bradycardia

Learning Objectives

- Apply the BLS, Primary, and Secondary Assessments sequence for a systematic evaluation of adult patients
- Recognize bradyarrhythmias that may result in cardiac arrest or complicate resuscitation outcome
- Perform early management of bradyarrhythmias that may result in cardiac arrest or complicate resuscitation outcome
- Model effective communication as a member or leader of a high-performance team
- Recognize the impact of team dynamics on overall team performance

General Debriefing Principles

- Use the table on the right to guide your debriefing.
- Debriefings are 4 to 6 minutes long (unless more time is needed).
- Address all objectives.
- Summarize take-home messages at the end of the debriefing.
- *Encourage* students to self-reflect, and engage all participants.
- *Avoid* mini-lectures, and prevent closed-ended questions from dominating the discussion.

Action	Gather	Analyze	Summarize
Assigns team roles and directs the team (effective team dynamics) - Assigns team roles and directs the team (effective team dynamics) - Directs the systematic approach - Directs team to apply monitor leads - Directs IV or IO access - Directs appropriate drug treatment or transcutaneous pacing - Directs reassessment of patient in response to treatments	**Student Observations** (primary is Team Leader and Timer/Recorder) - Can you describe the events from your perspective? - How did you think your treatments went? - Can you review the events of the scenario? *(directed to the Timer/Recorder)* - What could you have improved? - What did the team do well?	**Done Well** - How were you able to *[insert action here]*? - Why do you think you were able to *[insert action here]*? - Tell me a little more about how you *[insert action here]*.	**Student-Led Summary** - What are the main things you learned? - Can someone summarize the key points made? - What are the main take-home messages?
- Summarizes specific treatments - Verbalizes indications for advanced airway if needed	**Instructor Observations** - I noticed that *[insert action here]*. - I observed that *[insert action here]*. - I saw that *[insert action here]*.	**Needs Improvement** - Why do you think *[insert action here]* occurred? - How do you think *[insert action here]* could have been improved? - What was your thinking while *[insert action here]*? - What prevented you from *[insert action here]*?	**Instructor-Led Summary** - Let's summarize what we learned... - Here is what I think we learned... - The main take-home messages are...

Case 19: Emergency Department Unstable Bradycardia

Scenario Rating: 2

Lead-in: You are an emergency department provider in a medium-sized community hospital. You are assessing a woman with a history of peripheral vascular disease. She presents with a sensation of presyncope.

Vital Signs

Heart rate: 50/min
Blood pressure: 75/45 mm Hg
Respiratory rate: 20/min
SpO₂: 98% on room air
Temperature: 36.5°C
Weight:
Age: 79 years

Initial Information

- The patient began feeling dizzy, light-headed, weak, and faint 2 hours ago while watching TV.
- She has had no chest pain, dyspnea, or palpitations.
- Recently, she has been healthy with no fever, vomiting, diarrhea, dysuria, or recent changes to her medications.

What are your actions?

- Upon arrival in the acute care area of the emergency department, she is found to be hypotensive and bradycardic.
- An ECG shows a **second-degree type II AV block.**

What are your immediate actions?

Additional Information

- You attach a cardiac monitor/defibrillator, and a rhythm check finds a **narrow-complex bradycardia (second-degree type II AV block).**
- The patient appears pale and drowsy.

What are your actions?

- The patient has a history of peripheral vascular disease.
- She had claudication symptoms last year and underwent left femoral-popliteal bypass surgery. She has been asymptomatic since the procedure.
- The patient is also hypertensive and on maintenance medications.
- She takes aspirin 81 mg by mouth once daily, ramipril 10 mg by mouth once daily, and hydrochlorothiazide 25 mg by mouth twice daily.
- She has no allergies, and she has normal electrolytes, negative cardiac biomarkers, and a normal chest x-ray.

Additional Information (if needed)

- Attempts to use atropine to increase the heart rate are unsuccessful.
- The patient deteriorates into a third-degree AV block and requires transcutaneous pacing.

Adult Bradycardia Learning Station Checklist

Adult Bradycardia Algorithm

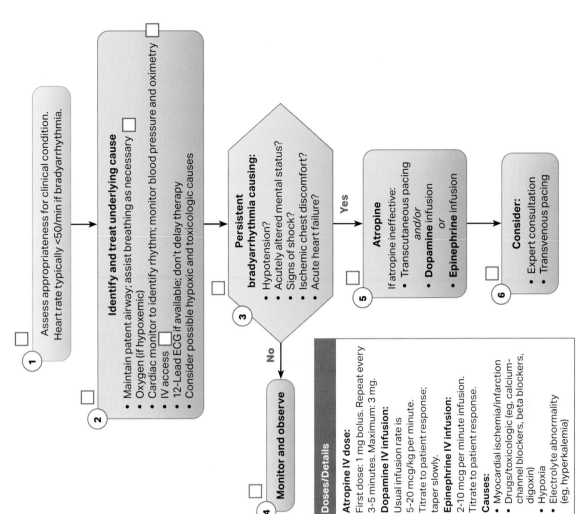

1 Assess appropriateness for clinical condition.
Heart rate typically <50/min if bradyarrhythmia.

2 **Identify and treat underlying cause**
- Maintain patent airway; assist breathing as necessary
- Oxygen (if hypoxemic)
- Cardiac monitor to identify rhythm; monitor blood pressure and oximetry
- IV access
- 12-Lead ECG if available; don't delay therapy
- Consider possible hypoxic and toxicologic causes

3 **Persistent bradyarrhythmia causing:**
- Hypotension?
- Acutely altered mental status?
- Signs of shock?
- Ischemic chest discomfort?
- Acute heart failure?

No → **4** **Monitor and observe**

Yes →

5 **Atropine**
If atropine ineffective:
- Transcutaneous pacing
and/or
- **Dopamine** infusion
or
- **Epinephrine** infusion

6 **Consider:**
- Expert consultation
- Transvenous pacing

Doses/Details

Atropine IV dose:
First dose: 1 mg bolus. Repeat every 3-5 minutes. Maximum: 3 mg.

Dopamine IV infusion:
Usual infusion rate is 5-20 mcg/kg per minute. Titrate to patient response; taper slowly.

Epinephrine IV infusion:
2-10 mcg per minute infusion. Titrate to patient response.

Causes:
- Myocardial ischemia/infarction
- Drugs/toxicologic (eg, calcium-channel blockers, beta blockers, digoxin)
- Hypoxia
- Electrolyte abnormality (eg, hyperkalemia)

Debriefing Tool

ACLS Sample Scenario: Bradycardia

Action	Gather	Analyze	Summarize
	Student Observations (primary is Team Leader and Timer/Recorder)	**Done Well**	**Student-Led Summary**
• Assigns team roles and directs the team (effective team dynamics)	• Can you describe the events from your perspective?	• How were you able to [insert action here]?	• What are the main things you learned?
• Directs the systematic approach	• How did you think your treatments went?	• Why do you think you were able to [insert action here]?	• Can someone summarize the key points made?
• Directs team to apply monitor leads	• Can you review the events of the scenario? (directed to the Timer/Recorder)	• Tell me a little more about how you [insert action here].	• What are the main take-home messages?
• Directs IV or IO access			
• Directs appropriate drug treatment or transcutaneous pacing	• What could you have improved?		
• Directs reassessment of patient in response to treatments	• What did the team do well?		
• Summarizes specific treatments	**Instructor Observations**	**Needs Improvement**	**Instructor-Led Summary**
• Verbalizes indications for advanced airway if needed	• I noticed that [insert action here].	• Why do you think [insert action here] occurred?	• Let's summarize what we learned…
	• I observed that [insert action here].	• How do you think [insert action here] could have been improved?	• Here is what I think we learned…
	• I saw that [insert action here].	• What was your thinking while [insert action here]?	• The main take-home messages are…
		• What prevented you from [insert action here]?	

Learning Objectives

- Apply the BLS, Primary, and Secondary Assessments sequence for a systematic evaluation of adult patients
- Recognize bradyarrhythmias that may result in cardiac arrest or complicate resuscitation outcome
- Perform early management of bradyarrhythmias that may result in cardiac arrest or complicate resuscitation outcome
- Model effective communication as a member or leader of a high-performance team
- Recognize the impact of team dynamics on overall team performance

General Debriefing Principles

- Use the table on the right to guide your debriefing.
- Debriefings are 4 to 6 minutes long (unless more time is needed).
- Address all objectives.
- Summarize take-home messages at the end of the debriefing.
- *Encourage* students to self-reflect, and engage all participants.
- *Avoid* mini-lectures, and prevent closed-ended questions from dominating the discussion.

Case 20: Emergency Department Unstable Bradycardia

Scenario Rating: 1

Lead-in: You are called to see a 78-year-old woman in the resuscitation bay of your emergency department. She presented to triage saying that she had light-headedness and shortness of breath. She had a witnessed syncopal episode at home, which prompted the visit to the emergency room.

Vital Signs

Heart rate: 29/min
Blood pressure: 75/34 mm Hg
Respiratory rate:
SpO$_2$: Unmeasurable
Temperature:
Weight:
Age:

Initial Information

- The patient appears to be very drowsy.
- She tells you that she has been feeling weak and tired for several days.
- Today, she stood up to go to the kitchen. In the kitchen, she felt light-headed and diaphoretic before losing consciousness.
- She continues to feel light-headed, dyspneic, and nauseated.
- She appears pale, diaphoretic, and drowsy.
- The monitor is sounding an alarm for slow heart rate and hypotension.
- A 12-lead ECG shows **third-degree heart block** at a rate of 29.

What are your initial actions?

Additional Information

Initial actions and treatments used with no effect on either heart rate or other symptoms:

- IV access
- Cardiac monitor
- Oxygen
- Atropine 1 mg IV × 2 doses

What is your next intervention?

Instructor notes: The student must move down the Adult Bradycardia Algorithm, choosing either transcutaneous pacing, dopamine infusion, or epinephrine infusion. The student should consider expert consultation as well as the preparation and execution of transvenous pacing.

Adult Bradycardia Learning Station Checklist

Adult Bradycardia Algorithm

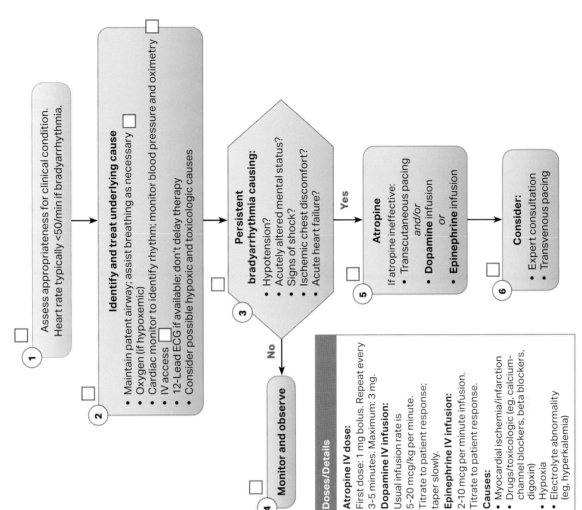

1
Assess appropriateness for clinical condition.
Heart rate typically <50/min if bradyarrhythmia.

2
Identify and treat underlying cause
- Maintain patent airway; assist breathing as necessary
- Oxygen (if hypoxemic)
- Cardiac monitor to identify rhythm; monitor blood pressure and oximetry
- IV access
- 12-Lead ECG if available; don't delay therapy
- Consider possible hypoxic and toxicologic causes

3
Persistent bradyarrhythmia causing:
- Hypotension?
- Acutely altered mental status?
- Signs of shock?
- Ischemic chest discomfort?
- Acute heart failure?

No → **4 Monitor and observe**

Yes →

5
Atropine
If atropine ineffective:
- Transcutaneous pacing
  and/or
- **Dopamine** infusion
  or
- **Epinephrine** infusion

6
Consider:
- Expert consultation
- Transvenous pacing

Doses/Details

Atropine IV dose:
First dose: 1 mg bolus. Repeat every 3-5 minutes. Maximum: 3 mg.

Dopamine IV infusion:
Usual infusion rate is 5-20 mcg/kg per minute. Titrate to patient response; taper slowly.

Epinephrine IV infusion:
2-10 mcg per minute infusion. Titrate to patient response.

Causes:
- Myocardial ischemia/infarction
- Drugs/toxicologic (eg, calcium-channel blockers, beta blockers, digoxin)
- Hypoxia
- Electrolyte abnormality (eg, hyperkalemia)

Debriefing Tool

ACLS Sample Scenario: Bradycardia

Learning Objectives

- Apply the BLS, Primary, and Secondary Assessments sequence for a systematic evaluation of adult patients
- Recognize bradyarrhythmias that may result in cardiac arrest or complicate resuscitation outcome
- Perform early management of bradyarrhythmias that may result in cardiac arrest or complicate resuscitation outcome
- Model effective communication as a member or leader of a high-performance team
- Recognize the impact of team dynamics on overall team performance

General Debriefing Principles

- Use the table on the right to guide your debriefing.
- Debriefings are 4 to 6 minutes long (unless more time is needed).
- Address all objectives.
- Summarize take-home messages at the end of the debriefing.
- **Encourage** students to self-reflect, and engage all participants.
- **Avoid** mini-lectures, and prevent closed-ended questions from dominating the discussion.

Action	Gather	Analyze	Summarize
	Student Observations (primary is Team Leader and Timer/Recorder)	**Done Well**	**Student-Led Summary**
- Assigns team roles and directs the team (effective team dynamics)	- Can you describe the events from your perspective?	- How were you able to [*insert action here*]?	- What are the main things you learned?
- Directs the systematic approach	- How did you think your treatments went?	- Why do you think you were able to [*insert action here*]?	- Can someone summarize the key points made?
- Directs team to apply monitor leads	- Can you review the events of the scenario? (*directed to the Timer/Recorder*)	- Tell me a little more about how you [*insert action here*].	- What are the main take-home messages?
- Directs IV or IO access	- What could you have improved?		
- Directs appropriate drug treatment or transcutaneous pacing	- What did the team do well?		
- Directs reassessment of patient in response to treatments			
- Summarizes specific treatments	**Instructor Observations**	**Needs Improvement**	**Instructor-Led Summary**
- Verbalizes indications for advanced airway if needed	- I noticed that [*insert action here*].	- Why do you think [*insert action here*] occurred?	- Let's summarize what we learned...
	- I observed that [*insert action here*].	- How do you think [*insert action here*] could have been improved?	- Here is what I think we learned...
	- I saw that [*insert action here*].	- What was your thinking while [*insert action here*]?	- The main take-home messages are...
		- What prevented you from [*insert action here*]?	

Case 21: In-Hospital—Cardiac Telemetry Unit Unstable Bradycardia

Scenario Rating: 1

Lead-in: You are a healthcare provider on a cardiac telemetry unit. You note on the monitor that your patient is experiencing bradycardia. You rapidly approach her room to see her clutching her chest and reaching out for help.

Vital Signs

Heart rate: 36/min
Blood pressure: 92/50 mm Hg
Respiratory rate: 20/min
SpO₂: 96% on 2 L/min via nasal cannula
Temperature:
Weight:
Age:

Initial Information

- Cardiac telemetry shows the patient has a narrow, slow **sinus bradycardia.**
- Her husband is at her bedside, holding her hand.

What are your next actions?

Additional Information

- She has a patent IV and reports extreme fatigue.
- She states that she has pressure in the middle of her chest.

What are your next actions?

Additional Information (if needed)

- You note that your patient's skin is ashen, and she says that her hands and feet feel very cold.
- Upon palpation, you note that her extremities are cool to the touch.

What are your next actions?

Adult Bradycardia Learning Station Checklist

Adult Bradycardia Algorithm

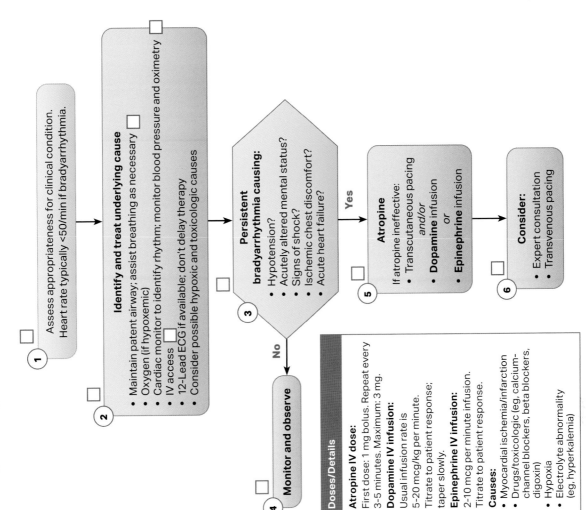

1 Assess appropriateness for clinical condition.
Heart rate typically <50/min if bradyarrhythmia.

2 Identify and treat underlying cause

- Maintain patent airway; assist breathing as necessary
- Oxygen (if hypoxemic)
- Cardiac monitor to identify rhythm; monitor blood pressure and oximetry
- IV access
- 12-Lead ECG if available; don't delay therapy
- Consider possible hypoxic and toxicologic causes

3 Persistent bradyarrhythmia causing:

- Hypotension?
- Acutely altered mental status?
- Signs of shock?
- Ischemic chest discomfort?
- Acute heart failure?

No → **4 Monitor and observe**

Yes →

5 Atropine
If atropine ineffective:
- Transcutaneous pacing
and/or
- **Dopamine** infusion
or
- **Epinephrine** infusion

6 Consider:
- Expert consultation
- Transvenous pacing

Doses/Details

Atropine IV dose:
First dose: 1 mg bolus. Repeat every 3-5 minutes. Maximum: 3 mg.

Dopamine IV infusion:
Usual infusion rate is 5-20 mcg/kg per minute.
Titrate to patient response; taper slowly.

Epinephrine IV infusion:
2-10 mcg per minute infusion. Titrate to patient response.

Causes:
- Myocardial ischemia/infarction
- Drugs/toxicologic (eg, calcium-channel blockers, beta blockers, digoxin)
- Hypoxia
- Electrolyte abnormality (eg, hyperkalemia)

Debriefing Tool

ACLS Sample Scenario: Bradycardia

Learning Objectives

- Apply the BLS, Primary, and Secondary Assessments sequence for a systematic evaluation of adult patients
- Recognize bradyarrhythmias that may result in cardiac arrest or complicate resuscitation outcome
- Perform early management of bradyarrhythmias that may result in cardiac arrest or complicate resuscitation outcome
- Model effective communication as a member or leader of a high-performance team
- Recognize the impact of team dynamics on overall team performance

General Debriefing Principles

- Use the table on the right to guide your debriefing.
- Debriefings are 4 to 6 minutes long (unless more time is needed).
- Address all objectives.
- Summarize take-home messages at the end of the debriefing.
- *Encourage* students to self-reflect, and engage all participants.
- *Avoid* mini-lectures, and prevent closed-ended questions from dominating the discussion.

Action	Gather	Analyze	Summarize
	Student Observations (primary is Team Leader and Timer/Recorder)	**Done Well**	**Student-Led Summary**
• Assigns team roles and directs the team (effective team dynamics)	• Can you describe the events from your perspective?	• How were you able to [*insert action here*]?	• What are the main things you learned?
• Directs the systematic approach	• How did you think your treatments went?	• Why do you think you were able to [*insert action here*]?	• Can someone summarize the key points made?
• Directs team to apply monitor leads	• Can you review the events of the scenario? (*directed to the Timer/ Recorder*)	• Tell me a little more about how you [*insert action here*].	• What are the main take-home messages?
• Directs IV or IO access	• What could you have improved?		
• Directs appropriate drug treatment or transcutaneous pacing	• What did the team do well?		
• Directs reassessment of patient in response to treatments			
• Summarizes specific treatments	**Instructor Observations**	**Needs Improvement**	**Instructor-Led Summary**
• Verbalizes indications for advanced airway if needed	• I noticed that [*insert action here*].	• Why do you think [*insert action here*] occurred?	• Let's summarize what we learned…
	• I observed that [*insert action here*].	• How do you think [*insert action here*] could have been improved?	• Here is what I think we learned…
	• I saw that [*insert action here*].	• What was your thinking while [*insert action here*]?	• The main take-home messages are…
		• What prevented you from [*insert action here*]?	

Case 22: In-Hospital Unstable Bradycardia

Scenario Rating: 2

Lead-in: A woman with a history of hypertension and atrial fibrillation is admitted to the hospital with a urinary tract infection and some confusion. Today, her initially slow heart rate and confusion have worsened.

Vital Signs
Heart rate: 20 to 30/min
Blood pressure: 70/30 mm Hg
Respiratory rate:
SpO₂:
Temperature:
Weight:
Age: 84 years

Initial Information
- The patient's monitor indicates a rhythm of **third-degree AV block**.
- The nurses assess her and find her to be confused and agitated.

What are your actions?

Additional Information
- A dose of atropine is given with little effect, and then pacing is successful.

Instructor notes: The student should describe how to perform pacing.

Additional Information (if needed)

Instructor notes: If the student asks, the patient is on both a β-blocker and a calcium channel blocker. Providing glucagon would be reasonable, but pacing would still be necessary to resolve the bradycardia.

The scenario should end with the student consulting cardiology and considering a temporary wire.

Adult Bradycardia Learning Station Checklist

Adult Bradycardia Algorithm

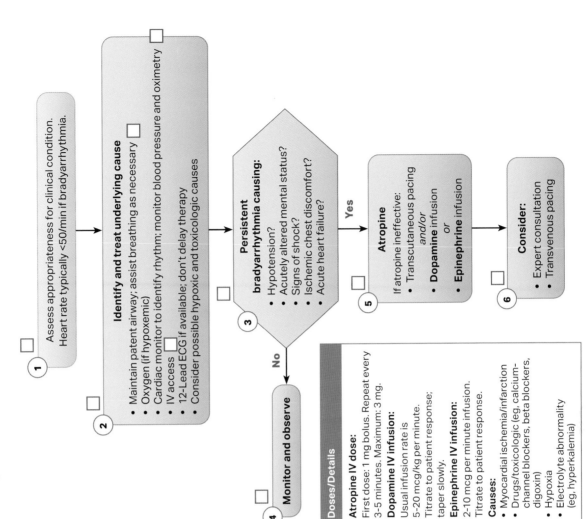

1
Assess appropriateness for clinical condition.
Heart rate typically <50/min if bradyarrhythmia.

2
Identify and treat underlying cause
- Maintain patent airway; assist breathing as necessary
- Oxygen (if hypoxemic)
- Cardiac monitor to identify rhythm; monitor blood pressure and oximetry
- IV access
- 12-Lead ECG if available; don't delay therapy
- Consider possible hypoxic and toxicologic causes

3
Persistent bradyarrhythmia causing:
- Hypotension?
- Acutely altered mental status?
- Signs of shock?
- Ischemic chest discomfort?
- Acute heart failure?

No →

4 Monitor and observe

Yes →

5
Atropine
If atropine ineffective:
- Transcutaneous pacing
and/or
- **Dopamine** infusion
or
- **Epinephrine** infusion

6
Consider:
- Expert consultation
- Transvenous pacing

Doses/Details

Atropine IV dose:
First dose: 1 mg bolus. Repeat every 3-5 minutes. Maximum: 3 mg.

Dopamine IV infusion:
Usual infusion rate is
5-20 mcg/kg per minute.
Titrate to patient response; taper slowly.

Epinephrine IV infusion:
2-10 mcg per minute infusion.
Titrate to patient response.

Causes:
- Myocardial ischemia/infarction
- Drugs/toxicologic (eg, calcium-channel blockers, beta blockers, digoxin)
- Hypoxia
- Electrolyte abnormality (eg, hyperkalemia)

© 2020 American Heart Association

Debriefing Tool

ACLS Sample Scenario: Bradycardia

Action	Gather	Analyze	Summarize
	Student Observations (primary is Team Leader and Timer/Recorder)	**Done Well**	**Student-Led Summary**
• Assigns team roles and directs the team (effective team dynamics)	• Can you describe the events from your perspective?	• How were you able to [insert action here]?	• What are the main things you learned?
• Directs the systematic approach	• How did you think your treatments went?	• Why do you think you were able to [insert action here]?	• Can someone summarize the key points made?
• Directs team to apply monitor leads	• Can you review the events of the scenario? (directed to the Timer/Recorder)	• Tell me a little more about how you [insert action here].	• What are the main take-home messages?
• Directs IV or IO access	• What could you have improved?		
• Directs appropriate drug treatment or transcutaneous pacing	• What did the team do well?		
• Directs reassessment of patient in response to treatments			
• Summarizes specific treatments	**Instructor Observations**	**Needs Improvement**	**Instructor-Led Summary**
• Verbalizes indications for advanced airway if needed	• I noticed that [insert action here].	• Why do you think [insert action here] occurred?	• Let's summarize what we learned…
	• I observed that [insert action here].	• How do you think [insert action here] could have been improved?	• Here is what I think we learned…
	• I saw that [insert action here].	• What was your thinking while [insert action here]?	• The main take-home messages are…
		• What prevented you from [insert action here]?	

Learning Objectives

- Apply the BLS, Primary, and Secondary Assessments sequence for a systematic evaluation of adult patients
- Recognize bradyarrhythmias that may result in cardiac arrest or complicate resuscitation outcome
- Perform early management of bradyarrhythmias that may result in cardiac arrest or complicate resuscitation outcome
- Model effective communication as a member or leader of a high-performance team
- Recognize the impact of team dynamics on overall team performance

General Debriefing Principles

- Use the table on the right to guide your debriefing.
- Debriefings are 4 to 6 minutes long (unless more time is needed).
- Address all objectives.
- Summarize take-home messages at the end of the debriefing.
- **Encourage** students to self-reflect, and engage all participants.
- **Avoid** mini-lectures, and prevent closed-ended questions from dominating the discussion.

Case 23: In-Hospital Unstable Bradycardia

Scenario Rating: 1

Lead-in: As you walk past the geriatric clinic, an elderly patient in front of you suddenly falls to the ground.

Vital Signs
Heart rate:
Blood pressure:
Respiratory rate:
SpO$_2$:
Temperature:
Weight:
Age:

Initial Information

- The patient is alert and oriented. He can follow all commands.
- He has a gash across his forehead that is bleeding.
- He speaks clearly and reports feeling tired and lethargic for the past week.
- He can move all his extremities and is in no discomfort.

What are your actions?

Additional Information

- You attach a cardiac monitor/defibrillator.
- A rhythm strip shows an atrial rate of 80/min and a regular narrow QRS at 50/min (**third-degree AV block**).
- The P waves and the QRS complex appear disassociated.

What are your actions?

Additional Information (if needed)

- The patient's wife states that he has been healthy.
- On a recent physical, no major health issues were noted.
- He does not take any prescription medications.

What are your next actions?

Adult Bradycardia Learning Station Checklist

Adult Bradycardia Algorithm

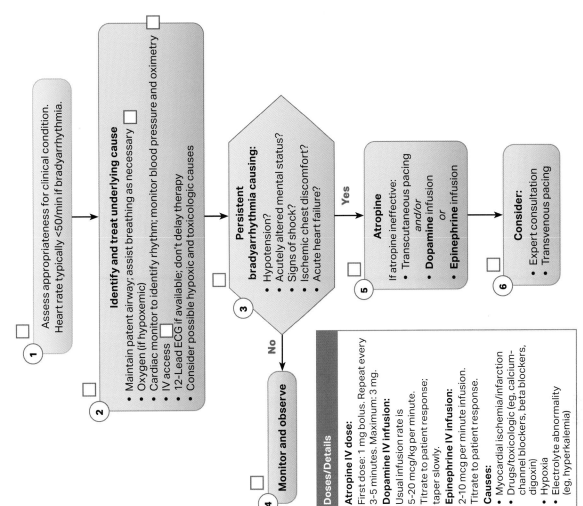

1
Assess appropriateness for clinical condition.
Heart rate typically <50/min if bradyarrhythmia.

2
Identify and treat underlying cause
- Maintain patent airway; assist breathing as necessary
- Oxygen (if hypoxemic)
- Cardiac monitor to identify rhythm; monitor blood pressure and oximetry
- IV access
- 12-Lead ECG if available; don't delay therapy
- Consider possible hypoxic and toxicologic causes

3
Persistent bradyarrhythmia causing:
- Hypotension?
- Acutely altered mental status?
- Signs of shock?
- Ischemic chest discomfort?
- Acute heart failure?

No →
4
Monitor and observe

Yes →
5
Atropine
If atropine ineffective:
- Transcutaneous pacing
and/or
- **Dopamine** infusion
or
- **Epinephrine** infusion

6
Consider:
- Expert consultation
- Transvenous pacing

Doses/Details

Atropine IV dose:
First dose: 1 mg bolus. Repeat every 3-5 minutes. Maximum: 3 mg.

Dopamine IV infusion:
Usual infusion rate is 5-20 mcg/kg per minute.
Titrate to patient response; taper slowly.

Epinephrine IV infusion:
2-10 mcg per minute infusion.
Titrate to patient response.

Causes:
- Myocardial ischemia/infarction
- Drugs/toxicologic (eg, calcium-channel blockers, beta blockers, digoxin)
- Hypoxia
- Electrolyte abnormality (eg, hyperkalemia)

Debriefing Tool

ACLS Sample Scenario: Bradycardia

Learning Objectives

- Apply the BLS, Primary, and Secondary Assessments sequence for a systematic evaluation of adult patients
- Recognize bradyarrhythmias that may result in cardiac arrest or complicate resuscitation outcome
- Perform early management of bradyarrhythmias that may result in cardiac arrest or complicate resuscitation outcome
- Model effective communication as a member or leader of a high-performance team
- Recognize the impact of team dynamics on overall team performance

General Debriefing Principles

- Use the table on the right to guide your debriefing.
- Debriefings are 4 to 6 minutes long (unless more time is needed).
- Address all objectives.
- Summarize take-home messages at the end of the debriefing.
- *Encourage* students to self-reflect, and engage all participants.
- *Avoid* mini-lectures, and prevent closed-ended questions from dominating the discussion.

Action	Gather	Analyze	Summarize
	Student Observations (primary is Team Leader and Timer/Recorder)	**Done Well**	**Student-Led Summary**
• Assigns team roles and directs the team (effective team dynamics)	• Can you describe the events from your perspective?	• How were you able to [insert action here]?	• What are the main things you learned?
• Directs the systematic approach	• How did you think your treatments went?	• Why do you think you were able to [insert action here]?	• Can someone summarize the key points made?
• Directs team to apply monitor leads	• Can you review the events of the scenario? (directed to the Timer/Recorder)	• Tell me a little more about how you [insert action here].	• What are the main take-home messages?
• Directs IV or IO access	• What could you have improved?		
• Directs appropriate drug treatment or transcutaneous pacing	• What did the team do well?		
• Directs reassessment of patient in response to treatments			
• Summarizes specific treatments	**Instructor Observations**	**Needs Improvement**	**Instructor-Led Summary**
• Verbalizes indications for advanced airway if needed	• I noticed that [insert action here].	• Why do you think [insert action here] occurred?	• Let's summarize what we learned...
	• I observed that [insert action here].	• How do you think [insert action here] could have been improved?	• Here is what I think we learned...
	• I saw that [insert action here].	• What was your thinking while [insert action here]?	• The main take-home messages are...
		• What prevented you from [insert action here]?	

Case 24: Out-of-Hospital Stable Tachycardia

Scenario Rating: 1

Lead-in: You are a paramedic and respond to a call for a patient with altered mental status.

Vital Signs

Heart rate: 116/min
Blood pressure: 134/82 mm Hg
Respiratory rate: 24/min
SpO₂: 94%
Temperature:
Weight:
Age: 73 years

Initial Information

- The patient feels weak and cannot get out of bed.
- His son says that the day before, his father briefly could not speak or understand words.
- About 3 weeks ago, the patient could not stand unaided because of weakness in his legs.
- He would not go to the emergency department in either case.
- He has a history of atrial fibrillation, hypertension, and diabetes.

What are your next actions?

Additional Information

- You attach a cardiac monitor/defibrillator.
- A rhythm check finds atrial fibrillation with rapid ventricular response.

What are your actions?

Adult Tachycardia With a Pulse Learning Station Checklist

Adult Tachycardia With a Pulse Algorithm

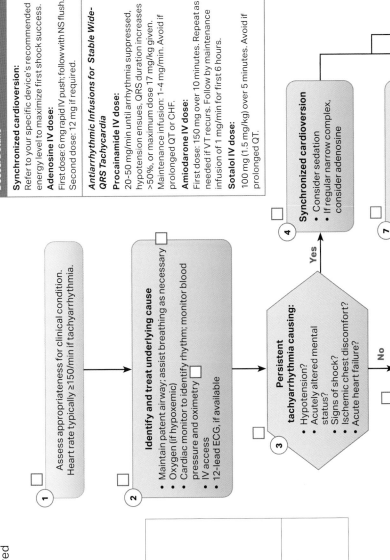

Doses/Details

Synchronized cardioversion:
Refer to your specific device's recommended energy level to maximize first shock success.

Adenosine IV dose:
First dose: 6 mg rapid IV push; follow with NS flush.
Second dose: 12 mg if required.

Antiarrhythmic Infusions for Stable Wide-QRS Tachycardia

Procainamide IV dose:
20-50 mg/min until arrhythmia suppressed, hypotension ensues, QRS duration increases >50%, or maximum dose 17 mg/kg given.
Maintenance infusion: 1-4 mg/min. Avoid if prolonged QT or CHF.

Amiodarone IV dose:
First dose: 150 mg over 10 minutes. Repeat as needed if VT recurs. Follow by maintenance infusion of 1 mg/min for first 6 hours.

Sotalol IV dose:
100 mg (1.5 mg/kg) over 5 minutes. Avoid if prolonged QT.

1
Assess appropriateness for clinical condition.
Heart rate typically ≥150/min if tachyarrhythmia.

2 **Identify and treat underlying cause**
- Maintain patent airway; assist breathing as necessary
- Oxygen (if hypoxemic)
- Cardiac monitor to identify rhythm; monitor blood pressure and oximetry
- IV access
- 12-lead ECG, if available

3 **Persistent tachyarrhythmia causing:**
- Hypotension?
- Acutely altered mental status?
- Signs of shock?
- Ischemic chest discomfort?
- Acute heart failure?

Yes →

4 **Synchronized cardioversion**
- Consider sedation
- If regular narrow complex, consider adenosine

No ↓

6 **Wide QRS?**
≥0.12 second

Yes →

7 **Consider**
- Adenosine only if regular and monomorphic
- Antiarrhythmic infusion
- Expert consultation

5 **If refractory, consider**
- Underlying cause
- Need to increase energy level for next cardioversion
- Addition of anti-arrhythmic drug
- Expert consultation

No ↓

8
- Vagal maneuvers (if regular)
- Adenosine (if regular)
- β-Blocker or calcium channel blocker
- Consider expert consultation

Debriefing Tool

ACLS Sample Scenario: Tachycardia

Learning Objectives

- Apply the BLS, Primary, and Secondary Assessments sequence for a systematic evaluation of adult patients
- Recognize tachyarrhythmias that may result in cardiac arrest or complicate resuscitation outcome
- Perform early management of tachyarrhythmias that may result in cardiac arrest or complicate resuscitation outcome
- Model effective communication as a member or leader of a high-performance team
- Recognize the impact of team dynamics on overall team performance

General Debriefing Principles

- Use the table on the right to guide your debriefing.
- Debriefings are 4 to 6 minutes long (unless more time is needed).
- Address all objectives.
- Summarize take-home messages at the end of the debriefing.
- **Encourage** students to self-reflect, and engage all participants.
- **Avoid** mini-lectures, and prevent closed-ended questions from dominating the discussion.

Action	Gather	Analyze	Summarize
	Student Observations (primary is Team Leader and Timer/Recorder)	**Done Well**	**Student-Led Summary**
• Assigns team roles and directs the team (effective team dynamics)	• Can you describe the events from your perspective?	• How were you able to [*insert action here*]?	• What are the main things you learned?
• Directs the systematic approach	• How did you think your treatments went?	• Why do you think you were able to [*insert action here*]?	• Can someone summarize the key points made?
• Directs team to apply monitor leads	• Can you review the events of the scenario? (*directed to the Timer/ Recorder*)	• Tell me a little more about how you [*insert action here*].	• What are the main take-home messages?
• Directs IV or IO access	• What could you have improved?		
• Directs appropriate drug treatment or synchronized/ unsynchronized cardioversion	• What did the team do well?		
• Directs reassessment of patient in response to treatments			
• Summarizes specific treatments	**Instructor Observations**	**Needs Improvement**	**Instructor-Led Summary**
• Verbalizes indications for advanced airway if needed	• I noticed that [*insert action here*].	• Why do you think [*insert action here*] occurred?	• Let's summarize what we learned...
	• I observed that [*insert action here*].	• How do you think [*insert action here*] could have been improved?	• Here is what I think we learned...
	• I saw that [*insert action here*].	• What was your thinking while [*insert action here*]?	• The main take-home messages are...
		• What prevented you from [*insert action here*]?	

Case 25: Out-of-Hospital Unstable Tachycardia

Scenario Rating: 2

Lead-in: You are in an advanced life support (ALS) ambulance dispatched to a patient with an unknown illness at home.

Vital Signs

Heart rate:
Blood pressure:
Respiratory rate: 22/min
SpO_2:
Temperature:
Weight:
Age: 68 years

Initial Information

- The woman is lying in the front doorway of her home.
- Her son helped her into the doorway to get some cool air (it is 30°F outside).
- She did not fall or injure herself.
- She is anxious, in mild respiratory distress, and grossly diaphoretic.
- She says she is short of breath; feels hot, dizzy, and nauseated; and can't get a deep breath.
- Her history includes obesity, non–insulin-dependent diabetes mellitus, and hypertension.

What are your initial actions?

Additional Information

- Your partner tries to obtain vital signs and finds the patient's respiratory rate is 22/min.
- Her carotid pulse is too fast to count, and he cannot obtain her blood pressure because of the absence of a radial pulse.
- She has no obvious dependent edema, and her neck veins are flat.
- Her lungs sounds are equal, with moderate rales present bilaterally.

What are your next actions?

Additional Information (if needed)

- After you attach the limb leads of the cardiac monitor, the patient appears in **monomorphic wide-complex (VT) tachycardia**.
- Peripheral IV access is not obtainable.
- Two attempts at cardioversion were unsuccessful; there is no change in rate or rhythm.
- An IO was placed, and she is receiving an amiodarone infusion.
- After 5 minutes of amiodarone, she is cardioverted a third time successfully to a normal sinus rhythm at 80/min.
- The vital signs then return toward normal.

Instructor notes: Local protocols may vary on the scope of this practice.

Adult Tachycardia With a Pulse Learning Station Checklist

Adult Tachycardia With a Pulse Algorithm

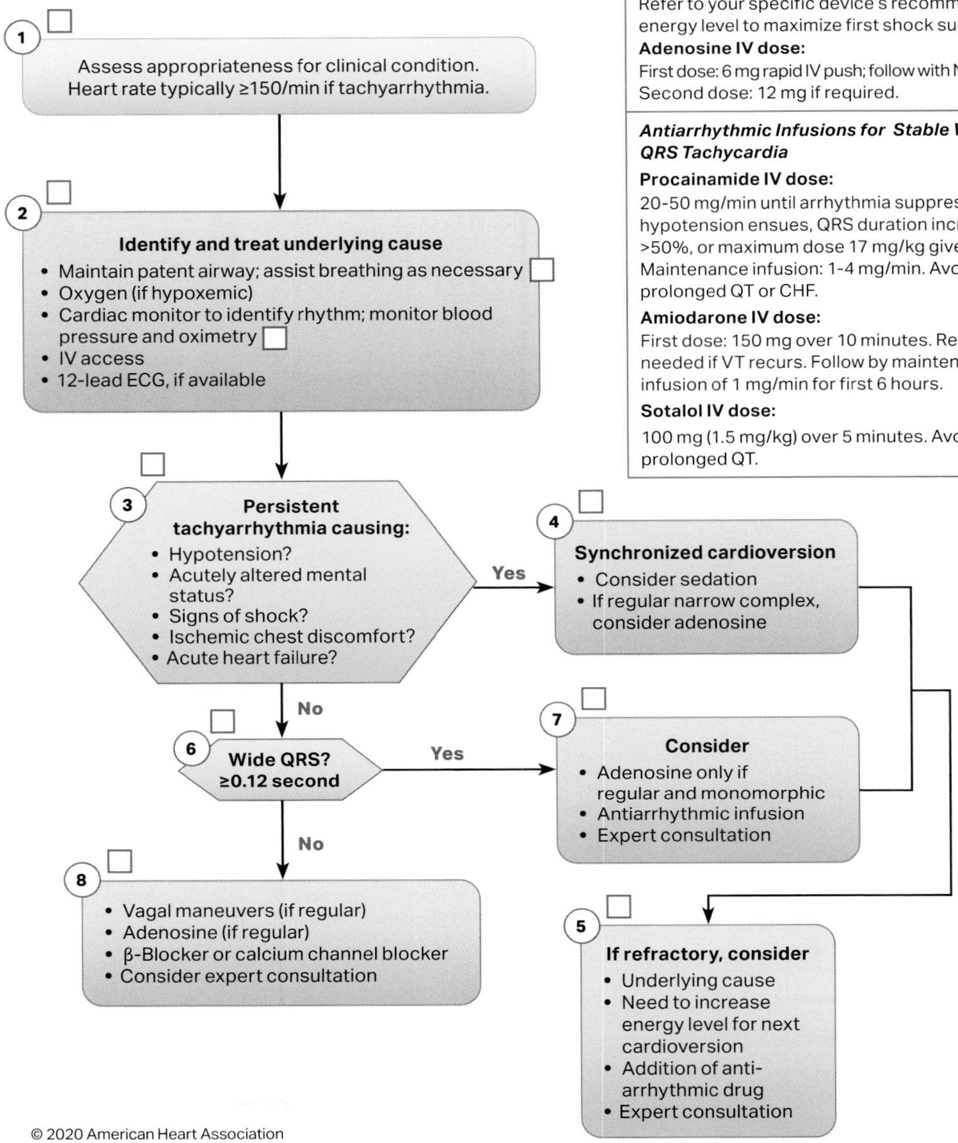

1
Assess appropriateness for clinical condition.
Heart rate typically ≥150/min if tachyarrhythmia.
2
Identify and treat underlying cause
• Maintain patent airway; assist breathing as necessary
• Oxygen (if hypoxemic)
• Cardiac monitor to identify rhythm; monitor blood pressure and oximetry
• IV access
• 12-lead ECG, if available
3
Persistent tachyarrhythmia causing:
• Hypotension?
• Acutely altered mental status?
• Signs of shock?
• Ischemic chest discomfort?
• Acute heart failure?
Yes
4
Synchronized cardioversion
• Consider sedation
• If regular narrow complex, consider adenosine
No
6
Wide QRS? ≥0.12 second
Yes
7
Consider
• Adenosine only if regular and monomorphic
• Antiarrhythmic infusion
• Expert consultation
No
8
• Vagal maneuvers (if regular)
• Adenosine (if regular)
• β-Blocker or calcium channel blocker
• Consider expert consultation
5
If refractory, consider
• Underlying cause
• Need to increase energy level for next cardioversion
• Addition of anti-arrhythmic drug
• Expert consultation

Doses/Details

Synchronized cardioversion:
Refer to your specific device's recommended energy level to maximize first shock success.

Adenosine IV dose:
First dose: 6 mg rapid IV push; follow with NS flush.
Second dose: 12 mg if required.

Antiarrhythmic Infusions for Stable Wide-QRS Tachycardia

Procainamide IV dose:
20-50 mg/min until arrhythmia suppressed, hypotension ensues, QRS duration increases >50%, or maximum dose 17 mg/kg given.
Maintenance infusion: 1-4 mg/min. Avoid if prolonged QT or CHF.

Amiodarone IV dose:
First dose: 150 mg over 10 minutes. Repeat as needed if VT recurs. Follow by maintenance infusion of 1 mg/min for first 6 hours.

Sotalol IV dose:
100 mg (1.5 mg/kg) over 5 minutes. Avoid if prolonged QT.

Debriefing Tool

ACLS Sample Scenario: Tachycardia

Learning Objectives

- Apply the BLS, Primary, and Secondary Assessments sequence for a systematic evaluation of adult patients
- Recognize tachyarrhythmias that may result in cardiac arrest or complicate resuscitation outcome
- Perform early management of tachyarrhythmias that may result in cardiac arrest or complicate resuscitation outcome
- Model effective communication as a member or leader of a high-performance team
- Recognize the impact of team dynamics on overall team performance

General Debriefing Principles

- Use the table on the right to guide your debriefing.
- Debriefings are 4 to 6 minutes long (unless more time is needed).
- Address all objectives.
- Summarize take-home messages at the end of the debriefing.
- *Encourage* students to self-reflect, and engage all participants.
- *Avoid* mini-lectures, and prevent closed-ended questions from dominating the discussion.

Action	Gather	Analyze	Summarize
	Student Observations (primary is Team Leader and Timer/Recorder)	**Done Well**	**Student-Led Summary**
• Assigns team roles and directs the team (effective team dynamics)	• Can you describe the events from your perspective?	• How were you able to [insert action here]?	• What are the main things you learned?
• Directs the systematic approach	• How did you think your treatments went?	• Why do you think you were able to [insert action here]?	• Can someone summarize the key points made?
• Directs team to apply monitor leads	• Can you review the events of the scenario? (directed to the Timer/Recorder)	• Tell me a little more about how you [insert action here].	• What are the main take-home messages?
• Directs IV or IO access	• What could you have improved?		
• Directs appropriate drug treatment or synchronized/ unsynchronized cardioversion	• What did the team do well?		
• Directs reassessment of patient in response to treatments			
• Summarizes specific treatments	**Instructor Observations**	**Needs Improvement**	**Instructor-Led Summary**
• Verbalizes indications for advanced airway if needed	• I noticed that [insert action here].	• Why do you think [insert action here] occurred?	• Let's summarize what we learned...
	• I observed that [insert action here].	• How do you think [insert action here] could have been improved?	• Here is what I think we learned...
	• I saw that [insert action here].	• What was your thinking while [insert action here]?	• The main take-home messages are...
		• What prevented you from [insert action here]?	

Case 26: Out-of-Hospital Unstable Tachycardia

Scenario Rating: 2

Lead-in: You are a paramedic who responds to a report of a woman who passed out in a gym.

Vital Signs
Heart rate:
Blood pressure:
Respiratory rate:
SpO₂:
Temperature:
Weight:
Age: 25 years

Initial Information
- The woman is lying on the floor, alert and oriented but pale and diaphoretic.
- Firefighters cannot obtain a blood pressure measurement.

What are your actions?

Additional Information
- You attach a cardiac monitor/defibrillator.
- A rhythm check finds a **narrow-complex tachycardia (SVT)** with a rate of 210/min.

What are your actions?

Additional Information (if needed)
- The patient is taking over-the-counter herbal appetite suppressants.
- She became dizzy while working out. No other medical history is available.

What are your next actions?

Adult Tachycardia With a Pulse Learning Station Checklist

Adult Tachycardia With a Pulse Algorithm

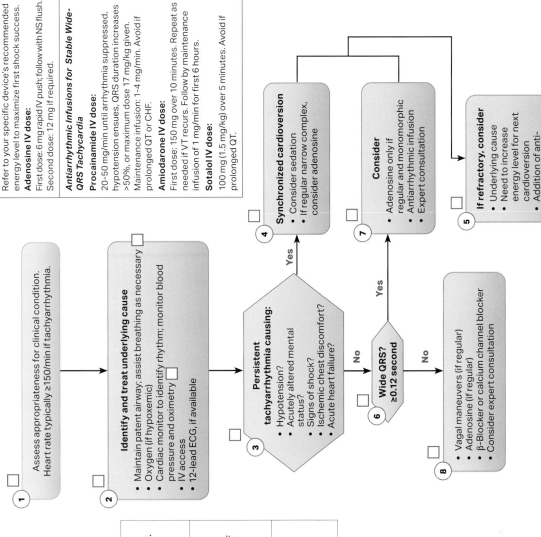

1
Assess appropriateness for clinical condition.
Heart rate typically ≥150/min if tachyarrhythmia.

2
Identify and treat underlying cause
- Maintain patent airway; assist breathing as necessary
- Oxygen (if hypoxemic)
- Cardiac monitor to identify rhythm; monitor blood pressure and oximetry
- IV access
- 12-lead ECG, if available

3
Persistent tachyarrhythmia causing:
- Hypotension?
- Acutely altered mental status?
- Signs of shock?
- Ischemic chest discomfort?
- Acute heart failure?

Yes →

4
Synchronized cardioversion
- Consider sedation
- If regular narrow complex, consider adenosine

No ↓

6
Wide QRS?
≥0.12 second

Yes →

7
Consider
- Adenosine only if regular and monomorphic
- Antiarrhythmic infusion
- Expert consultation

5
If refractory, consider
- Underlying cause
- Need to increase energy level for next cardioversion
- Addition of anti-arrhythmic drug
- Expert consultation

No ↓

8
- Vagal maneuvers (if regular)
- Adenosine (if regular)
- β-Blocker or calcium channel blocker
- Consider expert consultation

Doses/Details

Synchronized cardioversion:
Refer to your specific device's recommended energy level to maximize first shock success.

Adenosine IV dose:
First dose: 6 mg rapid IV push; follow with NS flush.
Second dose: 12 mg if required.

Antiarrhythmic Infusions for Stable Wide-QRS Tachycardia

Procainamide IV dose:
20-50 mg/min until arrhythmia suppressed, hypotension ensues, QRS duration increases >50%, or maximum dose 17 mg/kg given. Maintenance infusion: 1-4 mg/min. Avoid if prolonged QT or CHF.

Amiodarone IV dose:
First dose: 150 mg over 10 minutes. Repeat as needed if VT recurs. Follow by maintenance infusion of 1 mg/min for first 6 hours.

Sotalol IV dose:
100 mg (1.5 mg/kg) over 5 minutes. Avoid if prolonged QT.

Debriefing Tool

ACLS Sample Scenario: Tachycardia

Action	Gather	Analyze	Summarize
	Student Observations (primary is Team Leader and Timer/Recorder)	**Done Well**	**Student-Led Summary**
• Assigns team roles and directs the team (effective team dynamics)	• Can you describe the events from your perspective?	• How were you able to [*insert action here*]?	• What are the main things you learned?
• Directs the systematic approach	• How did you think your treatments went?	• Why do you think you were able to [*insert action here*]?	• Can someone summarize the key points made?
• Directs team to apply monitor leads	• Can you review the events of the scenario? (*directed to the Timer/ Recorder*)	• Tell me a little more about how you [*insert action here*].	• What are the main take-home messages?
• Directs IV or IO access			
• Directs appropriate drug treatment or synchronized/ unsynchronized cardioversion	• What could you have improved?		
• Directs reassessment of patient in response to treatments	• What did the team do well?		

Action	Gather	Analyze	Summarize
	Instructor Observations	**Needs Improvement**	**Instructor-Led Summary**
• Summarizes specific treatments	• I noticed that [*insert action here*].	• Why do you think [*insert action here*] occurred?	• Let's summarize what we learned…
• Verbalizes indications for advanced airway if needed	• I observed that [*insert action here*].	• How do you think [*insert action here*] could have been improved?	• Here is what I think we learned…
	• I saw that [*insert action here*].	• What was your thinking while [*insert action here*]?	• The main take-home messages are…
		• What prevented you from [*insert action here*]?	

Learning Objectives

- Apply the BLS, Primary, and Secondary Assessments sequence for a systematic evaluation of adult patients
- Recognize tachyarrhythmias that may result in cardiac arrest or complicate resuscitation outcome
- Perform early management of tachyarrhythmias that may result in cardiac arrest or complicate resuscitation outcome
- Model effective communication as a member or leader of a high-performance team
- Recognize the impact of team dynamics on overall team performance

General Debriefing Principles

- Use the table on the right to guide your debriefing.
- Debriefings are 4 to 6 minutes long (unless more time is needed).
- Address all objectives.
- Summarize take-home messages at the end of the debriefing.
- **Encourage** students to self-reflect, and engage all participants.
- **Avoid** mini-lectures, and prevent closed-ended questions from dominating the discussion.

Case 27: Emergency Department Unstable Tachycardia

Scenario Rating: 3

Lead-in: You are an emergency department care provider assessing a woman who reported multiple episodes of syncope and palpitations.

Vital Signs

Heart rate: 160/min
Blood pressure: 80/65 mm Hg
Respiratory rate: 16/min
SpO₂: 96%
Temperature: 36.3°C
Weight: 60 kg
Age: 35 years

Initial Information

- The patient has had these episodes for years, but they have become more frequent over the last few days.
- She states that she is feeling very weak.

What are your initial actions?

- The ECG shows **atrial fibrillation with Wolff-Parkinson-White** (irregular, wide-complex tachycardia).

Additional Information

- The patient has a medical history as a smoker, with no medications and no allergies.
- During the interview, her palpitations worsen and she becomes short of breath.
- Electrical cardioversion restores normal sinus rhythm.
- A follow-up ECG reveals normal sinus rhythm with signs of an accessory pathway (delta wave, short PR interval).

Instructor notes: If students deliver an AV nodal blocking agent (eg, calcium channel blocker, β-blocker, adenosine), the patient will deteriorate into a ventricular response of 300/min briefly before a VF arrest, which is resistant to all therapies.

Adult Tachycardia With a Pulse Learning Station Checklist

Adult Tachycardia With a Pulse Algorithm

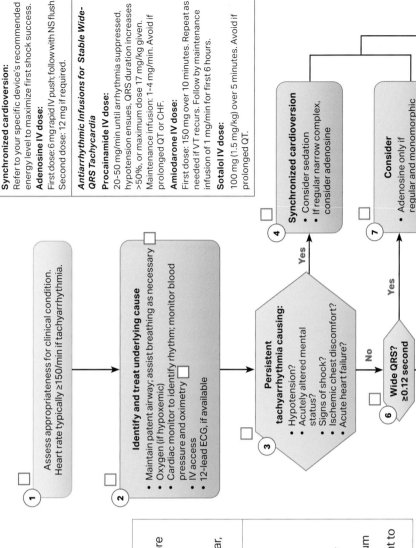

1 Assess appropriateness for clinical condition. Heart rate typically ≥150/min if tachyarrhythmia.

2 Identify and treat underlying cause
- Maintain patent airway; assist breathing as necessary
- Oxygen (if hypoxemic)
- Cardiac monitor to identify rhythm; monitor blood pressure and oximetry
- IV access
- 12-lead ECG, if available

3 Persistent tachyarrhythmia causing:
- Hypotension?
- Acutely altered mental status?
- Signs of shock?
- Ischemic chest discomfort?
- Acute heart failure?

Yes →

4 Synchronized cardioversion
- Consider sedation
- If regular narrow complex, consider adenosine

No →

6 Wide QRS? ≥0.12 second

Yes →

7 Consider
- Adenosine only if regular and monomorphic
- Antiarrhythmic infusion
- Expert consultation

No →

8
- Vagal maneuvers (if regular)
- Adenosine (if regular)
- β-Blocker or calcium channel blocker
- Consider expert consultation

5 If refractory, consider
- Underlying cause
- Need to increase energy level for next cardioversion
- Addition of anti-arrhythmic drug
- Expert consultation

Doses/Details

Synchronized cardioversion:
Refer to your specific device's recommended energy level to maximize first shock success.

Adenosine IV dose:
First dose: 6 mg rapid IV push; follow with NS flush.
Second dose: 12 mg if required.

Antiarrhythmic Infusions for Stable Wide-QRS Tachycardia

Procainamide IV dose:
20-50 mg/min until arrhythmia suppressed, hypotension ensues, QRS duration increases >50%, or maximum dose 17 mg/kg given. Maintenance infusion: 1-4 mg/min. Avoid if prolonged QT or CHF.

Amiodarone IV dose:
First dose: 150 mg over 10 minutes. Repeat as needed if VT recurs. Follow by maintenance infusion of 1 mg/min for first 6 hours.

Sotalol IV dose:
100 mg (1.5 mg/kg) over 5 minutes. Avoid if prolonged QT.

Debriefing Tool

ACLS Sample Scenario: Tachycardia

Learning Objectives

- Apply the BLS, Primary, and Secondary Assessments sequence for a systematic evaluation of adult patients
- Recognize tachyarrhythmias that may result in cardiac arrest or complicate resuscitation outcome
- Perform early management of tachyarrhythmias that may result in cardiac arrest or complicate resuscitation outcome
- Model effective communication as a member or leader of a high-performance team
- Recognize the impact of team dynamics on overall team performance

General Debriefing Principles

- Use the table on the right to guide your debriefing.
- Debriefings are 4 to 6 minutes long (unless more time is needed).
- Address all objectives.
- Summarize take-home messages at the end of the debriefing.
- *Encourage* students to self-reflect, and engage all participants.
- *Avoid* mini-lectures, and prevent closed-ended questions from dominating the discussion.

Action	Gather	Analyze	Summarize
- Assigns team roles and directs the team (effective team dynamics) - Directs the systematic approach - Directs team to apply monitor leads - Directs IV or IO access - Directs appropriate drug treatment or synchronized/ unsynchronized cardioversion - Directs reassessment of patient in response to treatments - Summarizes specific treatments - Verbalizes indications for advanced airway if needed	**Student Observations** (primary is Team Leader and Timer/Recorder) - Can you describe the events from your perspective? - How did you think your treatments went? - Can you review the events of the scenario? (*directed to the Timer/ Recorder*) - What could you have improved? - What did the team do well? **Instructor Observations** - I noticed that [*insert action here*]. - I observed that [*insert action here*]. - I saw that [*insert action here*].	**Done Well** - How were you able to [*insert action here*]? - Why do you think you were able to [*insert action here*]? - Tell me a little more about how you [*insert action here*]. **Needs Improvement** - Why do you think [*insert action here*] occurred? - How do you think [*insert action here*] could have been improved? - What was your thinking while [*insert action here*]? - What prevented you from [*insert action here*]?	**Student-Led Summary** - What are the main things you learned? - Can someone summarize the key points made? - What are the main take-home messages? **Instructor-Led Summary** - Let's summarize what we learned… - Here is what I think we learned… - The main take-home messages are…

Case 28: Emergency Department Unstable Tachycardia

Scenario Rating: 2

Lead-in: A woman presents to the emergency department. Her husband reports that she suddenly lost consciousness at dinner and was staring into space for 4 to 5 seconds.

Vital Signs
Heart rate:
Blood pressure:
Respiratory rate:
SpO₂:
Temperature:
Weight:
Age: 35 years

Initial Information

- The husband did not notice any seizure-like activity.
- The patient is a marathon runner and works as a schoolteacher.
- Over the past week, she developed nasal congestion and was prescribed clarithromycin for presumed sinusitis at a walk-in clinic.

What are your initial actions?

- She is placed on a cardiac monitor. Her physical and neurological exam is unremarkable.

Instructor notes: Show long QTc.

What are your actions?

Additional Information

- The nurse suddenly notices the patient is briefly unresponsive.
- The ECG monitor shows **polymorphic VT**, and the patient has a pulse.

What are your actions?

Adult Tachycardia With a Pulse Learning Station Checklist

Adult Tachycardia With a Pulse Algorithm

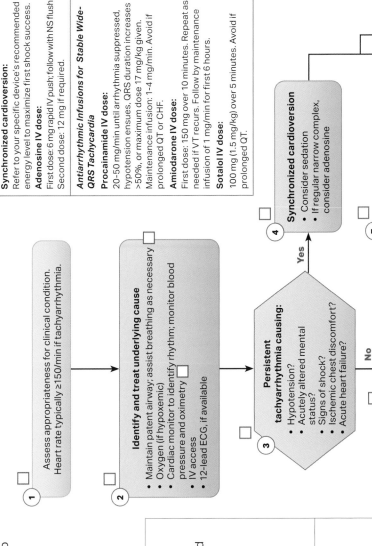

Doses/Details

Synchronized cardioversion:
Refer to your specific device's recommended energy level to maximize first shock success.

Adenosine IV dose:
First dose: 6 mg rapid IV push; follow with NS flush.
Second dose: 12 mg if required.

Antiarrhythmic Infusions for *Stable Wide-QRS Tachycardia*

Procainamide IV dose:
20-50 mg/min until arrhythmia suppressed, hypotension ensues, QRS duration increases >50%, or maximum dose 17 mg/kg given.
Maintenance infusion: 1-4 mg/min. Avoid if prolonged QT or CHF.

Amiodarone IV dose:
First dose: 150 mg over 10 minutes. Repeat as needed if VT recurs. Follow by maintenance infusion of 1 mg/min for first 6 hours.

Sotalol IV dose:
100 mg (1.5 mg/kg) over 5 minutes. Avoid if prolonged QT.

1 Assess appropriateness for clinical condition.
Heart rate typically ≥150/min if tachyarrhythmia.

2 Identify and treat underlying cause
- Maintain patent airway; assist breathing as necessary
- Oxygen (if hypoxemic)
- Cardiac monitor to identify rhythm; monitor blood pressure and oximetry
- IV access
- 12-lead ECG, if available

3 Persistent tachyarrhythmia causing:
- Hypotension?
- Acutely altered mental status?
- Signs of shock?
- Ischemic chest discomfort?
- Acute heart failure?

Yes → **4** Synchronized cardioversion
- Consider sedation
- If regular narrow complex, consider adenosine

No → **6** Wide QRS? ≥0.12 second

Yes → **7** Consider
- Adenosine only if regular and monomorphic
- Antiarrhythmic infusion
- Expert consultation

No → **8**
- Vagal maneuvers (if regular)
- Adenosine (if regular)
- β-Blocker or calcium channel blocker
- Consider expert consultation

5 If refractory, consider
- Underlying cause
- Need to increase energy level for next cardioversion
- Addition of anti-arrhythmic drug
- Expert consultation

Debriefing Tool

ACLS Sample Scenario: Tachycardia

Learning Objectives

- Apply the BLS, Primary, and Secondary Assessments sequence for a systematic evaluation of adult patients
- Recognize tachyarrhythmias that may result in cardiac arrest or complicate resuscitation outcome
- Perform early management of tachyarrhythmias that may result in cardiac arrest or complicate resuscitation outcome
- Model effective communication as a member or leader of a high-performance team
- Recognize the impact of team dynamics on overall team performance

General Debriefing Principles

- Use the table on the right to guide your debriefing.
- Debriefings are 4 to 6 minutes long (unless more time is needed).
- Address all objectives.
- Summarize take-home messages at the end of the debriefing.
- **Encourage** students to self-reflect, and engage all participants.
- **Avoid** mini-lectures, and prevent closed-ended questions from dominating the discussion.

Action	Gather	Analyze	Summarize
- Assigns team roles and directs the team (effective team dynamics) - Directs the systematic approach - Directs team to apply monitor leads - Directs IV or IO access - Directs appropriate drug treatment or synchronized/ unsynchronized cardioversion - Directs reassessment of patient in response to treatments - Summarizes specific treatments - Verbalizes indications for advanced airway if needed	**Student Observations** (primary is Team Leader and Timer/Recorder) - Can you describe the events from your perspective? - How did you think your treatments went? - Can you review the events of the scenario? *(directed to the Timer/ Recorder)* - What could you have improved? - What did the team do well?	**Done Well** - How were you able to [*insert action here*]? - Why do you think you were able to [*insert action here*]? - Tell me a little more about how you [*insert action here*].	**Student-Led Summary** - What are the main things you learned? - Can someone summarize the key points made? - What are the main take-home messages?
	Instructor Observations - I noticed that [*insert action here*]. - I observed that [*insert action here*]. - I saw that [*insert action here*].	**Needs Improvement** - Why do you think [*insert action here*] occurred? - How do you think [*insert action here*] could have been improved? - What was your thinking while [*insert action here*]? - What prevented you from [*insert action here*]?	**Instructor-Led Summary** - Let's summarize what we learned… - Here is what I think we learned… - The main take-home messages are…

Case 29: Emergency Department Stable Tachycardia

Scenario Rating: 1

Lead-in: You are working in the emergency department when EMS brings in a man who reports a "fast heart rate." At dinner, he noted palpitations, chest pressure, diaphoresis, and nausea.

Vital Signs
Heart rate: 155/min
Blood pressure: 136/45 mm Hg
Respiratory rate:
SpO₂: 97% on room air
Temperature:
Weight:
Age: 52 years

Initial Information
- The patient is anxious, diaphoretic, and holding his chest.

What are your actions?

Additional Information
- The patient is placed on a monitor, and the rhythm appears narrow and regular.

What are your actions now?

Additional Information (if needed)
- A trial of adenosine 6 mg slows down the heart rate to reveal **atrial flutter.**
- The patient starts on an IV calcium channel blocker and then is admitted to cardiology.

Additional Information (if needed)
- The patient says he recently had a 3-hour plane flight, and he has been training for a marathon and taking dietary supplements and "energy pills."
- He had a few cups of coffee at dinner.

Adult Tachycardia With a Pulse Learning Station Checklist

Adult Tachycardia With a Pulse Algorithm

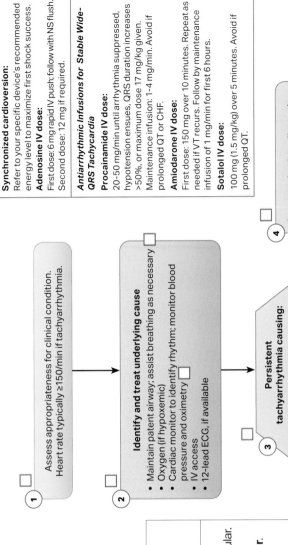

	Doses/Details
	Synchronized cardioversion: Refer to your specific device's recommended energy level to maximize first shock success. **Adenosine IV dose:** First dose: 6 mg rapid IV push; follow with NS flush. Second dose: 12 mg if required. ***Antiarrhythmic Infusions for Stable Wide-QRS Tachycardia*** **Procainamide IV dose:** 20-50 mg/min until arrhythmia suppressed, hypotension ensues, QRS duration increases >50%, or maximum dose 17 mg/kg given. Maintenance infusion: 1-4 mg/min. Avoid if prolonged QT or CHF. **Amiodarone IV dose:** First dose: 150 mg over 10 minutes. Repeat as needed if VT recurs. Follow by maintenance infusion of 1 mg/min for first 6 hours. **Sotalol IV dose:** 100 mg (1.5 mg/kg) over 5 minutes. Avoid if prolonged QT.

1 Assess appropriateness for clinical condition. Heart rate typically ≥150/min if tachyarrhythmia.

2 Identify and treat underlying cause
- Maintain patent airway; assist breathing as necessary
- Oxygen (if hypoxemic)
- Cardiac monitor to identify rhythm; monitor blood pressure and oximetry
- IV access
- 12-lead ECG, if available

3 Persistent tachyarrhythmia causing:
- Hypotension?
- Acutely altered mental status?
- Signs of shock?
- Ischemic chest discomfort?
- Acute heart failure?

Yes →

4 Synchronized cardioversion
- Consider sedation
- If regular narrow complex, consider adenosine

No →

6 Wide QRS? ≥0.12 second

Yes →

7 Consider
- Adenosine only if regular and monomorphic
- Antiarrhythmic infusion
- Expert consultation

No →

8
- Vagal maneuvers (if regular)
- Adenosine (if regular)
- β-Blocker or calcium channel blocker
- Consider expert consultation

5 If refractory, consider
- Underlying cause
- Need to increase energy level for next cardioversion
- Addition of anti-arrhythmic drug
- Expert consultation

Debriefing Tool

ACLS Sample Scenario: Tachycardia

Learning Objectives

- Apply the BLS, Primary, and Secondary Assessments sequence for a systematic evaluation of adult patients
- Recognize tachyarrhythmias that may result in cardiac arrest or complicate resuscitation outcome
- Perform early management of tachyarrhythmias that may result in cardiac arrest or complicate resuscitation outcome
- Model effective communication as a member or leader of a high-performance team
- Recognize the impact of team dynamics on overall team performance

General Debriefing Principles

- Use the table on the right to guide your debriefing.
- Debriefings are 4 to 6 minutes long (unless more time is needed).
- Address all objectives.
- Summarize take-home messages at the end of the debriefing.
- *Encourage* students to self-reflect, and engage all participants.
- *Avoid* mini-lectures, and prevent closed-ended questions from dominating the discussion.

Action	Gather	Analyze	Summarize
	Student Observations (primary is Team Leader and Timer/Recorder)	**Done Well**	**Student-Led Summary**
- Assigns team roles and directs the team (effective team dynamics)	- Can you describe the events from your perspective?	- How were you able to *[insert action here]*?	- What are the main things you learned?
- Directs the systematic approach	- How did you think your treatments went?	- Why do you think you were able to *[insert action here]*?	- Can someone summarize the key points made?
- Directs team to apply monitor leads	- Can you review the events of the scenario? *(directed to the Timer/Recorder)*	- Tell me a little more about how you *[insert action here]*.	- What are the main take-home messages?
- Directs IV or IO access	- What could you have improved?		
- Directs appropriate drug treatment or synchronized/unsynchronized cardioversion	- What did the team do well?		
- Directs reassessment of patient in response to treatments			
	Instructor Observations	**Needs Improvement**	**Instructor-Led Summary**
- Summarizes specific treatments	- I noticed that *[insert action here]*.	- Why do you think *[insert action here]* occurred?	- Let's summarize what we learned…
- Verbalizes indications for advanced airway if needed	- I observed that *[insert action here]*.	- How do you think *[insert action here]* could have been improved?	- Here is what I think we learned…
	- I saw that *[insert action here]*.	- What was your thinking while *[insert action here]*?	- The main take-home messages are…
		- What prevented you from *[insert action here]*?	

Case 30: In-Hospital—Acute Medical-Surgical Unit Stable Tachycardia

Scenario Rating: 1

Lead-in: You are a healthcare provider responding to a patient who feels like her "chest is going to explode."

Vital Signs

Heart rate: 123/min
Blood pressure: 123/78 mm Hg
Respiratory rate: 18/min
SpO₂:
Temperature:
Weight:
Age: 86 years

Initial Information

- The patient was admitted with exacerbation of asthma.
- Cardiac telemetry shows a narrow, rapid rhythm (**sinus tachycardia**).
- She is currently not using oxygen therapy.

What are your next actions?

Additional Information

- As you discuss what led to your patient's heart event, you notice that she has a nebulizer mask hanging over the oxygen flow meter.

What are your next actions?

Additional Information (if needed)

- Your patient says she has had many nebulizer treatments in the past, but she has never felt like this.
- She is frightened and anxious, and she is visibly shaking.

What are your next actions?

Adult Tachycardia With a Pulse Learning Station Checklist

Adult Tachycardia With a Pulse Algorithm

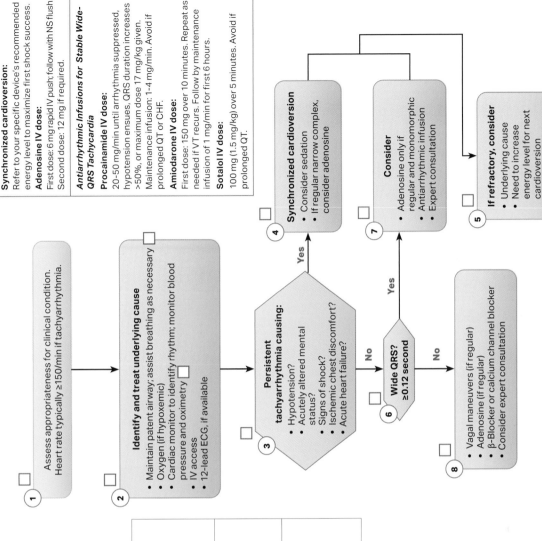

1
Assess appropriateness for clinical condition.
Heart rate typically ≥150/min if tachyarrhythmia.

2 Identify and treat underlying cause
- Maintain patent airway; assist breathing as necessary
- Oxygen (if hypoxemic)
- Cardiac monitor to identify rhythm; monitor blood pressure and oximetry
- IV access
- 12-lead ECG, if available

3 Persistent tachyarrhythmia causing:
- Hypotension?
- Acutely altered mental status?
- Signs of shock?
- Ischemic chest discomfort?
- Acute heart failure?

Yes →

4 Synchronized cardioversion
- Consider sedation
- If regular narrow complex, consider adenosine

No ↓

6 Wide QRS? ≥0.12 second

Yes →

7 Consider
- Adenosine only if regular and monomorphic
- Antiarrhythmic infusion
- Expert consultation

5 If refractory, consider
- Underlying cause
- Need to increase energy level for next cardioversion
- Addition of anti-arrhythmic drug
- Expert consultation

No ↓

8
- Vagal maneuvers (if regular)
- Adenosine (if regular)
- β-Blocker or calcium channel blocker
- Consider expert consultation

Doses/Details

Synchronized cardioversion:
Refer to your specific device's recommended energy level to maximize first shock success.

Adenosine IV dose:
First dose: 6 mg rapid IV push; follow with NS flush.
Second dose: 12 mg if required.

Antiarrhythmic Infusions for Stable Wide-QRS Tachycardia

Procainamide IV dose:
20-50 mg/min until arrhythmia suppressed, hypotension ensues, QRS duration increases >50%, or maximum dose 17 mg/kg given.
Maintenance infusion: 1-4 mg/min. Avoid if prolonged QT or CHF.

Amiodarone IV dose:
First dose: 150 mg over 10 minutes. Repeat as needed if VT recurs. Follow by maintenance infusion of 1 mg/min for first 6 hours.

Sotalol IV dose:
100 mg (1.5 mg/kg) over 5 minutes. Avoid if prolonged QT.

Debriefing Tool

ACLS Sample Scenario: Tachycardia

Learning Objectives

- Apply the BLS, Primary, and Secondary Assessments sequence for a systematic evaluation of adult patients
- Recognize tachyarrhythmias that may result in cardiac arrest or complicate resuscitation outcome
- Perform early management of tachyarrhythmias that may result in cardiac arrest or complicate resuscitation outcome
- Model effective communication as a member or leader of a high-performance team
- Recognize the impact of team dynamics on overall team performance

General Debriefing Principles

- Use the table on the right to guide your debriefing.
- Debriefings are 4 to 6 minutes long (unless more time is needed).
- Address all objectives.
- Summarize take-home messages at the end of the debriefing.
- **Encourage** students to self-reflect, and engage all participants.
- **Avoid** mini-lectures, and prevent closed-ended questions from dominating the discussion.

Action	Gather	Analyze	Summarize
• Assigns team roles and directs the team (effective team dynamics) • Directs the systematic approach • Directs team to apply monitor leads • Directs IV or IO access • Directs appropriate drug treatment or synchronized/ unsynchronized cardioversion • Directs reassessment of patient in response to treatments • Summarizes specific treatments • Verbalizes indications for advanced airway if needed	**Student Observations** (primary is Team Leader and Timer/Recorder) • Can you describe the events from your perspective? • How did you think your treatments went? • Can you review the events of the scenario? *(directed to the Timer/ Recorder)* • What could you have improved? • What did the team do well?	**Done Well** • How were you able to [*insert action here*]? • Why do you think you were able to [*insert action here*]? • Tell me a little more about how you [*insert action here*].	**Student-Led Summary** • What are the main things you learned? • Can someone summarize the key points made? • What are the main take-home messages?
	Instructor Observations • I noticed that [*insert action here*]. • I observed that [*insert action here*]. • I saw that [*insert action here*].	**Needs Improvement** • Why do you think [*insert action here*] occurred? • How do you think [*insert action here*] could have been improved? • What was your thinking while [*insert action here*]? • What prevented you from [*insert action here*]?	**Instructor-Led Summary** • Let's summarize what we learned… • Here is what I think we learned… • The main take-home messages are…

Case 31: In-Hospital Stable Tachycardia

Scenario Rating: 1

Lead-in: A man is recovering in the postanesthesia care unit after an elective inguinal hernia surgery. He reports feeling well. His blood pressure remains unchanged, but the nurse notices a sudden increase in his heart rate. You are asked to evaluate the patient.

Vital Signs

Heart rate: 140/min
Blood pressure: 110/60 mm Hg
Respiratory rate:
SpO₂:
Temperature:
Weight:
Age: 80 years

Initial Information

- The patient is alert and oriented.
- He is asymptomatic, and his lungs sound clear.

What are your actions?

Additional Information

- You attach a cardiac monitor/defibrillator.
- The ECG strip shows a **narrow-complex QRS tachycardia** with beat-to-beat variation in the respiratory rate interval.

What is the diagnosis? What are your actions?

Additional Information (if needed)

- As you wait for the medications, you notice that the patient has a regular heart rate of 84/min on the monitor.
- His bedside ECG confirms normal sinus rhythm.
- He remains asymptomatic.

What are your actions?

Adult Tachycardia With a Pulse Learning Station Checklist

Adult Tachycardia With a Pulse Algorithm

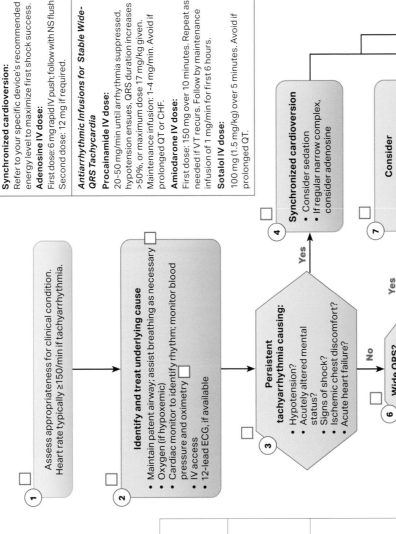

	Doses/Details
	Synchronized cardioversion: Refer to your specific device's recommended energy level to maximize first shock success.
	Adenosine IV dose: First dose: 6 mg rapid IV push; follow with NS flush. Second dose: 12 mg if required.
	Antiarrhythmic Infusions for Stable Wide-QRS Tachycardia
	Procainamide IV dose: 20-50 mg/min until arrhythmia suppressed, hypotension ensues, QRS duration increases >50%, or maximum dose 17 mg/kg given. Maintenance infusion: 1-4 mg/min. Avoid if prolonged QT or CHF.
	Amiodarone IV dose: First dose: 150 mg over 10 minutes. Repeat as needed if VT recurs. Follow by maintenance infusion of 1 mg/min for first 6 hours.
	Sotalol IV dose: 100 mg (1.5 mg/kg) over 5 minutes. Avoid if prolonged QT.

1
Assess appropriateness for clinical condition.
Heart rate typically ≥150/min if tachyarrhythmia.

2 Identify and treat underlying cause
- Maintain patent airway; assist breathing as necessary
- Oxygen (if hypoxemic)
- Cardiac monitor to identify rhythm; monitor blood pressure and oximetry
- IV access
- 12-lead ECG, if available

3 Persistent tachyarrhythmia causing:
- Hypotension?
- Acutely altered mental status?
- Signs of shock?
- Ischemic chest discomfort?
- Acute heart failure?

Yes →

4 Synchronized cardioversion
- Consider sedation
- If regular narrow complex, consider adenosine

No ↓

6 Wide QRS?
≥0.12 second

Yes →

7 Consider
- Adenosine only if regular and monomorphic
- Antiarrhythmic infusion
- Expert consultation

No ↓

8
- Vagal maneuvers (if regular)
- Adenosine (if regular)
- β-Blocker or calcium channel blocker
- Consider expert consultation

5 If refractory, consider
- Underlying cause
- Need to increase energy level for next cardioversion
- Addition of anti-arrhythmic drug
- Expert consultation

Debriefing Tool

ACLS Sample Scenario: Tachycardia

Action	Gather	Analyze	Summarize
	Student Observations (primary is Team Leader and Timer/Recorder)	**Done Well**	**Student-Led Summary**
• Assigns team roles and directs the team (effective team dynamics)	• Can you describe the events from your perspective?	• How were you able to [*insert action here*]?	• What are the main things you learned?
• Directs the systematic approach	• How did you think your treatments went?	• Why do you think you were able to [*insert action here*]?	• Can someone summarize the key points made?
• Directs team to apply monitor leads	• Can you review the events of the scenario? (*directed to the Timer/Recorder*)	• Tell me a little more about how you [*insert action here*].	• What are the main take-home messages?
• Directs IV or IO access	• What could you have improved?		
• Directs appropriate drug treatment or synchronized/unsynchronized cardioversion	• What did the team do well?		
• Directs reassessment of patient in response to treatments			
• Summarizes specific treatments	**Instructor Observations**	**Needs Improvement**	**Instructor-Led Summary**
• Verbalizes indications for advanced airway if needed	• I noticed that [*insert action here*].	• Why do you think [*insert action here*] occurred?	• Let's summarize what we learned…
	• I observed that [*insert action here*].	• How do you think [*insert action here*] could have been improved?	• Here is what I think we learned…
	• I saw that [*insert action here*].	• What was your thinking while [*insert action here*]?	• The main take-home messages are…
		• What prevented you from [*insert action here*]?	

Learning Objectives

- Apply the BLS, Primary, and Secondary Assessments sequence for a systematic evaluation of adult patients
- Recognize tachyarrhythmias that may result in cardiac arrest or complicate resuscitation outcome
- Perform early management of tachyarrhythmias that may result in cardiac arrest or complicate resuscitation outcome
- Model effective communication as a member or leader of a high-performance team
- Recognize the impact of team dynamics on overall team performance

General Debriefing Principles

- Use the table on the right to guide your debriefing.
- Debriefings are 4 to 6 minutes long (unless more time is needed).
- Address all objectives.
- Summarize take-home messages at the end of the debriefing.
- *Encourage* students to self-reflect, and engage all participants.
- *Avoid* mini-lectures, and prevent closed-ended questions from dominating the discussion.

Case 32: In-Hospital—Intermediate Medical-Surgical Unit
Unstable Tachycardia

Scenario Rating: 1

Lead-in: You are a healthcare provider on an intermediate medical-surgical unit caring for a motor vehicle crash trauma patient with a chest tube. His wife runs to the nurses' station, yelling that her husband needs help.

Vital Signs
Heart rate: 166/min
Blood pressure:
Respiratory rate: 24/min
SpO₂: 94% on 4 L/min via nasal cannula
Temperature:
Weight:
Age: 28 years

Initial Information
- The patient's cardiac telemetry shows a narrow, rapid rhythm (**SVT**).

What are your next actions?

Additional Information
- Using a Doppler, you find that his blood pressure is 86 mm Hg systolic.
- You note cutaneous vasoconstriction, and he is becoming less responsive to your voice and commands.

What are your next actions?

Additional Information (if needed)
- You assess that the chest tube is working, but the output has increased from minimal drainage to over 1500 mL.
- His respirations have now increased to 28/min, and his wife yells for you to do something.
- The cardiac rhythm continues to be narrow and rapid without ectopy.

What are your next actions?

Adult Tachycardia With a Pulse Learning Station Checklist

Adult Tachycardia With a Pulse Algorithm

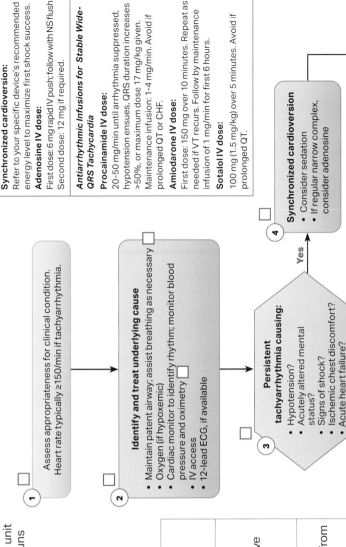

1 Assess appropriateness for clinical condition.
Heart rate typically ≥150/min if tachyarrhythmia.

2 **Identify and treat underlying cause**
- Maintain patent airway; assist breathing as necessary
- Oxygen (if hypoxemic)
- Cardiac monitor to identify rhythm; monitor blood pressure and oximetry
- IV access
- 12-lead ECG, if available

3 **Persistent tachyarrhythmia causing:**
- Hypotension?
- Acutely altered mental status?
- Signs of shock?
- Ischemic chest discomfort?
- Acute heart failure?

Yes → **4** **Synchronized cardioversion**
- Consider sedation
- If regular narrow complex, consider adenosine

No → **6** **Wide QRS? ≥0.12 second**

Yes → **7** **Consider**
- Adenosine only if regular and monomorphic
- Antiarrhythmic infusion
- Expert consultation

If refractory → **5** **If refractory, consider**
- Underlying cause
- Need to increase energy level for next cardioversion
- Addition of anti-arrhythmic drug
- Expert consultation

No → **8**
- Vagal maneuvers (if regular)
- Adenosine (if regular)
- β-Blocker or calcium channel blocker
- Consider expert consultation

Doses/Details

Synchronized cardioversion:
Refer to your specific device's recommended energy level to maximize first shock success.

Adenosine IV dose:
First dose: 6 mg rapid IV push; follow with NS flush.
Second dose: 12 mg if required.

Antiarrhythmic Infusions for Stable Wide-QRS Tachycardia

Procainamide IV dose:
20-50 mg/min until arrhythmia suppressed, hypotension ensues, QRS duration increases >50%, or maximum dose 17 mg/kg given.
Maintenance infusion: 1-4 mg/min. Avoid if prolonged QT or CHF.

Amiodarone IV dose:
First dose: 150 mg over 10 minutes. Repeat as needed if VT recurs. Follow by maintenance infusion of 1 mg/min for first 6 hours.

Sotalol IV dose:
100 mg (1.5 mg/kg) over 5 minutes. Avoid if prolonged QT.

© 2020 American Heart Association

147

Debriefing Tool

ACLS Sample Scenario: Tachycardia

Learning Objectives

- Apply the BLS, Primary, and Secondary Assessments sequence for a systematic evaluation of adult patients
- Recognize tachyarrhythmias that may result in cardiac arrest or complicate resuscitation outcome
- Perform early management of tachyarrhythmias that may result in cardiac arrest or complicate resuscitation outcome
- Model effective communication as a member or leader of a high-performance team
- Recognize the impact of team dynamics on overall team performance

General Debriefing Principles

- Use the table on the right to guide your debriefing.
- Debriefings are 4 to 6 minutes long (unless more time is needed).
- Address all objectives.
- Summarize take-home messages at the end of the debriefing.
- **Encourage** students to self-reflect, and engage all participants.
- **Avoid** mini-lectures, and prevent closed-ended questions from dominating the discussion.

Action	Gather	Analyze	Summarize
	Student Observations (primary is Team Leader and Timer/Recorder)	**Done Well**	**Student-Led Summary**
• Assigns team roles and directs the team (effective team dynamics) • Directs the systematic approach • Directs team to apply monitor leads • Directs IV or IO access • Directs appropriate drug treatment or synchronized/unsynchronized cardioversion • Directs reassessment of patient in response to treatments • Summarizes specific treatments • Verbalizes indications for advanced airway if needed	• Can you describe the events from your perspective? • How did you think your treatments went? • Can you review the events of the scenario? *(directed to the Timer/Recorder)* • What could you have improved? • What did the team do well?	• How were you able to *[insert action here]*? • Why do you think you were able to *[insert action here]*? • Tell me a little more about how you *[insert action here]*.	• What are the main things you learned? • Can someone summarize the key points made? • What are the main take-home messages?
	Instructor Observations	**Needs Improvement**	**Instructor-Led Summary**
	• I noticed that *[insert action here]*. • I observed that *[insert action here]*. • I saw that *[insert action here]*.	• Why do you think *[insert action here]* occurred? • How do you think *[insert action here]* could have been improved? • What was your thinking while *[insert action here]*? • What prevented you from *[insert action here]*?	• Let's summarize what we learned… • Here is what I think we learned… • The main take-home messages are…

Case 33: Out-of-Hospital Cardiac Arrest (VF/pVT)—Obstetrics

Scenario Rating: 3

Lead-in: You are a paramedic and respond to a patient in her third trimester of pregnancy; CPR is in progress.

Vital Signs
Heart rate:
Blood pressure:
Respiratory rate:
SpO₂:
Temperature:
Weight:
Age:

Initial Information

- The patient's husband says that his wife has had a high-risk pregnancy.
- She has been on bed rest since the 20th week of pregnancy and is currently in her 34th week.
- She reported increasing, severe shortness of breath, had a decreased level of consciousness, and became apneic and unresponsive before EMS arrived.

What are your initial actions?

- Cardiac arrest is confirmed by EMS, and CPR is started.
- Your partner is retrieving the monitor/defibrillator.

Additional Information

- The patient is pulseless and apneic, and the cardiac monitor shows **VF.**

What are your next actions?

- You have administered 1 shock, and CPR is being continued.
- You establish an IO.

What are your next actions?

- Intubation is complicated by the anatomical changes of pregnancy.
  - Consider placing an alternative airway, such as a laryngeal tube.
- During CPR, your partner should perform manual left uterine displacement to relieve aortocaval compression.

Post–Cardiac Arrest Care Algorithm

Instructor notes: The team continues high-quality chest compressions, the patient has ROSC, and the team initiates the Post–Cardiac Arrest Care Algorithm.

What are your next actions?

- Optimizing ventilation and oxygenation
- Hypotension management
- 12-lead ECG
- Rapid transport to the ED/cath lab (STEMI) or intensive care unit
- Advance notification to hospital to assemble the OB/GYN team

---

Adult Cardiac Arrest Learning Station Checklist (VF/pVT)

Adult Cardiac Arrest Algorithm

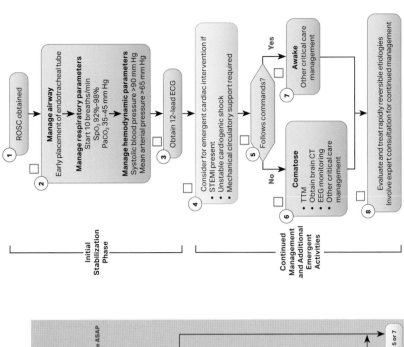

CPR Quality
- Push hard (at least 2 inches [5 cm]) and fast (100-120/min) and allow complete chest recoil.
- Minimize interruptions in compressions.
- Avoid excessive ventilation.
- Change compressor every 2 minutes, or sooner if fatigued.
- If no advanced airway, 30:2 compression-ventilation ratio.
- Quantitative waveform capnography
  - If PETCO₂ is low or decreasing, reassess CPR quality.

Reversible Causes
- Hypovolemia
- Hypoxia
- Hydrogen ion (acidosis)
- Hypo-/hyperkalemia
- Hypothermia
- Tension pneumothorax
- Tamponade, cardiac
- Toxins
- Thrombosis, pulmonary
- Thrombosis, coronary

© 2020 American Heart Association

Adult Post–Cardiac Arrest Care Learning Station Checklist

Adult Post–Cardiac Arrest Care Algorithm

1 ROSC obtained

Initial Stabilization Phase

2
- **Manage airway**
  Early placement of endotracheal tube
- **Manage respiratory parameters**
  Start 10 breaths/min
  SpO₂ 92%-98%
  PaCO₂ 35-45 mm Hg
- **Manage hemodynamic parameters**
  Systolic blood pressure >90 mm Hg
  Mean arterial pressure >65 mm Hg

3 Obtain 12-lead ECG

4
Consider for emergent cardiac intervention if
- STEMI present
- Unstable cardiogenic shock
- Mechanical circulatory support required

5 Follows commands?

Continued Management and Additional Emergent Activities

— No →

6 **Comatose**
- TTM
- Obtain brain CT
- EEG monitoring
- Other critical care management

— Yes →

7 **Awake**
Other critical care management

8
Evaluate and treat rapidly reversible etiologies
Involve expert consultation for continued management

H's and T's
- Hypovolemia
- Hypoxia
- Hydrogen ion (acidosis)
- Hypokalemia/hyperkalemia
- Hypothermia
- Tension pneumothorax
- Tamponade, cardiac
- Toxins
- Thrombosis, pulmonary
- Thrombosis, coronary

© 2020 American Heart Association

Cardiac Arrest in Pregnancy ACLS Learning Station Checklist

Consider etiology of arrest

Perform maternal interventions
- Perform airway management
- Administer 100% O₂, avoid excess ventilation
- Place IV above diaphragm
- If receiving IV magnesium, stop and give calcium chloride or gluconate

Perform obstetric interventions
- Provide continuous lateral uterine displacement
- Detach fetal monitors

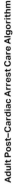

149

Debriefing Tool

ACLS Sample Scenario: Cardiac Arrest (VF/pVT/Asystole/PEA)

Learning Objectives

- Apply the BLS, Primary, and Secondary Assessments sequence for a systematic evaluation of adult patients
- Perform prompt, high-quality BLS, including prioritizing early chest compressions and integrating early AED use
- Recognize cardiac arrest
- Perform early management of cardiac arrest until termination of resuscitation or transfer of care, including post–cardiac arrest care
- Evaluate resuscitative efforts during a cardiac arrest through continuous assessment of CPR quality, monitoring the patient's physiologic response and delivering real-time feedback to the team
- Model effective communication as a member or leader of a high-performance team
- Recognize the impact of team dynamics on overall team performance

General Debriefing Principles

- Use the table on the right to guide your debriefing.
- Debriefings are 10 minutes long (unless more time is needed).
- Address all objectives.
- Summarize take-home messages at the end of the debriefing.
- **Encourage** students to self-reflect, and engage all participants.
- **Avoid** mini-lectures, and prevent closed-ended questions from dominating the discussion.

Action	Gather	Analyze	Summarize
• Assigns team roles and directs the team (effective team dynamics) • Directs the systematic approach • Directs team to administer 100% oxygen • Directs team to apply monitor leads • Directs IV or IO access • Directs appropriate defibrillation and drug treatment • Directs reassessment of patient in response to treatments • Summarizes specific treatments • Verbalizes indications for advanced airway if needed • Considers reversible causes • Directs post–cardiac arrest care	**Student Observations** (primary is Team Leader and Timer/Recorder) • Can you describe the events from your perspective? • How did you think your treatments went? • Can you review the events of the scenario? *(directed to the Timer/Recorder)* • What could you have improved? • What did the team do well?	**Done Well** • How were you able to [*insert action here*]? • Why do you think you were able to [*insert action here*]? • Tell me a little more about how you [*insert action here*].	**Student-Led Summary** • What are the main things you learned? • Can someone summarize the key points made? • What are the main take-home messages?
	Instructor Observations • I noticed that [*insert action here*]. • I observed that [*insert action here*]. • I saw that [*insert action here*].	**Needs Improvement** • Why do you think [*insert action here*] occurred? • How do you think [*insert action here*] could have been improved? • What was your thinking while [*insert action here*]? • What prevented you from [*insert action here*]?	**Instructor-Led Summary** • Let's summarize what we learned… • Here is what I think we learned… • The main take-home messages are…

Case 34: Out-of-Hospital Cardiac Arrest (VF/pVT)

Scenario Rating: 2

Lead-in: You are a paramedic and are 90 minutes into a 5-hour, early-morning flight. You and your coworkers hear someone loudly trying to wake a middle-aged man 4 rows in front of you. The flight attendants are trying to get him into the aisle when your group offers assistance.

Vital Signs
Heart rate:
Blood pressure:
Respiratory rate:
SpO₂:
Temperature:
Weight:
Age:

Initial Information

- As the group lays him down, you notice the man takes an agonal gasp.
- His wife says he has been complaining of indigestion for the past 8 hours and has been burping more than normal.
- The flight crew is trained in Hands-Only CPR.
- You and your team identify yourselves as medical providers and ask for an AED and the emergency medical kit.
  - The kit has some advanced-level items, including at least 2 doses of all ACLS cardiac arrest drugs, peripheral IV equipment, personal protective equipment, a bag-mask device, and a supraglottic airway that is size appropriate.

What are your initial actions?

Additional Information

- The patient is unresponsive, taking 2 to 3 agonal gasps per minute, and is pulseless, with skin becoming gray and mottled.
- The AED shocks on the first attempt.

What are your actions?

Additional Information (if needed)

- CPR continues, and the AED delivers a second shock. The patient receives 1 dose of epinephrine.
- In-flight medical consultation is available; the pilot told them of the situation, and they are available by radio for consultation.
- The pilot wants your opinion on the urgency to land. A smaller, more rural airstrip is within 15 minutes, and a larger urban airport is 25 minutes away.
- The pilot has received clearance from air traffic control to descend from 35 000 to 25 000 feet while you treat the patient.

Post-Cardiac Arrest Care Algorithm

Instructor notes: The team continues high-quality chest compressions, the patient has ROSC, and the team initiates the Post-Cardiac Arrest Care Algorithm.

What are your next actions?

- Optimizing ventilation and oxygenation
- Hypotension management
- 12-lead ECG
- Targeted temperature management if appropriate
- Transfer to cath lab (STEMI) or intensive care unit

Adult Cardiac Arrest Learning Station Checklist (VF/pVT)

Adult Cardiac Arrest Algorithm

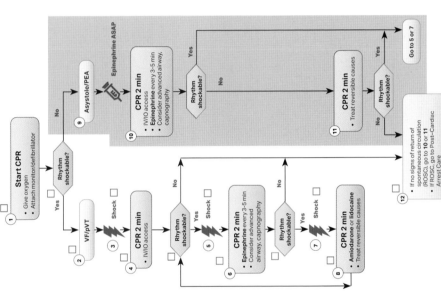

1. **Start CPR**
   - Give oxygen
   - Attach monitor/defibrillator

   Rhythm shockable?

2. **VF/pVT** (Yes)

3. **Shock**

4. **CPR 2 min**
   - IV/IO access

   Rhythm shockable? — No

5. **Shock** (Yes)

6. **CPR 2 min**
   - Epinephrine every 3-5 min
   - Consider advanced airway, capnography

   Rhythm shockable? — No

7. **Shock** (Yes)

8. **CPR 2 min**
   - Amiodarone or lidocaine
   - Treat reversible causes

9. **Asystole/PEA** (No)

   Epinephrine ASAP

10. **CPR 2 min**
    - IV/IO access
    - Epinephrine every 3-5 min
    - Consider advanced airway, capnography

    Rhythm shockable? — Yes → Go to 5 or 7

11. **CPR 2 min**
    - Treat reversible causes

    Rhythm shockable? — Yes → Go to 5 or 7; No

12. - If no signs of return of spontaneous circulation (ROSC), go to **10** or **11**
    - If ROSC, go to Post–Cardiac Arrest Care
    - Consider appropriateness of continued resuscitation

CPR Quality	Reversible Causes
• Push hard (at least 2 inches [5 cm]) and fast (100-120/min) and allow complete chest recoil. • Minimize interruptions in compressions. • Avoid excessive ventilation. • Change compressor every 2 minutes, or sooner if fatigued. • If no advanced airway, 30:2 compression-ventilation ratio. • Quantitative waveform capnography – If PETCO₂ is low or decreasing, reassess CPR quality.	• Hypovolemia • Hypoxia • Hydrogen ion (acidosis) • Hypo-/hyperkalemia • Hypothermia • Tension pneumothorax • Tamponade, cardiac • Toxins • Thrombosis, pulmonary • Thrombosis, coronary

---

Adult Post–Cardiac Arrest Care Learning Station Checklist

Adult Post–Cardiac Arrest Care Algorithm

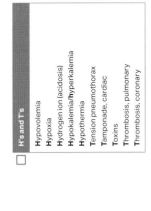

1. **ROSC obtained**

2. **Manage airway**
   Early placement of endotracheal tube

   Manage respiratory parameters
   Start 10 breaths/min
   SpO₂ 92%-98%
   PaCO₂ 35-45 mm Hg

   Manage hemodynamic parameters
   Systolic blood pressure >90 mm Hg
   Mean arterial pressure >65 mm Hg

3. **Obtain 12-lead ECG**

4. **Consider for emergent cardiac intervention if**
   - STEMI present
   - Unstable cardiogenic shock
   - Mechanical circulatory support required

5. **Follows commands?** — Yes / No

6. **Comatose** (No)
   - TTM
   - Obtain brain CT
   - EEG monitoring
   - Other critical care management

7. **Awake** (Yes)
   Other critical care management

8. Evaluate and treat rapidly reversible etiologies
   Involve expert consultation for continued management

Initial Stabilization Phase (steps 1-4)

Continued Management and Additional Emergent Activities (steps 6-8)

H's and T's
Hypovolemia Hypoxia Hydrogen ion (acidosis) Hypokalemia/**hyperkalemia** Hypothermia Tension pneumothorax Tamponade, cardiac Toxins Thrombosis, pulmonary Thrombosis, coronary

Debriefing Tool

ACLS Sample Scenario: Cardiac Arrest (VF/pVT/Asystole/PEA)

Learning Objectives

- Apply the BLS, Primary, and Secondary Assessments sequence for a systematic evaluation of adult patients
- Perform prompt, high-quality BLS, including prioritizing early chest compressions and integrating early AED use
- Recognize cardiac arrest
- Perform early management of cardiac arrest until termination of resuscitation or transfer of care, including post–cardiac arrest care
- Evaluate resuscitative efforts during a cardiac arrest through continuous assessment of CPR quality, monitoring the patient's physiologic response and delivering real-time feedback to the team
- Model effective communication as a member or leader of a high-performance team
- Recognize the impact of team dynamics on overall team performance

General Debriefing Principles

- Use the table on the right to guide your debriefing.
- Debriefings are 10 minutes long (unless more time is needed).
- Address all objectives.
- Summarize take-home messages at the end of the debriefing.
- **Encourage** students to self-reflect, and engage all participants.
- **Avoid** mini-lectures, and prevent closed-ended questions from dominating the discussion.

Action	Gather	Analyze	Summarize
	Student Observations (primary is Team Leader and Timer/Recorder)	**Done Well**	**Student-Led Summary**
• Assigns team roles and directs the team (effective team dynamics)	• Can you describe the events from your perspective?	• How were you able to [*insert action here*]?	• What are the main things you learned?
• Directs the systematic approach	• How did you think your treatments went?	• Why do you think you were able to [*insert action here*]?	• Can someone summarize the key points made?
• Directs team to administer 100% oxygen	• Can you review the events of the scenario? *(directed to the Timer/Recorder)*	• Tell me a little more about how you [*insert action here*].	• What are the main take-home messages?
• Directs team to apply monitor leads	• What could you have improved?		
• Directs IV or IO access	• What did the team do well?		
• Directs appropriate defibrillation and drug treatment			
• Directs reassessment of patient in response to treatments	**Instructor Observations**	**Needs Improvement**	**Instructor-Led Summary**
• Summarizes specific treatments	• I noticed that [*insert action here*].	• Why do you think [*insert action here*] occurred?	• Let's summarize what we learned…
• Verbalizes indications for advanced airway if needed	• I observed that [*insert action here*].	• How do you think [*insert action here*] could have been improved?	• Here is what I think we learned…
• Considers reversible causes	• I saw that [*insert action here*].	• What was your thinking while [*insert action here*]?	• The main take-home messages are…
• Directs post–cardiac arrest care		• What prevented you from [*insert action here*]?	

Case 35: Out-of-Hospital Cardiac Arrest—LVAD

Scenario Rating: 3

Lead-in: You are a paramedic who responds to a report of an unconscious person.

Vital Signs
Heart rate:
Blood pressure:
Respiratory rate:
SpO$_2$:
Temperature:
Weight:
Age: 67 years

Initial Information

- The unconscious man had a left ventricular assist device (LVAD) implanted 8 months ago.
- He has no pulse when first responders arrive, but his wife tells them not to perform chest compressions.
- The first responders also did not attach the AED.
- There is an alarm sounding from the LVAD's external machinery.

What are your actions?

Additional Information

- You attach a cardiac monitor/defibrillator. A rhythm check finds a **VF**.

What are your actions?

Additional Information (if needed)

Instructor notes: Auscultation of the chest (if performed) will reveal no machine sounds.

What are your next actions?

Adult Ventricular Assist Device Learning Station Checklist

Adult Ventricular Assist Device Algorithm

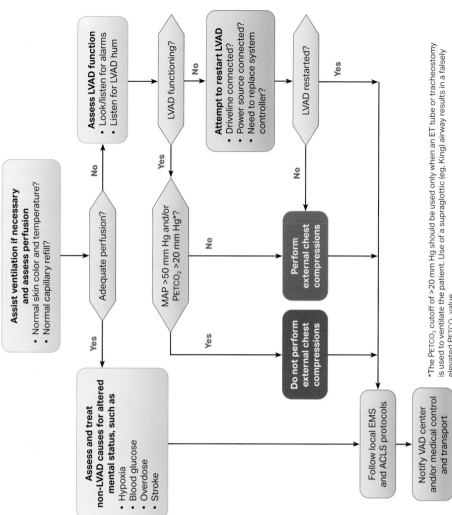

*The PETCO$_2$ cutoff of >20 mm Hg should be used only when an ET tube or tracheostomy is used to ventilate the patient. Use of a supraglottic (eg, King) airway results in a falsely elevated PETCO$_2$ value.

© 2020 American Heart Association

153

Debriefing Tool

ACLS Sample Scenario: Cardiac Arrest (VF/pVT/Asystole/PEA)

Learning Objectives

- Apply the BLS, Primary, and Secondary Assessments sequence for a systematic evaluation of adult patients
- Perform prompt, high-quality BLS, including prioritizing early chest compressions and integrating early AED use
- Recognize cardiac arrest
- Perform early management of cardiac arrest until termination of resuscitation or transfer of care, including post–cardiac arrest care
- Evaluate resuscitative efforts during a cardiac arrest through continuous assessment of CPR quality, monitoring the patient's physiologic response and delivering real-time feedback to the team
- Model effective communication as a member or leader of a high-performance team
- Recognize the impact of team dynamics on overall team performance

General Debriefing Principles

- Use the table on the right to guide your debriefing.
- Debriefings are 10 minutes long (unless more time is needed).
- Address all objectives.
- Summarize take-home messages at the end of the debriefing.
- *Encourage* students to self-reflect, and engage all participants.
- *Avoid* mini-lectures, and prevent closed-ended questions from dominating the discussion.

Action	Gather	Analyze	Summarize
- Assigns team roles and directs the team (effective team dynamics) - Directs the systematic approach - Directs team to administer 100% oxygen - Directs team to apply monitor leads - Directs IV or IO access - Directs appropriate defibrillation and drug treatment - Directs reassessment of patient in response to treatments - Summarizes specific treatments - Verbalizes indications for advanced airway if needed - Considers reversible causes - Directs post–cardiac arrest care	**Student Observations** (primary is Team Leader and Timer/Recorder) - Can you describe the events from your perspective? - How did you think your treatments went? - Can you review the events of the scenario? *(directed to the Timer/Recorder)* - What could you have improved? - What did the team do well?	**Done Well** - How were you able to *[insert action here]?* - Why do you think you were able to *[insert action here]?* - Tell me a little more about how you *[insert action here]*.	**Student-Led Summary** - What are the main things you learned? - Can someone summarize the key points made? - What are the main take-home messages?
	Instructor Observations - I noticed that *[insert action here]*. - I observed that *[insert action here]*. - I saw that *[insert action here]*.	**Needs Improvement** - Why do you think *[insert action here]* occurred? - How do you think *[insert action here]* could have been improved? - What was your thinking while *[insert action here]?* - What prevented you from *[insert action here]?*	**Instructor-Led Summary** - Let's summarize what we learned… - Here is what I think we learned… - The main take-home messages are…

154

Case 36: Out-of-Hospital—Outpatient Clinic Cardiac Arrest (PEA)

Scenario Rating: 2

Lead-in: You are a paramedic responding to an outpatient methadone clinic for a patient who is not breathing.

Vital Signs
Heart rate:
Blood pressure:
Respiratory rate:
SpO$_2$:
Temperature:
Weight:
Age:

Initial Information

- Clinic staff say that a patient came in for an appointment and became unresponsive in the waiting room.
- CPR is in progress, and an AED has been applied, but no shock was advised.

What are your initial actions?

- The patient is **pulseless** and apneic, and the cardiac monitor shows a **sinus tachycardia** (PEA).

What are your next actions?

Additional Information

- You have established an IV and administered epinephrine.
- Some vomitus is in the hypopharynx.

What are your next actions?

- The patient is highly susceptible for opioid overdose.
- He has an unmanageable BLS airway.

Instructor notes: The airway should be secured with an advanced airway. Naloxone will only reverse the respiratory suppression, not the systemic perfusion effects caused by hypoventilation and the subsequent oxygen desaturation. Patients with opioid-associated cardiac arrest are managed in accordance with standard ACLS practices.

Post-Cardiac Arrest Care Algorithm

- After 4 minutes of CPR, the patient has a weak pulse and a blood pressure of 82/53 mm Hg.

What are your next actions?

Instructor notes: The team continues high-quality chest compressions, the patient has ROSC, and the team initiates the Post-Cardiac Arrest Care Algorithm.

- Optimizing ventilation and oxygenation
- Hypotension management
- 12-lead ECG
- Targeted temperature management if appropriate
- Transfer to cath lab (STEMI) or intensive care unit

Adult Cardiac Arrest Learning Station Checklist (Asystole/PEA)

Adult Cardiac Arrest Algorithm

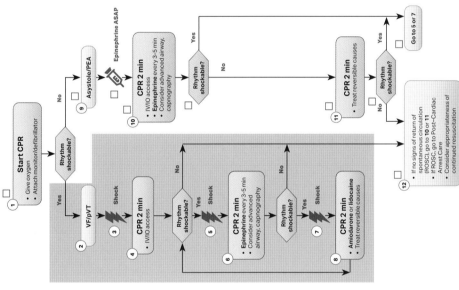

Adult Post-Cardiac Arrest Care Learning Station Checklist

Adult Post-Cardiac Arrest Care Algorithm

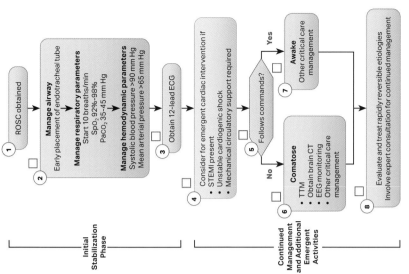

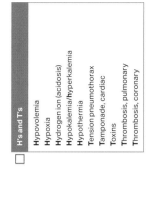

Debriefing Tool

ACLS Sample Scenario: Cardiac Arrest (VF/pVT/Asystole/PEA)

Action	Gather	Analyze	Summarize
• Assigns team roles and directs the team (effective team dynamics) • Directs the systematic approach • Directs team to administer 100% oxygen • Directs team to apply monitor leads • Directs IV or IO access • Directs appropriate defibrillation and drug treatment • Directs reassessment of patient in response to treatments • Summarizes specific treatments • Verbalizes indications for advanced airway if needed • Considers reversible causes • Directs post–cardiac arrest care	**Student Observations** (primary is Team Leader and Timer/Recorder) • Can you describe the events from your perspective? • How did you think your treatments went? • Can you review the events of the scenario? *(directed to the Timer/Recorder)* • What could you have improved? • What did the team do well? **Instructor Observations** • I noticed that *[insert action here]*. • I observed that *[insert action here]*. • I saw that *[insert action here]*.	**Done Well** • How were you able to *[insert action here]*? • Why do you think you were able to *[insert action here]*? • Tell me a little more about how you *[insert action here]*. **Needs Improvement** • Why do you think *[insert action here]* occurred? • How do you think *[insert action here]* could have been improved? • What was your thinking while *[insert action here]*? • What prevented you from *[insert action here]*?	**Student-Led Summary** • What are the main things you learned? • Can someone summarize the key points made? • What are the main take-home messages? **Instructor-Led Summary** • Let's summarize what we learned… • Here is what I think we learned… • The main take-home messages are…

Learning Objectives

- Apply the BLS, Primary, and Secondary Assessments sequence for a systematic evaluation of adult patients
- Perform prompt, high-quality BLS, including prioritizing early chest compressions and integrating early AED use
- Recognize cardiac arrest
- Perform early management of cardiac arrest until termination of resuscitation or transfer of care, including post–cardiac arrest care
- Evaluate resuscitative efforts during a cardiac arrest through continuous assessment of CPR quality, monitoring the patient's physiologic response and delivering real-time feedback to the team
- Model effective communication as a member or leader of a high-performance team
- Recognize the impact of team dynamics on overall team performance

General Debriefing Principles

- Use the table on the right to guide your debriefing.
- Debriefings are 10 minutes long (unless more time is needed).
- Address all objectives.
- Summarize take-home messages at the end of the debriefing.
- *Encourage* students to self-reflect, and engage all participants.
- *Avoid* mini-lectures, and prevent closed-ended questions from dominating the discussion.

Case 37: Emergency Department Cardiac Arrest—LVAD

Scenario Rating: 2

Lead-in: You are evaluating a left ventricular assist device (LVAD) patient in the emergency department who reports dizziness.

Vital Signs
Heart rate: 200/min
Blood pressure: 90/50 mm Hg
Respiratory rate:
SpO₂:
Temperature:
Weight:
Age:

Initial Information

- His initial ECG shows **wide-complex tachycardia** suspicious for VT.
- The nurses say they cannot obtain a pulse oximetry reading on the patient.

What are your initial actions?

- On initial assessment, the patient is awake and talking to you.
- He says that he has received 2 shocks from his automated implantable cardioverter defibrillator (AICD).
- While you assess him, he suddenly becomes unconscious with agonal respirations.
- As the patient becomes unconscious, his AICD delivers another shock and converts his rhythm to a paced rhythm at 80/min.

What are your actions?

Additional Information

- When you assess the motor of the LVAD, you can hear it humming. The patient remains unconscious with agonal respirations.

What are your next actions?

Post–Cardiac Arrest Care Algorithm

- After AICD defibrillation and fluid bolus, the patient regains spontaneous respirations, becomes responsive, and localizes to pain.

What are your next actions?

Instructor notes: The team continues high-quality chest compressions, the patient has ROSC, and the team initiates the Post–Cardiac Arrest Care Algorithm.

- Optimizing ventilation and oxygenation
- Hypotension management
- 12-lead ECG
- Targeted temperature management if appropriate
- Transfer to cath lab (STEMI) or intensive care unit

Note: May need Adult Cardiac Arrest Algorithm

Adult Ventricular Assist Device Learning Station Checklist

Adult Ventricular Assist Device Algorithm

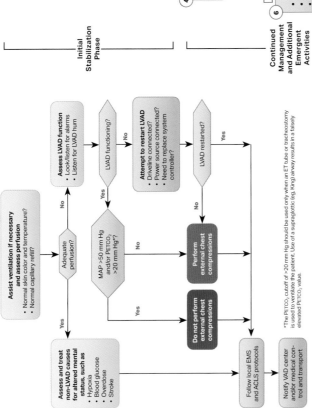

*The PetCO₂ cutoff of >20 mm Hg should be used only when an ET tube or tracheostomy is used to ventilate the patient. Use of a supraglottic (eg, King) airway results in a falsely elevated PetCO₂ value.

© 2020 American Heart Association

Adult Post–Cardiac Arrest Care Learning Station Checklist

Adult Post–Cardiac Arrest Care Algorithm

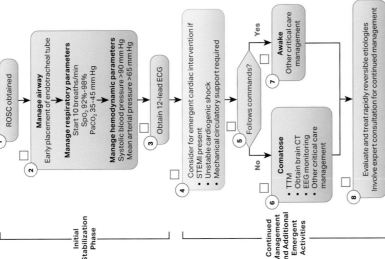

H's and T's
Hypovolemia
Hypoxia
Hydrogen ion (acidosis)
Hypokalemia/**hy**perkalemia
Hypothermia
Tension pneumothorax
Tamponade, cardiac
Toxins
Thrombosis, pulmonary
Thrombosis, coronary

© 2020 American Heart Association

Debriefing Tool

ACLS Sample Scenario: Cardiac Arrest (VF/pVT/Asystole/PEA)

Action	Gather	Analyze	Summarize
• Assigns team roles and directs the team (effective team dynamics)	**Student Observations** (primary is Team Leader and Timer/Recorder)	**Done Well**	**Student-Led Summary**
• Directs the systematic approach	• Can you describe the events from your perspective?	• How were you able to [insert action here]?	• What are the main things you learned?
• Directs team to administer 100% oxygen	• How did you think your treatments went?	• Why do you think you were able to [insert action here]?	• Can someone summarize the key points made?
• Directs team to apply monitor leads	• Can you review the events of the scenario? (directed to the Timer/ Recorder)	• Tell me a little more about how you [insert action here].	• What are the main take-home messages?
• Directs IV or IO access	• What could you have improved?		
• Directs appropriate defibrillation and drug treatment	• What did the team do well?		
• Directs reassessment of patient in response to treatments	**Instructor Observations**	**Needs Improvement**	**Instructor-Led Summary**
• Summarizes specific treatments	• I noticed that [insert action here].	• Why do you think [insert action here] occurred?	• Let's summarize what we learned…
• Verbalizes indications for advanced airway if needed	• I observed that [insert action here].	• How do you think [insert action here] could have been improved?	• Here is what I think we learned…
• Considers reversible causes	• I saw that [insert action here].	• What was your thinking while [insert action here]?	• The main take-home messages are…
• Directs post-cardiac arrest care		• What prevented you from [insert action here]?	

Learning Objectives

- Apply the BLS, Primary, and Secondary Assessments sequence for a systematic evaluation of adult patients
- Perform prompt, high-quality BLS, including prioritizing early chest compressions and integrating early AED use
- Recognize cardiac arrest
- Perform early management of cardiac arrest until termination of resuscitation or transfer of care, including post-cardiac arrest care
- Evaluate resuscitative efforts during a cardiac arrest through continuous assessment of CPR quality, monitoring the patient's physiologic response and delivering real-time feedback to the team
- Model effective communication as a member or leader of a high-performance team
- Recognize the impact of team dynamics on overall team performance

General Debriefing Principles

- Use the table on the right to guide your debriefing.
- Debriefings are 10 minutes long (unless more time is needed).
- Address all objectives.
- Summarize take-home messages at the end of the debriefing.
- *Encourage* students to self-reflect, and engage all participants.
- *Avoid* mini-lectures, and prevent closed-ended questions from dominating the discussion.

Case 38: Emergency Department Cardiac Arrest—OB

Scenario Rating: 3

Lead-in: EMS arrives in your emergency department with a woman who is in cardiac arrest. They were called to her home after she became acutely short of breath. She told the emergency call-taker that she is 30 weeks pregnant. The EMS crew arrived on scene to find the patient in extremis with severe shortness of breath and altered level of consciousness. She appeared ashen gray and diaphoretic.

Vital Signs

Heart rate: 140/min	Temperature: 36.5°C
Blood pressure: 70/30 mm Hg	Weight:
Respiratory rate: 35	Age: 28
SpO₂: 65%	

Initial Information

Emergency department providers note that the patient has an obvious gravid uterus with the fundus well above the umbilicus. She is barely conscious and in severe respiratory distress. She appears pale and is unable to answer any questions. When she is transferred to the resuscitation bay stretcher, she becomes apneic and pulseless.

What are your initial actions?

Instructor notes: Students are expected to begin CPR, with an assistant providing leftward displacement of the uterus. Focus on high-quality chest compressions while following ACLS algorithms. Immediately call for help, including OB/GYN and NICU, and provide anesthesia if available (potentially difficult airway). Preparations for a perimortem hysterotomy should be verbalized early, with a plan to proceed within 4 minutes if the patient is unresponsive to ACLS.

Additional Information

- Despite good-quality CPR, ACLS, fluid bolus, and leftward displacement of the uterus, the patient remains in cardiac arrest at 4 minutes into the resuscitation attempt.
- Unfortunately, the obstetrics team is delayed by another obstetrical emergency in the operating room.

What is your next intervention?

Instructor notes: Students should be able to verbalize that emergency hysterotomy is required to optimize outcomes for both the mother and the fetus. Resuscitation of the mother and infant (with 2 teams) should continue after the hysterotomy.

Post-Cardiac Arrest Care Algorithm

After the baby is surgically removed from the uterus, the patient has ROSC.

Updated vital signs

- Heart rate: 150/min
- Blood pressure: 70/45 mm Hg
- SpO₂: 75%
- Temperature: 35.8°C

The obstetrics team arrives to assist with posthysterotomy management.

What are your next interventions?

Instructor notes: Students should consider aggressive resuscitative efforts with blood products, crystalloid, and vasopressors. Potential cause of cardiac arrest should be considered: pulmonary embolism, myocardial infarction, amniotic fluid embolism.

The patient will require multidisciplinary critical care, including operative management of hysterotomy, hemorrhage control, and then investigation for cause of cardiac arrest.

Decisions on post-cardiac arrest management will be complex and must be made in conjunction with OB/GYN and critical care, with the most pressing concerns being targeted temperature management and hemostasis in the context of a potential pulmonary embolism.

Cardiac Arrest in Pregnancy In-Hospital ACLS Learning Station Checklist

Cardiac Arrest in Pregnancy In-Hospital ACLS Algorithm

1 — Continue BLS/ACLS
- High-quality CPR
- Defibrillation when indicated
- Other ACLS interventions (eg, epinephrine)

2 — Assemble maternal cardiac arrest team

3 — Consider etiology of arrest

4 — Perform maternal interventions
- Perform airway management
- Administer 100% O₂, avoid excess ventilation
- Place IV above diaphragm
- If receiving IV magnesium, stop and give calcium chloride or gluconate

5 — Continue BLS/ACLS
- High-quality CPR
- Defibrillation when indicated
- Other ACLS interventions (eg, epinephrine)

6 — Perform obstetric interventions
- Provide continuous lateral uterine displacement
- Detach fetal monitors
- Prepare for perimortem cesarean delivery

7 — Perform perimortem cesarean delivery
- If no ROSC in 5 minutes, consider immediate perimortem cesarean delivery

8 — Neonatal team to receive neonate

© 2020 American Heart Association

Adult Post-Cardiac Arrest Care Learning Station Checklist

Adult Post-Cardiac Arrest Care Algorithm

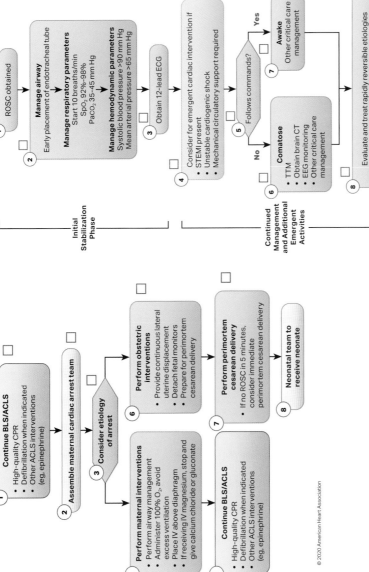

1 — ROSC obtained

2
- **Manage airway**
  Early placement of endotracheal tube
- **Manage respiratory parameters**
  Start 10 breaths/min
  SpO₂ 92%-98%
  PaCO₂ 35-45 mm Hg
- **Manage hemodynamic parameters**
  Systolic blood pressure >90 mm Hg
  Mean arterial pressure >65 mm Hg

3 — Obtain 12-lead ECG

4 — Consider for emergent cardiac intervention if
- STEMI present
- Unstable cardiogenic shock
- Mechanical circulatory support required

5 — Follows commands?
- No → **6 — Comatose**
  - TTM
  - Obtain brain CT
  - EEG monitoring
  - Other critical care management
- Yes → **7 — Awake**
  - Other critical care management

8 — Evaluate and treat rapidly reversible etiologies
Involve expert consultation for continued management

Initial Stabilization Phase

Continued Management and Additional Emergent Activities

H's and T's
- Hypovolemia
- Hypoxia
- Hydrogen ion (acidosis)
- Hypokalemia/**hyper**kalemia
- Hypothermia
- Tension pneumothorax
- Tamponade, cardiac
- Toxins
- Thrombosis, pulmonary
- Thrombosis, coronary

© 2020 American Heart Association

159

Debriefing Tool

ACLS Sample Scenario: Cardiac Arrest (VF/pVT/Asystole/PEA)

Learning Objectives

- Apply the BLS, Primary, and Secondary Assessments sequence for a systematic evaluation of adult patients
- Perform prompt, high-quality BLS, including prioritizing early chest compressions and integrating early AED use
- Recognize cardiac arrest
- Perform early management of cardiac arrest until termination of resuscitation or transfer of care, including post–cardiac arrest care
- Evaluate resuscitative efforts during a cardiac arrest through continuous assessment of CPR quality, monitoring the patient's physiologic response and delivering real-time feedback to the team
- Model effective communication as a member or leader of a high-performance team
- Recognize the impact of team dynamics on overall team performance

General Debriefing Principles

- Use the table on the right to guide your debriefing.
- Debriefings are 10 minutes long (unless more time is needed).
- Address all objectives.
- Summarize take-home messages at the end of the debriefing.
- *Encourage* students to self-reflect, and engage all participants.
- *Avoid* mini-lectures, and prevent closed-ended questions from dominating the discussion.

Action	Gather	Analyze	Summarize
	Student Observations (primary is Team Leader and Timer/Recorder)	**Done Well**	**Student-Led Summary**
• Assigns team roles and directs the team (effective team dynamics)	• Can you describe the events from your perspective?	• How were you able to *[insert action here]*?	• What are the main things you learned?
• Directs the systematic approach	• How did you think your treatments went?	• Why do you think you were able to *[insert action here]*?	• Can someone summarize the key points made?
• Directs team to administer 100% oxygen	• Can you review the events of the scenario? *(directed to the Timer/Recorder)*	• Tell me a little more about how you *[insert action here]*.	• What are the main take-home messages?
• Directs team to apply monitor leads	• What could you have improved?		
• Directs IV or IO access	• What did the team do well?		
• Directs appropriate defibrillation and drug treatment			
• Directs reassessment of patient in response to treatments	**Instructor Observations**	**Needs Improvement**	**Instructor-Led Summary**
• Summarizes specific treatments	• I noticed that *[insert action here]*.	• Why do you think *[insert action here]* occurred?	• Let's summarize what we learned…
• Verbalizes indications for advanced airway if needed	• I observed that *[insert action here]*.	• How do you think *[insert action here]* could have been improved?	• Here is what I think we learned…
• Considers reversible causes	• I saw that *[insert action here]*.	• What was your thinking while *[insert action here]*?	• The main take-home messages are…
• Directs post–cardiac arrest care		• What prevented you from *[insert action here]*?	

Case 39: Emergency Department Cardiac Arrest— PEA-Opioid Overdose

Scenario Rating: 2

Lead-in: EMS arrives in your emergency department with an unconscious man. EMS providers are ventilating him with a bag-mask device on arrival. The crew tells you that they were called by a passerby who found the patient lying unconscious on the street.

Vital Signs

Heart rate: 110/min
Blood pressure: 100/75 mm Hg
Respiratory rate: 6/min
SpO₂: 65%
Temperature: 36.5°C
Weight:
Age: 23

Initial Information

- The patient is unresponsive to voice and painful stimuli.
- The patient's pupils are pinpoint bilaterally.
- He has track marks on both arms and both feet.
- His respirations are infrequent and ineffective.
- He has snoring respirations with some upper airway obstruction.
- He has a thready pulse at approximately 110/min.

What are your initial actions?

Instructor notes: The student should open the airway (positioning with or without an OPA or NPA), place the patient on a monitor, provide oxygen, assess ventilation once the airway is open, and provide bag-mask ventilation as necessary. IV access should be established. The student may choose to administer naloxone. Naloxone 0.04 to 0.4 mg IV would be an appropriate initial dose, with repeat dosing after 2 to 3 minutes of no effect. Appropriate repeat dosing is 2 mg and then 4 mg, based on effect. The goal is to have effective ventilation and improved oxygen saturation.

Additional Information

- Despite the airway being opened, the patient's respirations remain slow and low volume.
- Level of consciousness and oxygen saturations are unchanged.
- Bradypnea progresses to apnea. Repeat pulse check finds no pulse.
- Monitor shows organized rhythm at 110/min.

What is your next intervention?

Instructor notes: Students must move down the PEA pathway on the Adult Cardiac Arrest Algorithm, beginning with start CPR, and focus on high-quality CPR. Students may consider administering naloxone. The benefit of naloxone in cardiac arrest is not clear. The ideal dose is not known, but 2 to 4 mg IV is reasonable.

Adult Cardiac Arrest Learning Station Checklist (Asystole/PEA)

Adult Cardiac Arrest Algorithm

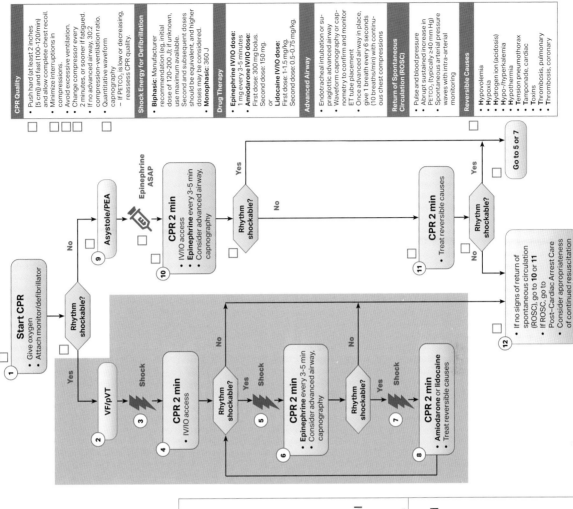

© 2020 American Heart Association

Debriefing Tool

ACLS Sample Scenario: Cardiac Arrest (VF/pVT/Asystole/PEA)

Learning Objectives

- Apply the BLS, Primary, and Secondary Assessments sequence for a systematic evaluation of adult patients
- Perform prompt, high-quality BLS, including prioritizing early chest compressions and integrating early AED use
- Recognize cardiac arrest
- Perform early management of cardiac arrest until termination of resuscitation or transfer of care, including post–cardiac arrest care
- Evaluate resuscitative efforts during a cardiac arrest through continuous assessment of CPR quality, monitoring the patient's physiologic response and delivering real-time feedback to the team
- Model effective communication as a member or leader of a high-performance team
- Recognize the impact of team dynamics on overall team performance

General Debriefing Principles

- Use the table on the right to guide your debriefing.
- Debriefings are 10 minutes long (unless more time is needed).
- Address all objectives.
- Summarize take-home messages at the end of the debriefing.
- *Encourage* students to self-reflect, and engage all participants.
- *Avoid* mini-lectures, and prevent closed-ended questions from dominating the discussion.

Action	Gather	Analyze	Summarize
	Student Observations (primary is Team Leader and Timer/Recorder)	**Done Well**	**Student-Led Summary**
• Assigns team roles and directs the team (effective team dynamics)	• Can you describe the events from your perspective?	• How were you able to [*insert action here*]?	• What are the main things you learned?
• Directs the systematic approach	• How did you think your treatments went?	• Why do you think you were able to [*insert action here*]?	• Can someone summarize the key points made?
• Directs team to administer 100% oxygen	• Can you review the events of the scenario? (*directed to the Timer/Recorder*)	• Tell me a little more about how you [*insert action here*].	• What are the main take-home messages?
• Directs team to apply monitor leads	• What could you have improved?		
• Directs IV or IO access	• What did the team do well?		
• Directs appropriate defibrillation and drug treatment			
• Directs reassessment of patient in response to treatments			
• Summarizes specific treatments	**Instructor Observations**	**Needs Improvement**	**Instructor-Led Summary**
• Verbalizes indications for advanced airway if needed	• I noticed that [*insert action here*].	• Why do you think [*insert action here*] occurred?	• Let's summarize what we learned…
• Considers reversible causes	• I observed that [*insert action here*].	• How do you think [*insert action here*] could have been improved?	• Here is what I think we learned…
• Directs post–cardiac arrest care	• I saw that [*insert action here*].	• What was your thinking while [*insert action here*]?	• The main take-home messages are…
		• What prevented you from [*insert action here*]?	

162

Case 40: In-Hospital—Cath Lab Cardiac Arrest (VF/pVT)

Scenario Rating: 1

Lead-in: A diabetic man is awaiting coronary angiography in the cath lab holding room when he develops sudden-onset crushing chest pain similar to what he had experienced the previous week.

Vital Signs
Heart rate:
Blood pressure:
Respiratory rate:
SpO₂:

Temperature:
Weight:
Age: 54 years

Initial Information

- His nurse gives him a sublingual nitroglycerin tablet, with prompt relief of symptoms.

What are your initial actions?

- His vital signs are stable.
- The nurse puts him on a cardiac monitor and goes to get the ECG equipment, but when she returns, he is unresponsive.
- The monitor now reveals **VF**.

What are your next actions?

Additional Information

Instructor notes: High-quality compressions should immediately be started and defibrillation pads placed. The patient should be shocked as soon as possible.

What are your next actions?

Instructor notes: After the second shock, 1 mg of epinephrine should be given and an antiarrhythmic drug may be considered for refractory VF.

Post-Cardiac Arrest Care Algorithm

Instructor notes: The team continues high-quality chest compressions, the patient has ROSC, and the team initiates the Post-Cardiac Arrest Care Algorithm.

What are your next actions?

- Optimizing ventilation and oxygenation
- Hypotension management
- 12-lead ECG
- Targeted temperature management if appropriate
- Transfer to cath lab (STEMI) or intensive care unit

Adult Cardiac Arrest Learning Station Checklist (VF/pVT)

Adult Cardiac Arrest Algorithm

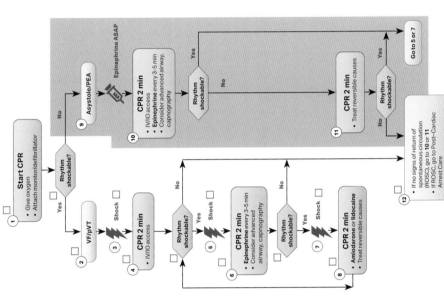

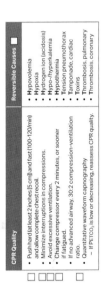

Adult Post-Cardiac Arrest Care Learning Station Checklist

Adult Post-Cardiac Arrest Care Algorithm

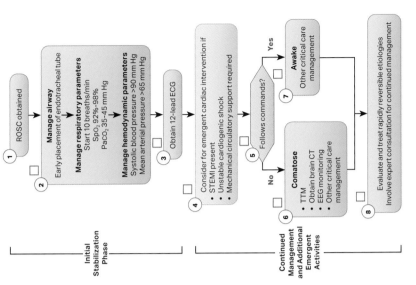

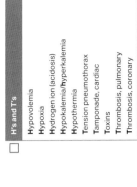

H's and T's

- Hypovolemia
- Hypoxia
- Hydrogen ion (acidosis)
- Hypokalemia/**hyperkalemia**
- Hypothermia
- Tension pneumothorax
- Tamponade, cardiac
- Toxins
- Thrombosis, pulmonary
- Thrombosis, coronary

Debriefing Tool

ACLS Sample Scenario: Cardiac Arrest (VF/pVT/Asystole/PEA)

Learning Objectives

- Apply the BLS, Primary, and Secondary Assessments sequence for a systematic evaluation of adult patients
- Perform prompt, high-quality BLS, including prioritizing early chest compressions and integrating early AED use
- Recognize cardiac arrest
- Perform early management of cardiac arrest until termination of resuscitation or transfer of care, including post–cardiac arrest care
- Evaluate resuscitative efforts during a cardiac arrest through continuous assessment of CPR quality, monitoring the patient's physiologic response and delivering real-time feedback to the team
- Model effective communication as a member or leader of a high-performance team
- Recognize the impact of team dynamics on overall team performance

General Debriefing Principles

- Use the table on the right to guide your debriefing.
- Debriefings are 10 minutes long (unless more time is needed).
- Address all objectives.
- Summarize take-home messages at the end of the debriefing.
- **Encourage** students to self-reflect, and engage all participants.
- **Avoid** mini-lectures, and prevent closed-ended questions from dominating the discussion.

Action	Gather	Analyze	Summarize
	Student Observations (primary is Team Leader and Timer/Recorder)	**Done Well**	**Student-Led Summary**
• Assigns team roles and directs the team (effective team dynamics)	• Can you describe the events from your perspective?	• How were you able to *[insert action here]*?	• What are the main things you learned?
• Directs the systematic approach	• How did you think your treatments went?	• Why do you think you were able to *[insert action here]*?	• Can someone summarize the key points made?
• Directs team to administer 100% oxygen	• Can you review the events of the scenario? *(directed to the Timer/ Recorder)*	• Tell me a little more about how you *[insert action here]*.	• What are the main take-home messages?
• Directs team to apply monitor leads	• What could you have improved?		
• Directs IV or IO access	• What did the team do well?		
• Directs appropriate defibrillation and drug treatment			
• Directs reassessment of patient in response to treatments	**Instructor Observations**	**Needs Improvement**	**Instructor-Led Summary**
• Summarizes specific treatments	• I noticed that *[insert action here]*.	• Why do you think *[insert action here]* occurred?	• Let's summarize what we learned...
• Verbalizes indications for advanced airway if needed	• I observed that *[insert action here]*.	• How do you think *[insert action here]* could have been improved?	• Here is what I think we learned...
• Considers reversible causes	• I saw that *[insert action here]*.	• What was your thinking while *[insert action here]*?	• The main take-home messages are...
• Directs post–cardiac arrest care		• What prevented you from *[insert action here]*?	

Case 41: In-Hospital—ICU Cardiac Arrest (VF/pVT)

Scenario Rating: 1

Lead-in: You are caring for a patient admitted from the emergency department after he collapsed in full arrest during a 15-km race. Bystanders called 9-1-1 and performed CPR until prehospital providers arrived.

Vital Signs

Heart rate: 48/min
Blood pressure: 126/80 mm Hg
Respiratory rate: 12/min
SpO₂:
Temperature: 37.2°C (99°F)
Weight:
Age:

Initial Information

- The patient has continuous cardiac, oximetry, and respiratory rate monitoring.
- Cardiac telemetry shows narrow rhythm (**sinus bradycardia**) without ectopy.
- You note a change in rhythm and rate at the nurses' station.
- Upon room entry, you see a wide, rapid rhythm (**VT**).
- Your patient is unresponsive, is not breathing, and has no palpable pulses.
- You and your colleagues begin CPR and notify the attending physicians and residents of your patient's status.

What is your initial action?

Additional Information

- You determine that the rhythm is pVT.
- A peer prepares to defibrillate while high-quality CPR and bag-mask ventilation with 100% oxygen are started immediately.
- Another team member is trying to establish IO access.

What are your next actions?

Additional Information (if needed)

- After appropriate shock delivery, CPR continues.
- Epinephrine is administered after the second shock, and antiarrhythmics are considered.

What should be considered as you continue to resuscitate your patient?

Post-Cardiac Arrest Care Algorithm

Instructor notes: The team continues high-quality chest compressions, the patient has ROSC, and the team initiates the Post-Cardiac Arrest Care Algorithm.

What are your next actions?

- Optimizing ventilation and oxygenation
- Hypotension management
- 12-lead ECG
- Targeted temperature management if appropriate
- Transfer to cath lab (STEMI) or intensive care unit

Adult Cardiac Arrest Learning Station Checklist (VF/pVT)

Adult Cardiac Arrest Algorithm

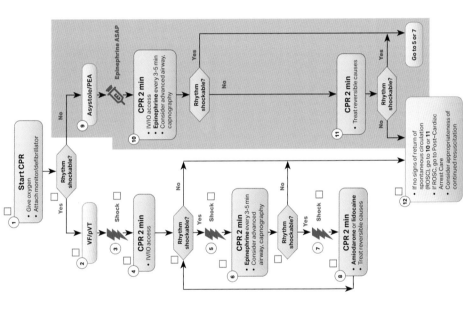

Adult Post–Cardiac Arrest Care Learning Station Checklist

Adult Post–Cardiac Arrest Care Algorithm

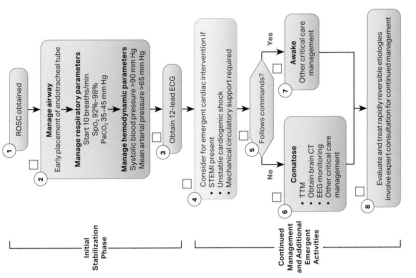

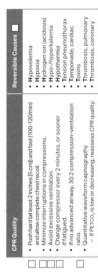

Debriefing Tool

ACLS Sample Scenario: Cardiac Arrest (VF/pVT/Asystole/PEA)

Learning Objectives

- Apply the BLS, Primary, and Secondary Assessments sequence for a systematic evaluation of adult patients
- Perform prompt, high-quality BLS, including prioritizing early chest compressions and integrating early AED use
- Recognize cardiac arrest
- Perform early management of cardiac arrest until termination of resuscitation or transfer of care, including post–cardiac arrest care
- Evaluate resuscitative efforts during a cardiac arrest through continuous assessment of CPR quality, monitoring the patient's physiologic response and delivering real-time feedback to the team
- Model effective communication as a member or leader of a high-performance team
- Recognize the impact of team dynamics on overall team performance

General Debriefing Principles

- Use the table on the right to guide your debriefing.
- Debriefings are 10 minutes long (unless more time is needed).
- Address all objectives.
- Summarize take-home messages at the end of the debriefing.
- **Encourage** students to self-reflect, and engage all participants.
- **Avoid** mini-lectures, and prevent closed-ended questions from dominating the discussion.

Action	Gather	Analyze	Summarize
	Student Observations (primary is Team Leader and Timer/Recorder)	**Done Well**	**Student-Led Summary**
• Assigns team roles and directs the team (effective team dynamics)	• Can you describe the events from your perspective?	• How were you able to *[insert action here]*?	• What are the main things you learned?
• Directs the systematic approach	• How did you think your treatments went?	• Why do you think you were able to *[insert action here]*?	• Can someone summarize the key points made?
• Directs team to administer 100% oxygen	• Can you review the events of the scenario? *(directed to the Timer/Recorder)*	• Tell me a little more about how you *[insert action here]*.	• What are the main take-home messages?
• Directs team to apply monitor leads	• What could you have improved?		
• Directs IV or IO access	• What did the team do well?		
• Directs appropriate defibrillation and drug treatment			
• Directs reassessment of patient in response to treatments	**Instructor Observations**	**Needs Improvement**	**Instructor-Led Summary**
• Summarizes specific treatments	• I noticed that *[insert action here]*.	• Why do you think *[insert action here]* occurred?	• Let's summarize what we learned…
• Verbalizes indications for advanced airway if needed	• I observed that *[insert action here]*.	• How do you think *[insert action here]* could have been improved?	• Here is what I think we learned…
• Considers reversible causes	• I saw that *[insert action here]*.	• What was your thinking while *[insert action here]*?	• The main take-home messages are…
• Directs post–cardiac arrest care		• What prevented you from *[insert action here]*?	

Case 42: In-Hospital Cardiac Arrest (PEA)

Scenario Rating: 3

Lead-in: A patient becomes unresponsive while checking in to a hospital dialysis unit. The Code Team is activated.

Vital Signs
Heart rate: 0/min
Blood pressure: 0/0 mm Hg
Respiratory rate:
SpO$_2$: 40% on room air
Temperature:
Weight:
Age: 52 years

Initial Information
- The patient has a history of hypertension and kidney disease.
- An initial assessment reveals she is not breathing and has no palpable pulse.

What are your actions?

Additional Information
- CPR is initiated, and she is placed on a monitor.
- The rhythm on the monitor demonstrates a wide-complex pattern.

What are your actions now?

- This is a case of PEA cardiac arrest.
- The Code Team establishes a definitive airway with bag-mask ventilation with 100% oxygen.
- IV access is obtained, and CPR is continued.
- IV epinephrine is given after the second cycle.

What are your next actions?

Additional Information (if needed)
Instructor notes: Hyperkalemia due to chronic renal failure is suspected and then treated (IV calcium chloride).

Adult Cardiac Arrest Learning Station Checklist (Asystole/PEA)

Adult Cardiac Arrest Algorithm

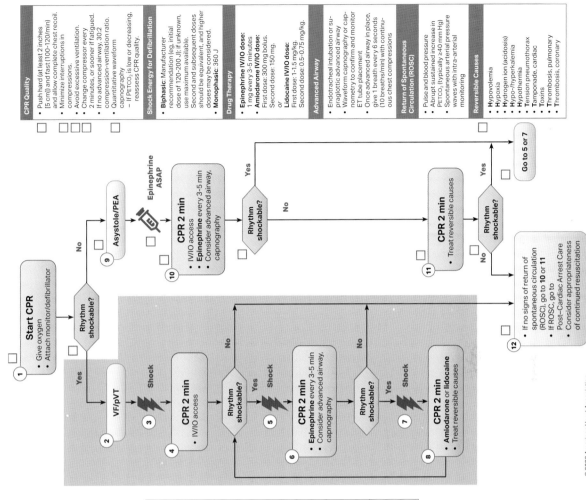

CPR Quality
- Push hard (at least 2 inches [5 cm]) and fast (100-120/min) and allow complete chest recoil.
- Minimize interruptions in compressions.
- Avoid excessive ventilation.
- Change compressor every 2 minutes, or sooner if fatigued.
- If no advanced airway, 30:2 compression-ventilation ratio.
- Quantitative waveform capnography
  – If PETCO$_2$ is low or decreasing, reassess CPR quality.

Shock Energy for Defibrillation
- **Biphasic:** Manufacturer recommendation (eg, initial dose of 120-200 J); if unknown, use maximum available. Second and subsequent doses should be equivalent, and higher doses may be considered.
- **Monophasic:** 360 J

Drug Therapy
- **Epinephrine IV/IO dose:** 1 mg every 3-5 minutes
- **Amiodarone IV/IO dose:** First dose: 300 mg bolus. Second dose: 150 mg.
or
- **Lidocaine IV/IO dose:** First dose: 1-1.5 mg/kg. Second dose: 0.5-0.75 mg/kg.

Advanced Airway
- Endotracheal intubation or supraglottic advanced airway
- Waveform capnography or capnometry to confirm and monitor ET tube placement
- Once advanced airway in place, give 1 breath every 6 seconds (10 breaths/min) with continuous chest compressions

Return of Spontaneous Circulation (ROSC)
- Pulse and blood pressure
- Abrupt sustained increase in PETCO$_2$ (typically ≥40 mm Hg)
- Spontaneous arterial pressure waves with intra-arterial monitoring

Reversible Causes
- Hypovolemia
- Hypoxia
- Hydrogen ion (acidosis)
- Hypo-/hyperkalemia
- Hypothermia
- Tension pneumothorax
- Tamponade, cardiac
- Toxins
- Thrombosis, pulmonary
- Thrombosis, coronary

Debriefing Tool

ACLS Sample Scenario: Cardiac Arrest (VF/pVT/Asystole/PEA)

Action	Gather	Analyze	Summarize
	Student Observations (primary is Team Leader and Timer/Recorder)	**Done Well**	**Student-Led Summary**
• Assigns team roles and directs the team (effective team dynamics)	• Can you describe the events from your perspective?	• How were you able to *[insert action here]*?	• What are the main things you learned?
• Directs the systematic approach	• How did you think your treatments went?	• Why do you think you were able to *[insert action here]*?	• Can someone summarize the key points made?
• Directs team to administer 100% oxygen	• Can you review the events of the scenario? *(directed to the Timer/Recorder)*	• Tell me a little more about how you *[insert action here]*.	• What are the main take-home messages?
• Directs team to apply monitor leads	• What could you have improved?		
• Directs IV or IO access	• What did the team do well?		
• Directs appropriate defibrillation and drug treatment			
• Directs reassessment of patient in response to treatments	**Instructor Observations**	**Needs Improvement**	**Instructor-Led Summary**
• Summarizes specific treatments	• I noticed that *[insert action here]*.	• Why do you think *[insert action here]* occurred?	• Let's summarize what we learned…
• Verbalizes indications for advanced airway if needed	• I observed that *[insert action here]*.	• How do you think *[insert action here]* could have been improved?	• Here is what I think we learned…
• Considers reversible causes	• I saw that *[insert action here]*.	• What was your thinking while *[insert action here]*?	• The main take-home messages are…
• Directs post–cardiac arrest care		• What prevented you from *[insert action here]*?	

Learning Objectives

- Apply the BLS, Primary, and Secondary Assessments sequence for a systematic evaluation of adult patients
- Perform prompt, high-quality BLS, including prioritizing early chest compressions and integrating early AED use
- Recognize cardiac arrest
- Perform early management of cardiac arrest until termination of resuscitation or transfer of care, including post–cardiac arrest care
- Evaluate resuscitative efforts during a cardiac arrest through continuous assessment of CPR quality, monitoring the patient's physiologic response and delivering real-time feedback to the team
- Model effective communication as a member or leader of a high-performance team
- Recognize the impact of team dynamics on overall team performance

General Debriefing Principles

- Use the table on the right to guide your debriefing.
- Debriefings are 10 minutes long (unless more time is needed).
- Address all objectives.
- Summarize take-home messages at the end of the debriefing.
- **Encourage** students to self-reflect, and engage all participants.
- **Avoid** mini-lectures, and prevent closed-ended questions from dominating the discussion.

Case 43: In-Hospital Cardiac Arrest (VF/pVT)

Scenario Rating: 2

Lead-in: A woman admitted with chest pain is now unresponsive with agonal respirations.

Vital Signs
Heart rate:
Blood pressure:
Respiratory rate:
SpO₂:

Temperature:
Weight:
Age: 65 years

Initial Information

- The patient has a history of hypercholesteremia and hypertension.
- She presented with shortness of breath and chest discomfort.
- About 6 hours after admission, she is found unresponsive with agonal respirations by a nurse, who calls you to the bedside.

What are your actions?

Additional Information

Instructor notes: Initial actions include calling a code, starting CPR, and attaching the defibrillator.

- Additional responders will be present after the call for help and can delegate tasks.
- Call a code while asking the nurse for the defibrillator to be attached and simultaneously having other responders begin chest compressions and ventilation with a bag-mask device.

What are your next actions?

- An ECG reveals **VF**.

Instructor notes: A shock should be given immediately after charging. Compressions should be resumed while charging.

What are your next actions?

Additional Information (if needed)

- The patient is defibrillated a second time for VF, and chest compressions are resumed.

What are your next actions?

Post–Cardiac Arrest Care Algorithm

Instructor notes: The team continues high-quality chest compressions, the patient has ROSC, and the team initiates the Post–Cardiac Arrest Care Algorithm.

What are your next actions?

- Optimizing ventilation and oxygenation
- Hypotension management
- 12-lead ECG
- Targeted temperature management if appropriate
- Transfer to cath lab (STEMI) or intensive care unit

Adult Cardiac Arrest Learning Station Checklist (VF/pVT)

Adult Cardiac Arrest Algorithm

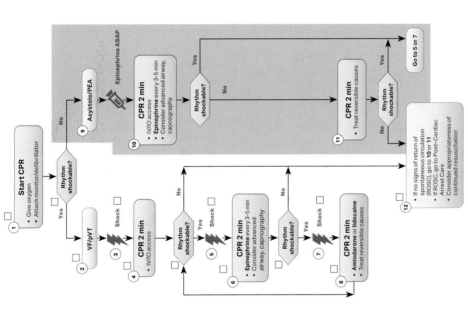

Adult Post–Cardiac Arrest Care Learning Station Checklist

Adult Post–Cardiac Arrest Care Algorithm

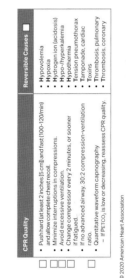

H's and T's

- Hypovolemia
- Hypoxia
- Hydrogen ion (acidosis)
- Hypokalemia/hyperkalemia
- Hypothermia
- Tension pneumothorax
- Tamponade, cardiac
- Toxins
- Thrombosis, pulmonary
- Thrombosis, coronary

Debriefing Tool

ACLS Sample Scenario: Cardiac Arrest (VF/pVT/Asystole/PEA)

Learning Objectives

- Apply the BLS, Primary, and Secondary Assessments sequence for a systematic evaluation of adult patients
- Perform prompt, high-quality BLS, including prioritizing early chest compressions and integrating early AED use
- Recognize cardiac arrest
- Perform early management of cardiac arrest until termination of resuscitation or transfer of care, including post-cardiac arrest care
- Evaluate resuscitative efforts during a cardiac arrest through continuous assessment of CPR quality, monitoring the patient's physiologic response and delivering real-time feedback to the team
- Model effective communication as a member or leader of a high-performance team
- Recognize the impact of team dynamics on overall team performance

General Debriefing Principles

- Use the table on the right to guide your debriefing.
- Debriefings are 10 minutes long (unless more time is needed).
- Address all objectives.
- Summarize take-home messages at the end of the debriefing.
- *Encourage* students to self-reflect, and engage all participants.
- *Avoid* mini-lectures, and prevent closed-ended questions from dominating the discussion.

Action	Gather	Analyze	Summarize
	Student Observations (primary is Team Leader and Timer/Recorder)	**Done Well**	**Student-Led Summary**
• Assigns team roles and directs the team (effective team dynamics)	• Can you describe the events from your perspective?	• How were you able to [*insert action here*]?	• What are the main things you learned?
• Directs the systematic approach	• How did you think your treatments went?	• Why do you think you were able to [*insert action here*]?	• Can someone summarize the key points made?
• Directs team to administer 100% oxygen	• Can you review the events of the scenario? (*directed to the Timer/ Recorder*)	• Tell me a little more about how you [*insert action here*].	• What are the main take-home messages?
• Directs team to apply monitor leads	• What could you have improved?		
• Directs IV or IO access	• What did the team do well?		
• Directs appropriate defibrillation and drug treatment			
• Directs reassessment of patient in response to treatments			
• Summarizes specific treatments	**Instructor Observations**	**Needs Improvement**	**Instructor-Led Summary**
• Verbalizes indications for advanced airway if needed	• I noticed that [*insert action here*].	• Why do you think [*insert action here*] occurred?	• Let's summarize what we learned…
• Considers reversible causes	• I observed that [*insert action here*].	• How do you think [*insert action here*] could have been improved?	• Here is what I think we learned…
• Directs post–cardiac arrest care	• I saw that [*insert action here*].	• What was your thinking while [*insert action here*]?	• The main take-home messages are…
		• What prevented you from [*insert action here*]?	

Case 44: In-Hospital—Obstetrics Cardiac Arrest (VF/pVT)

Scenario Rating: 3

Lead-in: You are an emergency physician who is called to obstetrics for a patient who is 36 weeks into pregnancy and in full cardiac arrest.

Vital Signs
Heart rate:
Blood pressure:
Respiratory rate:
SpO₂:

Temperature:
Weight:
Age: 29 years

Initial Information

- When you walk into the room, you see a woman with an obviously gravid uterus and an IV with a magnesium drip running.
- The respiratory therapist is providing bag-mask ventilation.
- The nurses are performing chest compressions.

What are your initial actions?

Additional Information

- After the patient is on the cardiac monitor, she is found to be in **VF**.
- The patient remains in VF, and emergency cesarean and NICU teams arrive within 3 minutes.
- Immediate defibrillation is performed and CPR is initiated.
- The OB/GYN physician performs an emergency cesarean delivery and delivers the infant while chest compressions are continued.
- The infant is warmed, stimulated, attended to by the NICU team, and begins crying.
- After 2 minutes of chest compressions, the patient remains in VF.

What are your next actions?

Additional Information (if needed)

Instructor notes: At 4 minutes after arrest, the student should consider stopping the magnesium drip and removing the IV tubing from the IV port, administering epinephrine, administering calcium, obtaining a second large-bore IV or IO access, and requesting the emergency cesarean delivery.

Once the cesarean delivery is performed, because the patient remains in VF, the patient should be defibrillated.

Post-Cardiac Arrest Care Algorithm

Instructor notes: The team continues high-quality chest compressions, the patient has ROSC, and the team initiates the Post-Cardiac Arrest Care Algorithm.

What are your next actions?

- Optimizing ventilation and oxygenation
- Hypotension management
- 12-lead ECG
- Targeted temperature management if appropriate
- Transfer to cath lab (STEMI) or intensive care unit

Cardiac Arrest in Pregnancy In-Hospital Learning Station Checklist

Cardiac Arrest in Pregnancy In-Hospital ACLS Algorithm

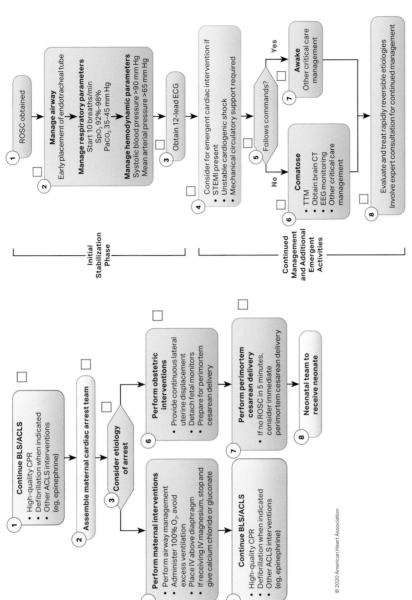

Adult Post–Cardiac Arrest Care Learning Station Checklist

Adult Post–Cardiac Arrest Care Algorithm

Debriefing Tool

ACLS Sample Scenario: Cardiac Arrest (VF/pVT/Asystole/PEA)

Learning Objectives

- Apply the BLS, Primary, and Secondary Assessments sequence for a systematic evaluation of adult patients
- Perform prompt, high-quality BLS, including prioritizing early chest compressions and integrating early AED use
- Recognize cardiac arrest
- Perform early management of cardiac arrest until termination of resuscitation or transfer of care, including post–cardiac arrest care
- Evaluate resuscitative efforts during a cardiac arrest through continuous assessment of CPR quality, monitoring the patient's physiologic response and delivering real-time feedback to the team
- Model effective communication as a member or leader of a high-performance team
- Recognize the impact of team dynamics on overall team performance

General Debriefing Principles

- Use the table on the right to guide your debriefing.
- Debriefings are 10 minutes long (unless more time is needed).
- Address all objectives.
- Summarize take-home messages at the end of the debriefing.
- **Encourage** students to self-reflect, and engage all participants.
- **Avoid** mini-lectures, and prevent closed-ended questions from dominating the discussion.

Action	Gather	Analyze	Summarize
	Student Observations (primary is Team Leader and Timer/Recorder)	**Done Well**	**Student-Led Summary**
• Assigns team roles and directs the team (effective team dynamics)	• Can you describe the events from your perspective?	• How were you able to [insert action here]?	• What are the main things you learned?
• Directs the systematic approach	• How did you think your treatments went?	• Why do you think you were able to [insert action here]?	• Can someone summarize the key points made?
• Directs team to administer 100% oxygen	• Can you review the events of the scenario? (directed to the Timer/Recorder)	• Tell me a little more about how you [insert action here].	• What are the main take-home messages?
• Directs team to apply monitor leads	• What could you have improved?		
• Directs IV or IO access	• What did the team do well?		
• Directs appropriate defibrillation and drug treatment			
• Directs reassessment of patient in response to treatments	**Instructor Observations**	**Needs Improvement**	**Instructor-Led Summary**
• Summarizes specific treatments	• I noticed that [insert action here].	• Why do you think [insert action here] occurred?	• Let's summarize what we learned…
• Verbalizes indications for advanced airway if needed	• I observed that [insert action here].	• How do you think [insert action here] could have been improved?	• Here is what I think we learned…
• Considers reversible causes	• I saw that [insert action here].	• What was your thinking while [insert action here]?	• The main take-home messages are…
• Directs post–cardiac arrest care		• What prevented you from [insert action here]?	

Case 45: In-Hospital—ICU Cardiac Arrest (PEA)

Scenario Rating: 2

Lead-in: A patient is admitted to the ICU with pneumonia/respiratory failure and is intubated and sedated. He is undergoing routine nursing care when he suddenly decompensates.

Vital Signs
Heart rate:
Blood pressure:
Respiratory rate:
SpO₂:
Temperature:
Weight:
Age: 80 years

Initial Information

- The patient suddenly develops **bradycardia**, and the arterial line tracing goes flat, indicating loss of blood pressure/pulse.

What are your actions?

Additional Information

- Call a code and begin chest compressions and bag-mask ventilation.
- The patient is in **PEA**.

What are your next actions?

Instructor notes: The student should discover that the patient had a PEA arrest from dislodgement of the endotracheal tube by seeking underlying and potentially reversible causes. Provide hints by stating that the patient is hard to ventilate.

Errors will include prolonged arrest management (repeated doses of epinephrine, chest compressions) without recognizing the malpositioned endotracheal tube. In addition, students may choose to perform bilateral needle decompressions and/or chest tubes, believing the patient has a pneumothorax. If this occurs, tell students after the case that pneumothorax is usually unilateral and that the most likely cause of bilateral absent breath sounds and difficult ventilation is a malpositioned tube.

End-tidal CO₂ would not register if used, and this could help identify the loss of airway as well. Pulse oximetry would not be registering a good saturation.

Adult Cardiac Arrest Learning Station Checklist (Asystole/PEA)

Adult Cardiac Arrest Algorithm

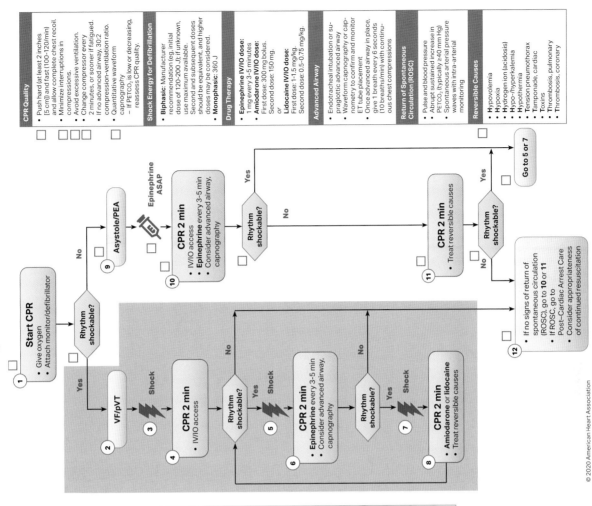

© 2020 American Heart Association

Debriefing Tool

ACLS Sample Scenario: Cardiac Arrest (VF/pVT/Asystole/PEA)

Learning Objectives

- Apply the BLS, Primary, and Secondary Assessments sequence for a systematic evaluation of adult patients
- Perform prompt, high-quality BLS, including prioritizing early chest compressions and integrating early AED use
- Recognize cardiac arrest
- Perform early management of cardiac arrest until termination of resuscitation or transfer of care, including post–cardiac arrest care
- Evaluate resuscitative efforts during a cardiac arrest through continuous assessment of CPR quality, monitoring the patient's physiologic response and delivering real-time feedback to the team
- Model effective communication as a member or leader of a high-performance team
- Recognize the impact of team dynamics on overall team performance

General Debriefing Principles

- Use the table on the right to guide your debriefing.
- Debriefings are 10 minutes long (unless more time is needed).
- Address all objectives.
- Summarize take-home messages at the end of the debriefing.
- **Encourage** students to self-reflect, and engage all participants.
- **Avoid** mini-lectures, and prevent closed-ended questions from dominating the discussion.

Action	Gather	Analyze	Summarize
• Assigns team roles and directs the team (effective team dynamics) • Directs the systematic approach • Directs team to administer 100% oxygen • Directs team to apply monitor leads • Directs IV or IO access • Directs appropriate defibrillation and drug treatment • Directs reassessment of patient in response to treatments • Summarizes specific treatments • Verbalizes indications for advanced airway if needed • Considers reversible causes • Directs post–cardiac arrest care	**Student Observations** (primary is Team Leader and Timer/Recorder) • Can you describe the events from your perspective? • How did you think your treatments went? • Can you review the events of the scenario? *(directed to the Timer/Recorder)* • What could you have improved? • What did the team do well?	**Done Well** • How were you able to *[insert action here]*? • Why do you think you were able to *[insert action here]*? • Tell me a little more about how you *[insert action here]*.	**Student-Led Summary** • What are the main things you learned? • Can someone summarize the key points made? • What are the main take-home messages?
	Instructor Observations • I noticed that *[insert action here]*. • I observed that *[insert action here]*. • I saw that *[insert action here]*.	**Needs Improvement** • Why do you think *[insert action here]* occurred? • How do you think *[insert action here]* could have been improved? • What was your thinking while *[insert action here]*? • What prevented you from *[insert action here]*?	**Instructor-Led Summary** • Let's summarize what we learned… • Here is what I think we learned… • The main take-home messages are…

Case 46: In-Hospital—Postsurgery Cardiac Arrest (Asystole)

Scenario Rating: 3

Lead-in: The patient is postoperative day 4 from coronary artery bypass graft surgery. He is found unresponsive by his nurse, and a code is called.

Vital Signs
Heart rate:
Blood pressure:
Respiratory rate:
SpO₂:
Temperature:
Weight:
Age: 55 years

Initial Information
- The patient is unresponsive, apneic, and pulseless.

What are your actions?

Additional Information
- The patient is hooked up to the monitor.
- The initial rhythm on the monitor is asystole, confirmed in 2 leads.
- Chest compressions are started, and bag-mask ventilation is initiated.

What are your next actions?

Instructor notes: This patient has an underlying pericardial tamponade, which is one of the T's that can cause asystole. The risk factor is the recent coronary artery bypass graft surgery. If the student asks for an ultrasound at the bedside, a large pericardial effusion will be present. The scenario will end when a pericardiocentesis is performed and/or the cardiothoracic surgeon is asked to perform a thoracotomy after the pericardial tamponade is identified.

Adult Cardiac Arrest Learning Station Checklist (Asystole/PEA)

Adult Cardiac Arrest Algorithm

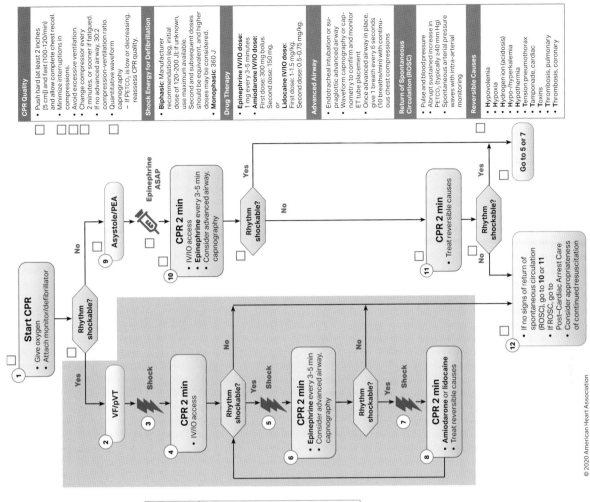

© 2020 American Heart Association

Debriefing Tool

ACLS Sample Scenario: Cardiac Arrest (VF/pVT/Asystole/PEA)

Learning Objectives

- Apply the BLS, Primary, and Secondary Assessments sequence for a systematic evaluation of adult patients
- Perform prompt, high-quality BLS, including prioritizing early chest compressions and integrating early AED use
- Recognize cardiac arrest
- Perform early management of cardiac arrest until termination of resuscitation or transfer of care, including post–cardiac arrest care
- Evaluate resuscitative efforts during a cardiac arrest through continuous assessment of CPR quality, monitoring the patient's physiologic response and delivering real-time feedback to the team
- Model effective communication as a member or leader of a high-performance team
- Recognize the impact of team dynamics on overall team performance

General Debriefing Principles

- Use the table on the right to guide your debriefing.
- Debriefings are 10 minutes long (unless more time is needed).
- Address all objectives.
- Summarize take-home messages at the end of the debriefing.
- *Encourage* students to self-reflect, and engage all participants.
- *Avoid* mini-lectures, and prevent closed-ended questions from dominating the discussion.

Action	Gather	Analyze	Summarize
	Student Observations (primary is Team Leader and Timer/Recorder)	**Done Well**	**Student-Led Summary**
• Assigns team roles and directs the team (effective team dynamics)	• Can you describe the events from your perspective?	• How were you able to *[insert action here]*?	• What are the main things you learned?
• Directs the systematic approach	• How did you think your treatments went?	• Why do you think you were able to *[insert action here]*?	• Can someone summarize the key points made?
• Directs team to administer 100% oxygen	• Can you review the events of the scenario? *(directed to the Timer/Recorder)*	• Tell me a little more about how you *[insert action here]*.	• What are the main take-home messages?
• Directs team to apply monitor leads			
• Directs IV or IO access	• What could you have improved?		
• Directs appropriate defibrillation and drug treatment	• What did the team do well?		
• Directs reassessment of patient in response to treatments	**Instructor Observations**	**Needs Improvement**	**Instructor-Led Summary**
• Summarizes specific treatments	• I noticed that *[insert action here]*.	• Why do you think *[insert action here]* occurred?	• Let's summarize what we learned…
• Verbalizes indications for advanced airway if needed	• I observed that *[insert action here]*.	• How do you think *[insert action here]* could have been improved?	• Here is what I think we learned…
• Considers reversible causes	• I saw that *[insert action here]*.	• What was your thinking while *[insert action here]*?	• The main take-home messages are…
• Directs post–cardiac arrest care		• What prevented you from *[insert action here]*?	

Case 47: In-Hospital—Cardiac Arrest (Post-CABG)

Scenario Rating: 3

Lead-in: A Code Blue is called in the cardiac surgery ICU. The team arrives to find a woman in cardiac arrest. She is 1 day postoperative for coronary artery bypass graft surgery.

Vital Signs

Heart rate: N/A
Blood pressure: Unmeasurable
Respiratory rate: Apneic
SpO$_2$: No reading possible
Temperature: 37.2°C
Weight:
Age: 68

Initial Information

The patient is in a monitored unit. She has been extubated for 12 hours and had been off all vasopressor medications. Before the arrest, she had complained of sudden shortness of breath and some chest discomfort. The monitor shows a narrow, organized rhythm at 120/min.

What are your initial actions?

Instructor notes: This patient, like many others in the cardiac surgery ICU, will have invasive monitoring in place. Begin BLS actions, including CPR and assessment of rhythm. Potential causes, including ventricular fibrillation, hypovolemia, cardiac tamponade, and tension pneumothorax, need to be considered early.

The student needs to call for help early in this scenario, anticipating the potential need for a resternotomy. A cardiac surgeon should be summoned to the bedside as soon as possible, and the sternotomy kit should be present and ready at the bedside. The timing of resternotomy first vs CPR first is controversial. It is reasonable for the student to begin CPR if resternotomy is not immediately available despite the acknowledged risk of disruption of the surgical site and injury caused by chest compressions.

Additional Information

The patient is found to have ventricular fibrillation on the second round of CPR that was done while the sternotomy kit is being sought.

Instructor notes: Students are expected to follow the Adult Cardiac Arrest Algorithm and treat the ventricular fibrillation with chest compressions and defibrillation.

Additional Information (if needed)

After 2 rounds of CPR, the rhythm deteriorates to a slow PEA. The sternotomy kit is at the bedside.

Instructor notes: The priority should be on considering emergency resternotomy. Factors involved in the decision include the training and experience of team members involved in the resuscitation, time until a surgical specialist is due to arrive, and suspected cause of the cardiac arrest.

As soon as the chest is open, direct cardiac massage can be facilitated, pericardial tamponade relieved, and sites of bleeding assessed. Internal cardioversion can be considered if ventricular fibrillation recurs. Alternative causes of arrest should be sought if there is no obvious cause identified after the chest is open.

Consider a fluid bolus. Consider epinephrine per the PEA pathway on the Adult Cardiac Arrest Algorithm.

What are your next actions?

- After the student opens the chest, a moderate amount of blood is removed from the pericardial space. The patient has ROSC.
- The surgeon arrives and takes the patient to the OR for further assessment and management.

Adult Cardiac Arrest Learning Station Checklist (VF/pVT/Asystole/PEA)

Adult Cardiac Arrest Algorithm

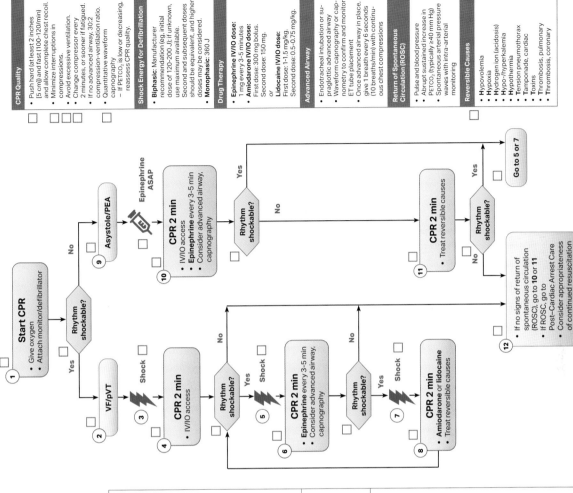

CPR Quality
- Push hard (at least 2 inches [5 cm]) and fast (100-120/min) and allow complete chest recoil.
- Minimize interruptions in compressions.
- Avoid excessive ventilation.
- Change compressor every 2 minutes, or sooner if fatigued.
- If no advanced airway, 30:2 compression-ventilation ratio.
- Quantitative waveform capnography
  - If PETCO$_2$ is low or decreasing, reassess CPR quality.

Shock Energy for Defibrillation
- **Biphasic:** Manufacturer recommendation (eg, initial dose of 120-200 J); if unknown, use maximum available. Second and subsequent doses should be equivalent, and higher doses may be considered.
- **Monophasic:** 360 J

Drug Therapy
- **Epinephrine IV/IO dose:** 1 mg every 3-5 minutes
- **Amiodarone IV/IO dose:** First dose: 300 mg bolus. Second dose: 150 mg.
or
- **Lidocaine IV/IO dose:** First dose: 1-1.5 mg/kg. Second dose: 0.5-0.75 mg/kg.

Advanced Airway
- Endotracheal intubation or supraglottic advanced airway
- Waveform capnography or capnometry to confirm and monitor ET tube placement
- Once advanced airway in place, give 1 breath every 6 seconds (10 breaths/min) with continuous chest compressions

Return of Spontaneous Circulation (ROSC)
- Pulse and blood pressure
- Abrupt sustained increase in PETCO$_2$ (typically ≥40 mm Hg)
- Spontaneous arterial pressure waves with intra-arterial monitoring

Reversible Causes
- Hypovolemia
- Hypoxia
- Hydrogen ion (acidosis)
- Hypo-/hyperkalemia
- Hypothermia
- Tension pneumothorax
- Tamponade, cardiac
- Toxins
- Thrombosis, pulmonary
- Thrombosis, coronary

1 Start CPR
- Give oxygen
- Attach monitor/defibrillator

Rhythm shockable?

Yes → **2** VF/pVT
No → **9** Asystole/PEA

3 Shock

4 CPR 2 min
- IV/IO access

Rhythm shockable? No / Yes

5 Shock

6 CPR 2 min
- Epinephrine every 3-5 min
- Consider advanced airway, capnography

Rhythm shockable? No / Yes

7 Shock

8 CPR 2 min
- Amiodarone or lidocaine
- Treat reversible causes

Epinephrine ASAP

10 CPR 2 min
- IV/IO access
- Epinephrine every 3-5 min
- Consider advanced airway, capnography

Rhythm shockable? Yes / No

11 CPR 2 min
- Treat reversible causes

Rhythm shockable? Yes → Go to 5 or 7
No

12
- If no signs of return of spontaneous circulation (ROSC), go to 10 or 11
- If ROSC, go to Post-Cardiac Arrest Care
- Consider appropriateness of continued resuscitation

© 2020 American Heart Association

177

Debriefing Tool

ACLS Sample Scenario: Cardiac Arrest (VF/pVT/Asystole/PEA)

Learning Objectives

- Apply the BLS, Primary, and Secondary Assessments sequence for a systematic evaluation of adult patients
- Perform prompt, high-quality BLS, including prioritizing early chest compressions and integrating early AED use
- Recognize cardiac arrest
- Perform early management of cardiac arrest until termination of resuscitation or transfer of care, including post–cardiac arrest care
- Evaluate resuscitative efforts during a cardiac arrest through continuous assessment of CPR quality, monitoring the patient's physiologic response and delivering real-time feedback to the team
- Model effective communication as a member or leader of a high-performance team
- Recognize the impact of team dynamics on overall team performance

General Debriefing Principles

- Use the table on the right to guide your debriefing.
- Debriefings are 10 minutes long (unless more time is needed).
- Address all objectives.
- Summarize take-home messages at the end of the debriefing.
- **Encourage** students to self-reflect, and engage all participants.
- **Avoid** mini-lectures, and prevent closed-ended questions from dominating the discussion.

Action	Gather	Analyze	Summarize
Assigns team roles and directs the team (effective team dynamics)	**Student Observations** (primary is Team Leader and Timer/Recorder)	**Done Well**	**Student-Led Summary**
• Directs the systematic approach	• Can you describe the events from your perspective?	• How were you able to [insert action here]?	• What are the main things you learned?
• Directs team to administer 100% oxygen	• How did you think your treatments went?	• Why do you think you were able to [insert action here]?	• Can someone summarize the key points made?
• Directs team to apply monitor leads	• Can you review the events of the scenario? (directed to the Timer/Recorder)	• Tell me a little more about how you [insert action here].	• What are the main take-home messages?
• Directs IV or IO access	• What could you have improved?		
• Directs appropriate defibrillation and drug treatment	• What did the team do well?		
• Directs reassessment of patient in response to treatments	**Instructor Observations**	**Needs Improvement**	**Instructor-Led Summary**
• Summarizes specific treatments	• I noticed that [insert action here].	• Why do you think [insert action here] occurred?	• Let's summarize what we learned…
• Verbalizes indications for advanced airway if needed	• I observed that [insert action here].	• How do you think [insert action here] could have been improved?	• Here is what I think we learned…
• Considers reversible causes	• I saw that [insert action here].	• What was your thinking while [insert action here]?	• The main take-home messages are…
• Directs post–cardiac arrest care		• What prevented you from [insert action here]?	

Case 48: Out-of-Hospital Megacode Practice—Tachycardia (SVT)
(Unstable Tachycardia > VF > Asystole > PCAC)

Scenario Rating: 2

Lead-in: You are a paramedic and arrive on the scene to find a man in respiratory arrest at a restaurant after he reportedly choked on his dinner.

Vital Signs

Heart rate: 140/min
Blood pressure: 62/P mm Hg
Respiratory rate: 0/min
SpO₂: 88%

Temperature:
Weight:
Age: 82 years

Initial Assessment

- The patient is cyanotic, warm, and dry, and EMS responders are ventilating him.

What are your initial actions?

Instructor notes: This man had an anoxic event from a choking. The case focus, however, is the sustained apnea.

The student should begin to take a history, start an IV, and attach monitor electrodes or pads to the patient. The focus should be on recognizing the periarrest state and improving perfusion to prevent cardiac arrest.

Adult Tachycardia With a Pulse Algorithm (SVT)

Instructor notes: The student is presented with apnea. A critical action is noting that the obstruction is resolved because ventilation can be administered through bag-mask ventilation.

The anoxic event has caused perfusion changes that put the patient in a periarrest state. The monitor shows a **narrow-complex tachycardia**.

The student should recognize that the tachycardia is a symptom of the preceding event and focus his or her efforts on oxygenation and ventilation.

Adult Cardiac Arrest Algorithm (VF)

Instructor notes: The patient suddenly develops VF. The student will follow the VF/pVT pathway of the Adult Cardiac Arrest Algorithm.

Now the student Team Leader will assign team functions and monitor for high-quality CPR.

The case should continue through safe defibrillation, administration of epinephrine, and consideration of an antiarrhythmic drug.

Adult Cardiac Arrest Algorithm (Asystole)

Instructor notes: The patient is now in asystole. The student continues to monitor high-quality CPR and follows the asystole pathway of the Adult Cardiac Arrest Algorithm.

Consider reversible causes.

Post–Cardiac Arrest Care Algorithm

Instructor notes: The team continues high-quality chest compressions, the patient has ROSC, and the team initiates the Post–Cardiac Arrest Care Algorithm.

Megacode Practice Learning Station Checklist: Case 48
Tachycardia → VF → Asystole → PCAC

Student Name _____ Date of Test _____

Critical Performance Steps	Check if done correctly
Team Leader	
Assigns team member roles	

	Compression rate 100-120/min	Compression depth of ≥2 inches	Chest compression fraction >80%	Chest recoil (optional)	Ventilation (optional)
Ensures high-quality CPR at all times	☐	☐	☐	☐	☐

Critical Performance Steps	Check if done correctly
Ensures that team members communicate well	
Tachycardia Management	
Starts oxygen if needed, places monitor, starts IV	
Places monitor leads in proper position	
Recognizes unstable tachycardia	
Recognizes symptoms due to respiratory arrest (choking)	
VF Management	
Recognizes VF	
Clears before analyze and shock	
Immediately resumes CPR after shocks	
Appropriate airway management	
Appropriate cycles of drug-rhythm check/shock-CPR	
Administers appropriate drug(s) and doses	
Asystole Management	
Recognizes asystole	
Verbalizes potential reversible causes of asystole (H's and T's)	
Administers appropriate drug(s) and doses	
Immediately resumes CPR after rhythm and pulse checks	
Post–Cardiac Arrest Care	
Identifies ROSC	
Ensures BP and 12-lead ECG are performed, O₂ saturation is monitored, verbalizes need for endotracheal intubation and waveform capnography, and orders laboratory tests	
Considers targeted temperature management	

STOP TEST

Test Results	Circle **PASS** or **NR** to indicate pass or needs remediation:	**PASS**	**NR**

Instructor Initials _____ Instructor Number _____ Date _____

Learning Station Competency
☐ Bradycardia ☐ Tachycardia ☐ Cardiac Arrest/Post–Cardiac Arrest Care ☐ Megacode Practice

Debriefing Tool

ACLS Sample Scenario: Megacode Practice Learning Station

Action	Gather	Analyze	Summarize
	Student Observations (primary is Team Leader and Timer/Recorder)	**Done Well**	**Student-Led Summary**
• Assigns team roles and directs the team (effective team dynamics)	• Can you describe the events from your perspective?	• How were you able to [insert action here]?	• What are the main things you learned?
• Directs the systematic approach	• How did you think your treatments went?	• Why do you think you were able to [insert action here]?	• Can someone summarize the key points made?
• Directs team to administer 100% oxygen	• Can you review the events of the scenario? (directed to the Timer/Recorder)	• Tell me a little more about how you [insert action here].	• What are the main take-home messages?
• Directs team to apply monitor leads	• What could you have improved?		
• Directs IV or IO access	• What did the team do well?		
• Directs appropriate defibrillation and drug treatment			
• Directs reassessment of patient in response to treatments	**Instructor Observations**	**Needs Improvement**	**Instructor-Led Summary**
• Summarizes specific treatments	• I noticed that [insert action here].	• Why do you think [insert action here] occurred?	• Let's summarize what we learned...
• Verbalizes indications for advanced airway if needed	• I observed that [insert action here].	• How do you think [insert action here] could have been improved?	• Here is what I think I we learned...
• Considers reversible causes	• I saw that [insert action here].	• What was your thinking while [insert action here]?	• The main take-home messages are...
• Directs post-cardiac arrest care		• What prevented you from [insert action here]?	

Learning Objectives

- Apply the BLS, Primary, and Secondary Assessments sequence for a systematic evaluation of adult patients
- Perform prompt, high-quality BLS, including prioritizing early chest compressions and integrating early AED use
- Recognize respiratory arrest
- Perform early management of respiratory arrest
- Recognize bradyarrhythmias and tachyarrhythmias that may result in cardiac arrest or complicate resuscitation outcome
- Perform early management of bradyarrhythmias and tachyarrhythmias that may result in cardiac arrest or complicate resuscitation outcome
- Discuss early recognition and management of ACS, including appropriate disposition
- Discuss early recognition and management of stroke, including appropriate disposition
- Recognize cardiac arrest
- Perform early management of cardiac arrest until termination of resuscitation or transfer of care, including post-cardiac arrest care
- Evaluate resuscitative efforts during a cardiac arrest through continuous assessment of CPR quality, monitoring the patient's physiologic response and delivering real-time feedback to the team
- Model effective communication as a member or leader of a high-performance team
- Recognize the impact of team dynamics on overall team performance

General Debriefing Principles

- Use the table on the right to guide your debriefing.
- Debriefings are 10 minutes long (unless more time is needed).
- Address all objectives.
- Summarize take-home messages at the end of the debriefing.
- *Encourage* students to self-reflect, and engage all participants.
- *Avoid* mini-lectures, and prevent closed-ended questions from dominating the discussion.

Case 49: Out-of-Hospital Megacode Practice—Unstable Tachycardia (VT), Cardioversion (Unstable VT > VF > PEA > PCAC)

Scenario Rating: 2

Lead-in: You are a paramedic, and you arrive on scene to find a man in severe distress with crushing chest pain.

Vital Signs

Heart rate: Impalpable
Blood pressure: 64/P mm Hg
Respiratory rate: 28/min
SpO₂: 89%

Temperature:
Weight:
Age: 45 years

Initial Assessment

- The patient is pale, sweating profusely, and cool.

What are your initial actions?

Instructor notes: This man is presenting with signs of a severe myocardial infarction. The case focus, however, is the signs of poor perfusion. The student should begin to take a history and attach monitor electrodes or pads to the patient. The patient is in **VT** with a pulse. The focus should be on preparing for immediate synchronized cardioversion. Treatment should not be delayed to accommodate IV and preshock medication.

Adult Tachycardia With a Pulse Algorithm (VT)

Instructor notes: The student is presented with unstable VT with pulses and needs to follow the unstable VT with pulses pathway of the Adult Tachycardia With a Pulse Algorithm.

A critical action is noting that synchronized cardioversion is the necessary intervention in this periarrest state. Obtaining a 12-lead ECG or starting an IV will delay the necessary intervention.

The student should recognize that the tachycardia is the likely cause of the symptoms and focus his or her efforts on correcting the underlying rhythm.

Adult Cardiac Arrest Algorithm (VF)

Instructor notes: The patient should suddenly develop VF. The student will follow the VF/pVT pathway of the Adult Cardiac Arrest Algorithm.

Now the student Team Leader will assign team functions and monitor for high-quality CPR. The case should continue through safe defibrillation, administration of a vasopressor, and consideration of an antiarrhythmic drug.

Adult Cardiac Arrest Algorithm (PEA)

Instructor notes: The patient is now in PEA. The student continues to monitor high-quality CPR and follows the PEA pathway of the Adult Cardiac Arrest Algorithm.

Post-Cardiac Arrest Care Algorithm

Instructor notes: The team continues high-quality chest compressions, the patient has ROSC, and the team initiates the Post-Cardiac Arrest Care Algorithm.

Megacode Practice Learning Station Checklist: Case 49/52/57/60/62
Tachycardia → VF → PEA → PCAC

Student Name _____ Date of Test _____

Critical Performance Steps							Check if done correctly
Team Leader							
Assigns team member roles							
Ensures high-quality CPR at all times	Compression rate 100-120/min ☐	Compression depth of ≥2 inches ☐	Chest compression fraction >80% ☐	Chest recoil (optional) ☐	Ventilation (optional) ☐		
Ensures that team members communicate well							
Tachycardia Management							
Starts oxygen if needed, places monitor, starts IV							
Places monitor leads in proper position							
Recognizes unstable tachycardia							
Performs immediate synchronized cardioversion							
VF Management							
Recognizes VF							
Clears before analyze and shock							
Immediately resumes CPR after shocks							
Appropriate airway management							
Appropriate cycles of drug–rhythm check/shock-CPR							
Administers appropriate drug(s) and doses							
PEA Management							
Recognizes PEA							
Verbalizes potential reversible causes of PEA (H's and T's)							
Administers appropriate drug(s) and doses							
Immediately resumes CPR after rhythm and pulse checks							
Post–Cardiac Arrest Care							
Identifies ROSC							
Ensures BP and 12-lead ECG are performed, O₂ saturation is monitored, verbalizes need for endotracheal intubation and waveform capnography, and orders laboratory tests							
Considers targeted temperature management							

STOP TEST

Test Results	Circle **PASS** or **NR** to indicate pass or needs remediation:	**PASS**	**NR**

Instructor Initials _____ Instructor Number _____ Date _____

Learning Station Competency
☐ Bradycardia ☐ Tachycardia ☐ Cardiac Arrest/Post–Cardiac Arrest Care ☐ Megacode Practice

Debriefing Tool

ACLS Sample Scenario: Megacode Practice Learning Station

Learning Objectives

- Apply the BLS, Primary, and Secondary Assessments sequence for a systematic evaluation of adult patients
- Perform prompt, high-quality BLS, including prioritizing early chest compressions and integrating early AED use
- Recognize respiratory arrest
- Perform early management of respiratory arrest
- Recognize bradyarrhythmias and tachyarrhythmias that may result in cardiac arrest or complicate resuscitation outcome
- Perform early management of bradyarrhythmias and tachyarrhythmias that may result in cardiac arrest or complicate resuscitation outcome
- Discuss early recognition and management of ACS, including appropriate disposition
- Discuss early recognition and management of stroke, including appropriate disposition
- Recognize cardiac arrest
- Perform early management of cardiac arrest until termination of resuscitation or transfer of care, including post–cardiac arrest care
- Evaluate resuscitative efforts during a cardiac arrest through continuous assessment of CPR quality, monitoring the patient's physiologic response and delivering real-time feedback to the team
- Model effective communication as a member or leader of a high-performance team
- Recognize the impact of team dynamics on overall team performance

General Debriefing Principles

- Use the table on the right to guide your debriefing.
- Debriefings are 10 minutes long (unless more time is needed).
- Address all objectives.
- Summarize take-home messages at the end of the debriefing.
- *Encourage* students to self-reflect, and engage all participants.
- *Avoid* mini-lectures, and prevent closed-ended questions from dominating the discussion.

Action	Gather	Analyze	Summarize
	Student Observations (primary is Team Leader and Timer/Recorder)	**Done Well**	**Student-Led Summary**
• Assigns team roles and directs the team (effective team dynamics)	• Can you describe the events from your perspective?	• How were you able to [insert action here]?	• What are the main things you learned?
• Directs the systematic approach	• How did you think your treatments went?	• Why do you think you were able to [insert action here]?	• Can someone summarize the key points made?
• Directs team to administer 100% oxygen	• Can you review the events of the scenario? (directed to the Timer/Recorder)	• Tell me a little more about how you [insert action here].	• What are the main take-home messages?
• Directs team to apply monitor leads	• What could you have improved?		
• Directs IV or IO access	• What did the team do well?		
• Directs appropriate defibrillation and drug treatment			
• Directs reassessment of patient in response to treatments			
• Summarizes specific treatments	**Instructor Observations**	**Needs Improvement**	**Instructor-Led Summary**
• Verbalizes indications for advanced airway if needed	• I noticed that [insert action here].	• Why do you think [insert action here] occurred?	• Let's summarize what we learned…
• Considers reversible causes	• I observed that [insert action here].	• How do you think [insert action here] could have been improved?	• Here is what I think we learned…
• Directs post–cardiac arrest care	• I saw that [insert action here].	• What was your thinking while [insert action here]?	• The main take-home messages are…
		• What prevented you from [insert action here]?	

Case 50: Out-of-Hospital Megacode Practice—Unstable Bradycardia (Unstable Bradycardia > pVT > Asystole > PCAC)

Scenario Rating: 2

Lead-in: You are a paramedic and arrive on the scene to find a man presenting with chest pain and lethargy.

Vital Signs

Heart rate: 50/min
Blood pressure: 82/P mm Hg
Respiratory rate: 20/min
SpO$_2$: 91%
Temperature:
Weight:
Age: 57 years

Initial Assessment

- The patient is pale and diaphoretic with cold and clammy skin.

What are your initial actions?

Instructor notes: This man is presenting with signs of chest pain that may be caused by either the rhythm or by an underlying cardiac event. The case focus should be initiating treatment to prevent the patient from going into cardiac arrest while determining the rhythm by 12-lead ECG. The student should begin to take a history and attach monitor electrodes or pads to the patient. The patient presents with a **wide-complex bradycardic** rhythm.

Adult Bradycardia Algorithm

Instructor notes: The student is presented with bradycardia and needs to follow the Adult Bradycardia Algorithm. A critical action is obtaining a 12-lead ECG to determine the underlying cause of the rhythm. This patient's 12-lead ECG shows a **confirmed inferior wall STEMI.**

The student should recognize that the preferred means to correct the rhythm is transcutaneous pacing and focus his or her efforts on correcting the underlying rhythm.

Adult Cardiac Arrest Algorithm (pVT)

Instructor notes: The patient should suddenly develop pVT. The student will follow the VF/pVT pathway of the Adult Cardiac Arrest Algorithm.

Now, the student Team Leader will assign team functions and monitor for high-quality CPR. The case should continue through safe defibrillation, administration of a vasopressor, and consideration of an antiarrhythmic drug.

Adult Cardiac Arrest Algorithm (Asystole)

Instructor notes: The patient is now in asystole. The student continues to monitor high-quality CPR and follows the asystole pathway of the Adult Cardiac Arrest Algorithm.

Post-Cardiac Arrest Care Algorithm

Instructor notes: The team continues high-quality chest compressions, the patient has ROSC, and the team initiates the Post-Cardiac Arrest Care Algorithm.

Megacode Practice Learning Station Checklist: Case 50

Bradycardia → Pulseless VT → Asystole → PCAC

Student Name _____ Date of Test _____

Critical Performance Steps						Check if done correctly
Team Leader						
Assigns team member roles						
Ensures high-quality CPR at all times	Compression rate 100-120/min ☐	Compression depth of ≥2 inches ☐	Chest compression fraction >80% ☐	Chest recoil (optional) ☐	Ventilation (optional) ☐	
Ensures that team members communicate well						
Bradycardia Management						
Starts oxygen if needed, places monitor, starts IV						
Places monitor leads in proper position						
Recognizes symptomatic bradycardia						
Administers correct dose of atropine						
Prepares for second-line treatment						
Pulseless VT Management						
Recognizes pVT						
Clears before analyze and shock						
Immediately resumes CPR after shocks						
Appropriate airway management						
Appropriate cycles of drug–rhythm check/shock–CPR						
Administers appropriate drug(s) and doses						
Asystole Management						
Recognizes asystole						
Verbalizes potential reversible causes of asystole (H's and T's)						
Administers appropriate drug(s) and doses						
Immediately resumes CPR after rhythm and pulse checks						
Post-Cardiac Arrest Care						
Identifies ROSC						
Ensures BP and 12-lead ECG are performed, O$_2$ saturation is monitored, verbalizes need for endotracheal intubation and waveform capnography, and orders laboratory tests						
Considers targeted temperature management						

STOP TEST

Test Results	Circle **PASS** or **NR** to indicate pass or needs remediation:	PASS	NR

Instructor Initials _____ Instructor Number _____ Date _____

Learning Station Competency
☐ Bradycardia ☐ Tachycardia ☐ Cardiac Arrest/Post–Cardiac Arrest Care ☐ Megacode Practice

Debriefing Tool

ACLS Sample Scenario: Megacode Practice Learning Station

Learning Objectives

- Apply the BLS, Primary, and Secondary Assessments sequence for a systematic evaluation of adult patients
- Perform prompt, high-quality BLS, including prioritizing early chest compressions and integrating early AED use
- Recognize respiratory arrest
- Perform early management of respiratory arrest
- Recognize bradyarrhythmias and tachyarrhythmias that may result in cardiac arrest or complicate resuscitation outcome
- Perform early management of bradyarrhythmias and tachyarrhythmias that may result in cardiac arrest or complicate resuscitation outcome
- Discuss early recognition and management of ACS, including appropriate disposition
- Discuss early recognition and management of stroke, including appropriate disposition
- Recognize cardiac arrest
- Perform early management of cardiac arrest until termination of resuscitation or transfer of care, including post–cardiac arrest care
- Evaluate resuscitative efforts during a cardiac arrest through continuous assessment of CPR quality, monitoring the patient's physiologic response and delivering real-time feedback to the team
- Model effective communication as a member or leader of a high-performance team
- Recognize the impact of team dynamics on overall team performance

General Debriefing Principles

- Use the table on the right to guide your debriefing.
- Debriefings are 10 minutes long (unless more time is needed).
- Address all objectives.
- Summarize take-home messages at the end of the debriefing.
- **Encourage** students to self-reflect, and engage all participants.
- **Avoid** mini-lectures, and prevent closed-ended questions from dominating the discussion.

Action	Gather	Analyze	Summarize
	Student Observations (primary is Team Leader and Timer/Recorder)	**Done Well**	**Student-Led Summary**
• Assigns team roles and directs the team (effective team dynamics)	• Can you describe the events from your perspective?	• How were you able to *[insert action here]*?	• What are the main things you learned?
• Directs the systematic approach	• How did you think your treatments went?	• Why do you think you were able to *[insert action here]*?	• Can someone summarize the key points made?
• Directs team to administer 100% oxygen	• Can you review the events of the scenario? *(directed to the Timer/Recorder)*	• Tell me a little more about how you *[insert action here]*.	• What are the main take-home messages?
• Directs team to apply monitor leads	• What could you have improved?		
• Directs IV or IO access	• What did the team do well?		
• Directs appropriate defibrillation and drug treatment	**Instructor Observations**	**Needs Improvement**	**Instructor-Led Summary**
• Directs reassessment of patient in response to treatments	• I noticed that *[insert action here]*.	• Why do you think *[insert action here]* occurred?	• Let's summarize what we learned…
• Summarizes specific treatments	• I observed that *[insert action here]*.	• How do you think *[insert action here]* could have been improved?	• Here is what I think we learned…
• Verbalizes indications for advanced airway if needed	• I saw that *[insert action here]*.	• What was your thinking while *[insert action here]*?	• The main take-home messages are…
• Considers reversible causes		• What prevented you from *[insert action here]*?	
• Directs post–cardiac arrest care			

Case 51: Out-of-Hospital Megacode Practice—STEMI/Unstable Bradycardia (Unstable Bradycardia > pVT > PEA > PCAC)

Scenario Rating: 3

Lead-in: You are a paramedic, in the ambulance with your EMT partner. You are dispatched to a local church service to help a woman with an altered level of consciousness.

Vital Signs
Heart rate: 40/min
Blood pressure: 80/46 mm Hg
Respiratory rate:
SpO$_2$: 94% on room air
Temperature:
Weight:
Age: 60 years

Initial Assessment

- You arrive at the scene to find a fire engine already on scene, and 2 firefighters are waiting to assist with equipment.
- One of the firefighters says that the patient is hard to arouse and she looks really sick.
- You arrive at the patient, who is supine on a bench, with several parishioners nearby.
- She opens her eyes to loud voices but appears very confused.
- Witnesses state that she just slumped over without warning. .

What are your initial actions?

- The patient has no respiratory distress, her skin is cold and clammy, and her lungs are clear.
- While you are acquiring a 12-lead ECG, family members state that she has a history of non-insulin-dependent diabetes mellitus and gastroesophageal reflux disease and a family history of cardiac problems.
- The 12-lead ECG shows a **sinus bradycardia** at 40/min, with ST elevation in leads III and aVF, and V$_4$R shows ST elevation as well.

Adult Bradycardia Algorithm

Instructor notes: The Team Leader should recognize the bradycardia as symptomatic and verbalize the need for atropine.

While you are initiating an IV, the patient starts having agonal respirations and becomes unresponsive.

She is now pulseless, and the limb leads **show monomorphic VT.**

Adult Cardiac Arrest Algorithm (pVT)

Instructor notes: After high-quality CPR, 3 shocks, placement of an advanced airway, a dose of epinephrine, and 300 mg amiodarone, the monitor shows a rhythm consistent with the one originally noted (sinus bradycardia with ST elevation in lead III) before arrest occurred, but no pulse is present (**PEA**).

Adult Cardiac Arrest Algorithm (PEA)

Instructor notes: After another minute of CPR, the quantitative capnography reading goes from 18 mm Hg to 55 mm Hg. Rhythm and pulse checks reveal that the patient has ROSC.

Post-Cardiac Arrest Care Algorithm

Instructor notes: Further assessment after ROSC reveals that the patient has a Glasgow Coma Scale score of 3; she is apneic, and ventilation is being assisted through an advanced airway, with a capnography reading of 44 mm Hg.

Her blood pressure is 88/50 mm Hg, and her finger-stick glucose is 285 mg/dL (15.8 mmol/L).

The nearest hospital is 12 minutes from the scene, and a cardiac arrest receiving center is 30 minutes from the scene.

Megacode Practice Learning Station Checklist: Case 51/54 Bradycardia → Pulseless VT → PEA → PCAC

Student Name _____   Date of Test _____

Critical Performance Steps	Compression rate 100–120/min	Compression depth of ≥2 inches	Chest compression fraction >80%	Chest recoil (optional)	Ventilation (optional)	Check if done correctly
Team Leader						
Assigns team member roles						
Ensures high-quality CPR at all times	☐	☐	☐	☐	☐	
Ensures that team members communicate well						
Bradycardia Management						
Starts oxygen if needed, places monitor, starts IV						
Places monitor leads in proper position						
Recognizes symptomatic bradycardia						
Administers correct dose of atropine						
Prepares for second-line treatment						
Pulseless VT Management						
Recognizes pVT						
Clears before analyze and shock						
Immediately resumes CPR after shocks						
Appropriate airway management						
Appropriate cycles of drug-rhythm check/shock-CPR						
Administers appropriate drug(s) and doses						
PEA Management						
Recognizes PEA						
Verbalizes potential reversible causes of PEA (H's and T's)						
Administers appropriate drug(s) and doses						
Immediately resumes CPR after rhythm and pulse checks						
Post-Cardiac Arrest Care						
Identifies ROSC						
Ensures BP and 12-lead ECG are performed, O$_2$ saturation is monitored, verbalizes need for endotracheal intubation and waveform capnography, and orders laboratory tests						
Considers targeted temperature management						

STOP TEST

Test Results	Circle **PASS** or **NR** to indicate pass or needs remediation:	PASS	NR

Instructor Initials _____   Instructor Number _____   Date _____

Learning Station Competency
☐ Bradycardia   ☐ Tachycardia   ☐ Cardiac Arrest/Post-Cardiac Arrest Care   ☐ Megacode Practice

Debriefing Tool

ACLS Sample Scenario: Megacode Practice Learning Station

Learning Objectives

- Apply the BLS, Primary, and Secondary Assessments sequence for a systematic evaluation of adult patients
- Perform prompt, high-quality BLS, including prioritizing early chest compressions and integrating early AED use
- Recognize respiratory arrest
- Perform early management of respiratory arrest
- Recognize bradyarrhythmias and tachyarrhythmias that may result in cardiac arrest or complicate resuscitation outcome
- Perform early management of bradyarrhythmias and tachyarrhythmias that may result in cardiac arrest or complicate resuscitation outcome
- Discuss early recognition and management of ACS, including appropriate disposition
- Discuss early recognition and management of stroke, including appropriate disposition
- Recognize cardiac arrest
- Perform early management of cardiac arrest until termination of resuscitation or transfer of care, including post-cardiac arrest care
- Evaluate resuscitative efforts during a cardiac arrest through continuous assessment of CPR quality, monitoring the patient's physiologic response and delivering real-time feedback to the team
- Model effective communication as a member or leader of a high-performance team
- Recognize the impact of team dynamics on overall team performance

General Debriefing Principles

- Use the table on the right to guide your debriefing.
- Debriefings are 10 minutes long (unless more time is needed).
- Address all objectives.
- Summarize take-home messages at the end of the debriefing.
- *Encourage* students to self-reflect, and engage all participants.
- *Avoid* mini-lectures, and prevent closed-ended questions from dominating the discussion.

Action	Gather	Analyze	Summarize
	Student Observations (primary is Team Leader and Timer/Recorder)	**Done Well**	**Student-Led Summary**
• Assigns team roles and directs the team (effective team dynamics) • Directs the systematic approach • Directs team to administer 100% oxygen • Directs team to apply monitor leads • Directs IV or IO access • Directs appropriate defibrillation and drug treatment • Directs reassessment of patient in response to treatments • Summarizes specific treatments • Verbalizes indications for advanced airway if needed • Considers reversible causes • Directs post-cardiac arrest care	• Can you describe the events from your perspective? • How did you think your treatments went? • Can you review the events of the scenario? *(directed to the Timer/Recorder)* • What could you have improved? • What did the team do well?	• How were you able to *[insert action here]*? • Why do you think you were able to *[insert action here]*? • Tell me a little more about how you *[insert action here]*.	• What are the main things you learned? • Can someone summarize the key points made? • What are the main take-home messages?
	Instructor Observations	**Needs Improvement**	**Instructor-Led Summary**
	• I noticed that *[insert action here]*. • I observed that *[insert action here]*. • I saw that *[insert action here]*.	• Why do you think *[insert action here]* occurred? • How do you think *[insert action here]* could have been improved? • What was your thinking while *[insert action here]*? • What prevented you from *[insert action here]*?	• Let's summarize what we learned... • Here is what I think we learned... • The main take-home messages are...

Case 52: Out-of-Hospital Megacode Practice—Unstable Ventricular Tachycardia (Unstable Tachycardia > VF > PEA > PCAC)

Scenario Rating: 2

Lead-in: You are the paramedic on an ALS engine with 3 EMTs, dispatched to the home of a man with chest discomfort. An ALS ambulance has also been dispatched. You arrive to find 2 family members trying to help the man, who is clutching his chest.

Vital Signs

Heart rate:
Blood pressure: 80/60 mm Hg
Respiratory rate:
SpO$_2$: 96% on room air

Temperature:
Weight:
Age: 48 years

Initial Assessment

- The patient's wife says he had 2 stents placed 2 days ago.
- They are on the front porch of the house, and the ambulance should arrive in 3 minutes.

What are your initial actions?

- The patient is sitting up on a lawn chair, awake and oriented, and in obvious distress.
- He is breathing with normal effort and has a weak radial pulse that is too fast to count.
- The ECG monitor with limb leads shows **monomorphic wide-complex tachycardia** at 170/min.
- Your coworkers are acquiring a 12-lead ECG as you prepare for treatment.

Adult Tachycardia With a Pulse Algorithm

Instructor notes: The student should order the crew to administer oxygen as another student attempts IV access and prepare for emergency cardioversion.

Before cardioversion, the patient becomes unresponsive, and there is a rhythm change to **VF**.

Adult Cardiac Arrest Algorithm (VF)

Instructor notes: CPR should be initiated immediately after assessing for cardiac arrest. Immediate defibrillation is carried out and CPR is initiated. After 2 minutes, another rhythm check is performed (still VF), defibrillation is attempted, and then CPR is resumed.

During this 2-minute cycle, the IV is in place and epinephrine is administered. At the end of this 2-minute cycle, another rhythm check is done (still VF) and another shock is given. CPR is resumed, and an advanced airway is placed, with a capnography reading of 18 mm Hg. Amiodarone 300 mg is administered.

After 2 minutes, another rhythm check is done (still VF), followed by another shock, and then more CPR is given. After this cycle, another rhythm check shows an **organized wide-complex rhythm** at a rate of 50/min, but no pulse is present.

Adult Cardiac Arrest Algorithm (PEA)

Instructor notes: CPR continues, with another dose of epinephrine being administered. During this cycle, the team should consider potential causes of the arrest.

After 90 seconds of CPR, the capnography reading spikes to 65 mm Hg. CPR is interrupted for a rhythm check and then a pulse check, and strong pulses are detected at the carotid and radial areas.

Post–Cardiac Arrest Care Algorithm

Instructor notes: The patient has pulses but has no effort to breathe. Ventilation should continue at 10/min or be guided by capnography (reading currently 52 mm Hg). Blood pressure is 86/56 mm Hg. A finger-stick glucose test is performed, with a reading of 140 mg/dL (7.8 mmol/L).

The patient does not respond to any stimuli. The nearest emergency department is 7 minutes from the scene, and a cardiac arrest receiving facility is 18 minutes from the scene.

Megacode Practice Learning Station Checklist: Case 49/52/57/60/62

Tachycardia → VF → PEA → PCAC

Student Name _____ Date of Test _____

Critical Performance Steps						Check if done correctly
Team Leader						
Assigns team member roles						
Ensures high-quality CPR at all times	Compression rate 100-120/min ☐	Compression depth of ≥2 inches ☐	Chest compression fraction >80% ☐	Chest recoil (optional) ☐	Ventilation (optional) ☐	
Ensures that team members communicate well						
Tachycardia Management						
Starts oxygen if needed, places monitor, starts IV						
Places monitor leads in proper position						
Recognizes unstable tachycardia						
Performs immediate synchronized cardioversion						
VF Management						
Recognizes VF						
Clears before analyze and shock						
Immediately resumes CPR after shocks						
Appropriate airway management						
Appropriate cycles of drug-rhythm check/shock-CPR						
Administers appropriate drug(s) and doses						
PEA Management						
Recognizes PEA						
Verbalizes potential reversible causes of PEA (H's and T's)						
Administers appropriate drug(s) and doses						
Immediately resumes CPR after rhythm and pulse checks						
Post–Cardiac Arrest Care						
Identifies ROSC						
Ensures BP and 12-lead ECG are performed, O$_2$ saturation is monitored, verbalizes need for endotracheal intubation and waveform capnography, and orders laboratory tests						
Considers targeted temperature management						

STOP TEST

Test Results	Circle **PASS** or **NR** to indicate pass or needs remediation:	PASS	NR

Instructor Initials _____ Instructor Number _____ Date _____

Learning Station Competency
☐ Bradycardia ☐ Tachycardia ☐ Cardiac Arrest/Post–Cardiac Arrest Care ☐ Megacode Practice

Debriefing Tool

ACLS Sample Scenario: Megacode Practice Learning Station

Action	Gather	Analyze	Summarize
	Student Observations (primary is Team Leader and Timer/Recorder)	**Done Well**	**Student-Led Summary**
• Assigns team roles and directs the team (effective team dynamics)	• Can you describe the events from your perspective?	• How were you able to [insert action here]?	• What are the main things you learned?
• Directs the systematic approach	• How did you think your treatments went?	• Why do you think you were able to [insert action here]?	• Can someone summarize the key points made?
• Directs team to administer 100% oxygen	• Can you review the events of the scenario? (directed to the Timer/Recorder)	• Tell me a little more about how you [insert action here].	• What are the main take-home messages?
• Directs team to apply monitor leads	• What could you have improved?		
• Directs IV or IO access	• What did the team do well?		
• Directs appropriate defibrillation and drug treatment			
• Directs reassessment of patient in response to treatments	**Instructor Observations**	**Needs Improvement**	**Instructor-Led Summary**
• Summarizes specific treatments	• I noticed that [insert action here].	• Why do you think [insert action here] occurred?	• Let's summarize what we learned…
• Verbalizes indications for advanced airway if needed	• I observed that [insert action here].	• How do you think [insert action here] could have been improved?	• Here is what I think we learned…
• Considers reversible causes	• I saw that [insert action here].	• What was your thinking while [insert action here]?	• The main take-home messages are…
• Directs post–cardiac arrest care		• What prevented you from [insert action here]?	

Learning Objectives

- Apply the BLS, Primary, and Secondary Assessments sequence for a systematic evaluation of adult patients
- Perform prompt, high-quality BLS, including prioritizing early chest compressions and integrating early AED use
- Recognize respiratory arrest
- Perform early management of respiratory arrest
- Recognize bradyarrhythmias and tachyarrhythmias that may result in cardiac arrest or complicate resuscitation outcome
- Perform early management of bradyarrhythmias and tachyarrhythmias that may result in cardiac arrest or complicate resuscitation outcome
- Discuss early recognition and management of ACS, including appropriate disposition
- Discuss early recognition and management of stroke, including appropriate disposition
- Recognize cardiac arrest
- Perform early management of cardiac arrest until termination of resuscitation or transfer of care, including post–cardiac arrest care
- Evaluate resuscitative efforts during a cardiac arrest through continuous assessment of CPR quality, monitoring the patient's physiologic response and delivering real-time feedback to the team
- Model effective communication as a member or leader of a high-performance team
- Recognize the impact of team dynamics on overall team performance

General Debriefing Principles

- Use the table on the right to guide your debriefing.
- Debriefings are 10 minutes long (unless more time is needed).
- Address all objectives.
- Summarize take-home messages at the end of the debriefing.
- *Encourage* students to self-reflect, and engage all participants.
- *Avoid* mini-lectures, and prevent closed-ended questions from dominating the discussion.

Case 53: Out-of-Hospital Megacode Practice—Unstable Tachycardia (Unstable Tachycardia > VF > Asystole > PCAC)

Scenario Rating: 2

Lead-in: You are a paramedic treating a woman who collapsed after reporting nausea and dizziness.

Vital Signs

Heart rate:
Blood pressure:
Respiratory rate:
SpO₂:

Temperature:
Weight:
Age: 63 years

Initial Assessment

- The patient is lying on the floor.
- She is cyanotic and taking agonal respirations.

What are your initial actions?

Instructor notes: First responders are assembling the bag-mask device when you walk into the room. The student should ensure that the patient is being properly ventilated by first responders.

The student can choose to continue ventilation with the bag-mask device or to insert an advanced airway. Advanced airway insertion will require the use of waveform capnography.

The student should start an IV and attach monitor electrodes or pads to the patient. The ECG is **sinus tachycardia with multiple PVCs.**

Adult Tachycardia With a Pulse Algorithm

Instructor notes: The patient suddenly develops a **wide-complex tachycardia.** The radial pulse disappears; however, the student can still feel a carotid pulse.

The student should deliver immediate electrical cardioversion. Blood pressure is 78/56 mm Hg. Consideration of drug therapy should not delay cardioversion.

Adult Cardiac Arrest Algorithm (VF)

Instructor notes: After a single cardioversion attempt, the patient develops **VF.** The student will follow the VF/pVT pathway of the Adult Cardiac Arrest Algorithm. The student should assign team functions and monitor for high-quality CPR. The case should continue through safe defibrillation, administration of epinephrine, and consideration of an antiarrhythmic drug.

Adult Cardiac Arrest Algorithm (Asystole)

Instructor notes: Before the student can administer an antiarrhythmic drug, the patient develops **asystole.**

The student continues to monitor high-quality CPR and follows the asystole pathway of the Adult Cardiac Arrest Algorithm. The student should consider the H's and T's.

Post-Cardiac Arrest Care Algorithm

Instructor notes: After the second dose of epinephrine, the ECG displays an organized rhythm. The rate increases, and the patient has ROSC. The student should initiate the Post-Cardiac Arrest Care Algorithm.

Megacode Practice Learning Station Checklist: Case 53
Tachycardia → VF → Asystole → PCAC

Student Name _____ Date of Test _____

Critical Performance Steps						Check if done correctly
Team Leader						
Assigns team member roles						
	Compression rate 100-120/min	Compression depth of ≥2 inches	Chest compression fraction >80%	Chest recoil (optional)	Ventilation (optional)	
Ensures high-quality CPR at all times	☐	☐	☐	☐	☐	
Ensures that team members communicate well						
Tachycardia Management						
Starts oxygen if needed, places monitor, starts IV						
Places monitor leads in proper position						
Recognizes unstable tachycardia						
Recognizes symptoms due to tachycardia						
Performs immediate synchronized cardioversion						
VF Management						
Recognizes VF						
Clears before analyze and shock						
Immediately resumes CPR after shocks						
Appropriate airway management						
Appropriate cycles of drug–rhythm check/shock–CPR						
Administers appropriate drug(s) and doses						
Asystole Management						
Recognizes asystole						
Verbalizes potential reversible causes of asystole (H's and T's)						
Administers appropriate drug(s) and doses						
Immediately resumes CPR after rhythm and pulse checks						
Post-Cardiac Arrest Care						
Identifies ROSC						
Ensures BP and 12-lead ECG are performed, O₂ saturation is monitored, verbalizes need for endotracheal intubation and waveform capnography, and orders laboratory tests						
Considers targeted temperature management						

STOP TEST

Test Results	Circle **PASS** or **NR** to indicate pass or needs remediation:	**PASS**	**NR**

Instructor Initials _____ Instructor Number _____ Date _____

Learning Station Competency
☐ Bradycardia ☐ Tachycardia ☐ Cardiac Arrest/Post–Cardiac Arrest Care ☐ Megacode Practice

Debriefing Tool

ACLS Sample Scenario: Megacode Practice Learning Station

Learning Objectives

- Apply the BLS, Primary, and Secondary Assessments sequence for a systematic evaluation of adult patients
- Perform prompt, high-quality BLS, including prioritizing early chest compressions and integrating early AED use
- Recognize respiratory arrest
- Perform early management of respiratory arrest
- Recognize bradyarrhythmias and tachyarrhythmias that may result in cardiac arrest or complicate resuscitation outcome
- Perform early management of bradyarrhythmias and tachyarrhythmias that may result in cardiac arrest or complicate resuscitation outcome
- Discuss early recognition and management of ACS, including appropriate disposition
- Discuss early recognition and management of stroke, including appropriate disposition
- Recognize cardiac arrest
- Perform early management of cardiac arrest until termination of resuscitation or transfer of care, including post-cardiac arrest care
- Evaluate resuscitative efforts during a cardiac arrest through continuous assessment of CPR quality, monitoring the patient's physiologic response and delivering real-time feedback to the team
- Model effective communication as a member or leader of a high-performance team
- Recognize the impact of team dynamics on overall team performance

General Debriefing Principles

- Use the table on the right to guide your debriefing.
- Debriefings are 10 minutes long (unless more time is needed).
- Address all objectives.
- Summarize take-home messages at the end of the debriefing.
- *Encourage* students to self-reflect, and engage all participants.
- *Avoid* mini-lectures, and prevent closed-ended questions from dominating the discussion.

Action	Gather	Analyze	Summarize
	Student Observations (primary is Team Leader and Timer/Recorder)	**Done Well**	**Student-Led Summary**
• Assigns team roles and directs the team (effective team dynamics)	• Can you describe the events from your perspective?	• How were you able to [insert action here]?	• What are the main things you learned?
• Directs the systematic approach	• How did you think your treatments went?	• Why do you think you were able to [insert action here]?	• Can someone summarize the key points made?
• Directs team to administer 100% oxygen	• Can you review the events of the scenario? (directed to the Timer/Recorder)	• Tell me a little more about how you [insert action here].	• What are the main take-home messages?
• Directs team to apply monitor leads	• What could you have improved?		
• Directs IV or IO access	• What did the team do well?		
• Directs appropriate defibrillation and drug treatment			
• Directs reassessment of patient in response to treatments			
• Summarizes specific treatments	**Instructor Observations**	**Needs Improvement**	**Instructor-Led Summary**
• Verbalizes indications for advanced airway if needed	• I noticed that [insert action here].	• Why do you think [insert action here] occurred?	• Let's summarize what we learned…
• Considers reversible causes	• I observed that [insert action here].	• How do you think [insert action here] could have been improved?	• Here is what I think we learned…
• Directs post-cardiac arrest care	• I saw that [insert action here].	• What was your thinking while [insert action here]?	• The main take-home messages are…
		• What prevented you from [insert action here]?	

Megacode Practice Learning Station Checklist: Case 51/54

Bradycardia → Pulseless VT → PEA → PCAC

Student Name _____   Date of Test _____

Critical Performance Steps					Check if done correctly
Team Leader					
Assigns team member roles					
Ensures high-quality CPR at all times	Compression rate 100–120/min ☐	Compression depth of ≥2 inches ☐	Chest compression fraction >80% ☐	Chest recoil (optional) ☐ Ventilation (optional) ☐	
Ensures that team members communicate well					
Bradycardia Management					
Starts oxygen if needed, places monitor, starts IV					
Places monitor leads in proper position					
Recognizes symptomatic bradycardia					
Administers correct dose of atropine					
Prepares for second-line treatment					
Pulseless VT Management					
Recognizes pVT					
Clears before analyze and shock					
Immediately resumes CPR after shocks					
Appropriate airway management					
Appropriate cycles of drug–rhythm check/shock–CPR					
Administers appropriate drug(s) and doses					
PEA Management					
Recognizes PEA					
Verbalizes potential reversible causes of PEA (H's and T's)					
Administers appropriate drug(s) and doses					
Immediately resumes CPR after rhythm and pulse checks					
Post-Cardiac Arrest Care					
Identifies ROSC					
Ensures BP and 12-lead ECG are performed, O$_2$ saturation is monitored, verbalizes need for endotracheal intubation and waveform capnography, and orders laboratory tests					
Considers targeted temperature management					

STOP TEST

Test Results	Circle **PASS** or **NR** to indicate pass or needs remediation:	PASS	NR

Instructor Initials _____   Instructor Number _____   Date _____

Learning Station Competency
☐ Bradycardia ☐ Tachycardia ☐ Cardiac Arrest/Post–Cardiac Arrest Care ☐ Megacode Practice

---

Case 54: Out-of-Hospital Megacode Practice—Unstable Bradycardia (Unstable Bradycardia > pVT > PEA > PCAC)

Scenario Rating: 3

Lead-in: You are a paramedic treating a man with chest pain.

Vital Signs
Heart rate: 120/min
Blood pressure: 110/50 mm Hg
Respiratory rate: 18/min
SpO$_2$: 90% on room air
Temperature:
Weight:
Age: 54 years

Initial Assessment

What are your initial actions?

Instructor notes: This student begins with the Acute Coronary Syndromes Algorithm. The 12-lead ECG shows evidence of an **anterior-wall STEMI**. The student should begin to take a history, start an IV, and administer aspirin. Shortly after the student administers nitroglycerin, the patient loses consciousness.

Adult Bradycardia Algorithm

Instructor notes: The ECG displays **sinus bradycardia** at a rate of 40/min. There is no radial pulse, but the student can still feel a carotid pulse.

The student should follow the Adult Bradycardia Algorithm and be prepared to administer a single dose of atropine while preparing for transcutaneous pacing.

Adult Cardiac Arrest Algorithm (pVT)

Instructor notes: Before the student can begin transcutaneous pacing, the patient develops **VF**. The student will follow the VF/pVT pathway of the Adult Cardiac Arrest Algorithm. The student should assign team functions and monitor for high-quality CPR. The case should continue through safe defibrillation, administration of a vasopressor, and consideration of an antiarrhythmic drug.

Adult Cardiac Arrest Algorithm (PEA)

Instructor notes: After receiving the vasopressor, the patient develops an **organized rhythm that is slow**. There is no pulse. The patient is now in PEA. The student continues to monitor high-quality CPR and follows the PEA pathway of the Adult Cardiac Arrest Algorithm. The student should consider the H's and T's.

Post–Cardiac Arrest Care Algorithm

Instructor notes: After the student verifies that the patient is being adequately ventilated, the heart rate increases and the student can now detect a carotid pulse. The patient has ROSC.

The student should initiate the Post–Cardiac Arrest Care Algorithm.

191

Debriefing Tool

ACLS Sample Scenario: Megacode Practice Learning Station

Learning Objectives

- Apply the BLS, Primary, and Secondary Assessments sequence for a systematic evaluation of adult patients
- Perform prompt, high-quality BLS, including prioritizing early chest compressions and integrating early AED use
- Recognize respiratory arrest
- Perform early management of respiratory arrest
- Recognize bradyarrhythmias and tachyarrhythmias that may result in cardiac arrest or complicate resuscitation outcome
- Perform early management of bradyarrhythmias and tachyarrhythmias that may result in cardiac arrest or complicate resuscitation outcome
- Discuss early recognition and management of ACS, including appropriate disposition
- Discuss early recognition and management of stroke, including appropriate disposition
- Recognize cardiac arrest
- Perform early management of cardiac arrest until termination of resuscitation or transfer of care, including post–cardiac arrest care
- Evaluate resuscitative efforts during a cardiac arrest through continuous assessment of CPR quality, monitoring the patient's physiologic response and delivering real-time feedback to the team
- Model effective communication as a member or leader of a high-performance team
- Recognize the impact of team dynamics on overall team performance

General Debriefing Principles

- Use the table on the right to guide your debriefing.
- Debriefings are 10 minutes long (unless more time is needed).
- Address all objectives.
- Summarize take-home messages at the end of the debriefing.
- *Encourage* students to self-reflect, and engage all participants.
- *Avoid* mini-lectures, and prevent closed-ended questions from dominating the discussion.

Action	Gather	Analyze	Summarize
	Student Observations	**Done Well**	**Student-Led Summary**
- Assigns team roles and directs the team (effective team dynamics)	(primary is Team Leader and Timer/Recorder)	- How were you able to *[insert action here]*?	- What are the main things you learned?
- Directs the systematic approach	- Can you describe the events from your perspective?	- Why do you think you were able to *[insert action here]*?	- Can someone summarize the key points made?
- Directs team to administer 100% oxygen	- How did you think your treatments went?	- Tell me a little more about how you *[insert action here]*.	- What are the main take-home messages?
- Directs team to apply monitor leads	- Can you review the events of the scenario? *(directed to the Timer/Recorder)*		
- Directs IV or IO access	- What could you have improved?		
- Directs appropriate defibrillation and drug treatment	- What did the team do well?		
- Directs reassessment of patient in response to treatments	**Instructor Observations**	**Needs Improvement**	**Instructor-Led Summary**
- Summarizes specific treatments	- I noticed that *[insert action here]*.	- Why do you think *[insert action here]* occurred?	- Let's summarize what we learned…
- Verbalizes indications for advanced airway if needed	- I observed that *[insert action here]*.	- How do you think *[insert action here]* could have been improved?	- Here is what I think we learned…
- Considers reversible causes	- I saw that *[insert action here]*.	- What was your thinking while *[insert action here]*?	- The main take-home messages are…
- Directs post–cardiac arrest care		- What prevented you from *[insert action here]*?	

Megacode Practice Learning Station Checklist: Case 55/58
Tachycardia → Pulseless VT → PEA → PCAC

Student Name _____   Date of Test _____

Critical Performance Steps						Check if done correctly
Team Leader						
Assigns team member roles						
Ensures high-quality CPR at all times	Compression rate 100–120/min ☐	Compression depth of ≥2 inches ☐	Chest compression fraction >80% ☐	Chest recoil (optional) ☐	Ventilation (optional) ☐	
Ensures that team members communicate well						
Tachycardia Management						
Starts oxygen if needed, places monitor, starts IV						
Places monitor leads in proper position						
Recognizes unstable tachycardia						
Recognizes symptoms due to tachycardia						
Performs immediate synchronized cardioversion						
Pulseless VT Management						
Recognizes pulseless VT						
Clears before analyze and shock						
Immediately resumes CPR after shocks						
Appropriate airway management						
Appropriate cycles of drug–rhythm check/shock–CPR						
Administers appropriate drug(s) and doses						
PEA Management						
Recognizes PEA						
Verbalizes potential reversible causes of PEA (H's and T's)						
Administers appropriate drug(s) and doses						
Immediately resumes CPR after rhythm and pulse checks						
Post–Cardiac Arrest Care						
Identifies ROSC						
Ensures BP and 12-lead ECG are performed, O₂ saturation is monitored, verbalizes need for endotracheal intubation and waveform capnography, and orders laboratory tests						
Considers targeted temperature management						

STOP TEST

Test Results	Circle **PASS** or **NR** to indicate pass or needs remediation:	PASS	NR

Instructor Initials _____ Instructor Number _____ Date _____

Learning Station Competency
☐ Bradycardia ☐ Tachycardia ☐ Cardiac Arrest/Post–Cardiac Arrest Care ☐ Megacode Practice

---

Case 55: Out-of-Hospital Megacode Practice—Unstable Tachycardia (SVT) (Unstable Tachycardia > pVT > PEA > PCAC)

Scenario Rating: 2

Lead-in: You are a paramedic treating a man with an altered mental status.

Vital Signs
Heart rate:
Blood pressure: 80 mm Hg palpated
Respiratory rate: 22/min
SpO₂:
Temperature:
Weight:
Age: 57 years

Initial Assessment

- The patient was working in the yard and told his wife he was feeling dizzy.
- He sat on the porch and soon had noticeable changes in mental status.

What are your initial actions?

- Both radial and brachial pulses are too weak to reliably count.

Adult Tachycardia With a Pulse Algorithm

Instructor notes: The ECG shows **atrial fibrillation with multiple PVCs**. The student should follow the Adult Tachycardia With a Pulse Algorithm.

The student should begin to take a history, start an IV, and prepare sedation for cardioversion.

Adult Cardiac Arrest Algorithm (pVT)

Instructor notes: Before the student can administer the sedation, the patient loses consciousness. The ECG displays **VT**. There is no pulse.

The student will follow the VF/pVT pathway of the Adult Cardiac Arrest Algorithm. The student should assign team functions and monitor for high-quality CPR.

The case should continue through safe defibrillation, administration of epinephrine, and consideration of an antiarrhythmic drug.

Adult Cardiac Arrest Algorithm (PEA)

Instructor notes: After the administration of the vasopressor, the patient develops an **organized rhythm that is fast**. There is no pulse. The patient is now in PEA.

The student continues to monitor high-quality CPR and follows the PEA pathway of the Adult Cardiac Arrest Algorithm. The student should consider the H's and T's.

Post–Cardiac Arrest Care Algorithm

Instructor notes: After administering a fluid bolus, the student can now detect a carotid pulse. The patient has ROSC.

The student should initiate the Post–Cardiac Arrest Care Algorithm.

Debriefing Tool

ACLS Sample Scenario: Megacode Practice Learning Station

Learning Objectives

- Apply the BLS, Primary, and Secondary Assessments sequence for a systematic evaluation of adult patients
- Perform prompt, high-quality BLS, including prioritizing early chest compressions and integrating early AED use
- Recognize respiratory arrest
- Perform early management of respiratory arrest
- Recognize bradyarrhythmias and tachyarrhythmias that may result in cardiac arrest or complicate resuscitation outcome
- Perform early management of bradyarrhythmias and tachyarrhythmias that may result in cardiac arrest or complicate resuscitation outcome
- Discuss early recognition and management of ACS, including appropriate disposition
- Discuss early recognition and management of stroke, including appropriate disposition
- Recognize cardiac arrest
- Perform early management of cardiac arrest until termination of resuscitation or transfer of care, including post–cardiac arrest care
- Evaluate resuscitative efforts during a cardiac arrest through continuous assessment of CPR quality, monitoring the patient's physiologic response and delivering real-time feedback to the team
- Model effective communication as a member or leader of a high-performance team
- Recognize the impact of team dynamics on overall team performance

General Debriefing Principles

- Use the table on the right to guide your debriefing.
- Debriefings are 10 minutes long (unless more time is needed).
- Address all objectives.
- Summarize take-home messages at the end of the debriefing.
- **Encourage** students to self-reflect, and engage all participants.
- **Avoid** mini-lectures, and prevent closed-ended questions from dominating the discussion.

Action	Gather	Analyze	Summarize
	Student Observations (primary is Team Leader and Timer/ Recorder)	**Done Well**	**Student-Led Summary**
• Assigns team roles and directs the team (effective team dynamics)	• Can you describe the events from your perspective?	• How were you able to *[insert action here]*?	• What are the main things you learned?
• Directs the systematic approach	• How did you think your treatments went?	• Why do you think you were able to *[insert action here]*?	• Can someone summarize the key points made?
• Directs team to administer 100% oxygen	• Can you review the events of the scenario? *(directed to the Timer/Recorder)*	• Tell me a little more about how you *[insert action here]*.	• What are the main take-home messages?
• Directs team to apply monitor leads	• What could you have improved?		
• Directs IV or IO access	• What did the team do well?		
• Directs appropriate defibrillation and drug treatment			
• Directs reassessment of patient in response to treatments	**Instructor Observations**	**Needs Improvement**	**Instructor-Led Summary**
• Summarizes specific treatments	• I noticed that *[insert action here]*.	• Why do you think *[insert action here]* occurred?	• Let's summarize what we learned…
• Verbalizes indications for advanced airway if needed	• I observed that *[insert action here]*.	• How do you think *[insert action here]* could have been improved?	• Here is what I think we learned…
• Considers reversible causes	• I saw that *[insert action here]*.	• What was your thinking while *[insert action here]*?	• The main take-home messages are…
• Directs post–cardiac arrest care		• What prevented you from *[insert action here]*?	

Case 56: Emergency Department Megacode Practice—Unstable Bradycardia

(Unstable Bradycardia > VF > Asystole > PCAC)

Scenario Rating: 2

Lead-in: You receive a 5-minute notification of an inbound woman reporting nausea and vomiting, abdominal pain, and low blood pressure. By report, the patient is placed on oxygen and vital signs are obtained.

Vital Signs
Heart rate: 43/min
Blood pressure: 70 mm Hg/palp
Respiratory rate: 14/min
SpO₂: 95% on 100% oxygen

Temperature:
Weight:
Age: 75 years

Initial Assessment

What are your initial actions upon arrival?

Instructor notes: The initial differential diagnosis is broad: acute coronary syndrome, abdominal aortic aneurysm, and sepsis syndrome. The initial focus will be the bradycardia.

A history is obtained that indicates hypertension, hyperlipidemia, and previous NSTE-ACS with stents twice. Symptoms begin just before the EMS call.

An IV is started and the patient is placed on a monitor with pacer pads. Her vital signs are similar to her prehospital vital signs. The ECG shows a **second-degree type I AV block.**

Adult Bradycardia Algorithm

Instructor notes: The student should recognize unstable bradycardia and follow the Adult Bradycardia Algorithm. The critical action is to note the abnormal heart rate and hypotension. The bradycardia is narrow complex without ST changes.

The patient is unstable and given IV atropine (0.5 mg) twice without change in heart rate or blood pressure. While the dopamine infusion is being prepared, the patient becomes unresponsive.

What is the next action?

Adult Cardiac Arrest Algorithm (VF)

Instructor notes: The monitor demonstrates **VF.** The patient has no pulse. CPR is started. The VF/pVT pathway should be followed. The patient is shocked twice. Epinephrine is given. An advanced airway is obtained.

During rhythm check, the monitor shows **asystole.** No pulse or spontaneous respirations are confirmed.

Adult Cardiac Arrest Algorithm (Asystole)

Instructor notes: CPR is continued. Ventilation at 100% oxygen continues. Another dose of epinephrine is given.

Post-Cardiac Arrest Care Algorithm

Instructor notes: The team continues high-quality chest compressions, waveform capnography jumps to 52 mm Hg, and compressions are paused for rhythm and pulse checks that reveal a sinus tachycardia at 126/min.

Initiate the Post-Cardiac Arrest Care Algorithm.

Megacode Practice Learning Station Checklist: Case 56/59

Bradycardia → VF → Asystole → PCAC

Student Name _____   Date of Test _____

Critical Performance Steps						Check if done correctly
Team Leader						
Assigns team member roles						
Ensures high-quality CPR at all times	Compression rate 100–120/min ☐	Compression depth of ≥2 inches ☐	Chest compression fraction >80% ☐	Chest recoil (optional) ☐	Ventilation (optional) ☐	
Ensures that team members communicate well						
Bradycardia Management						
Starts oxygen if needed, places monitor, starts IV						
Places monitor leads in proper position						
Recognizes symptomatic bradycardia						
Administers correct dose of atropine						
Prepares for second-line treatment						
VF Management						
Recognizes VF						
Clears before analyze and shock						
Immediately resumes CPR after shocks						
Appropriate airway management						
Appropriate cycles of drug–rhythm check/shock–CPR						
Administers appropriate drug(s) and doses						
Asystole Management						
Recognizes asystole						
Verbalizes potential reversible causes of asystole (H's and T's)						
Administers appropriate drug(s) and doses						
Immediately resumes CPR after rhythm and pulse checks						
Post–Cardiac Arrest Care						
Identifies ROSC						
Ensures BP and 12-lead ECG are performed, O₂ saturation is monitored, verbalizes need for endotracheal intubation and waveform capnography, and orders laboratory tests						
Considers targeted temperature management						

STOP TEST

Test Results	Circle **PASS** or **NR** to indicate pass or needs remediation:	**PASS**	**NR**

Instructor Initials _____ Instructor Number _____ Date _____

Learning Station Competency
☐ Bradycardia ☐ Tachycardia ☐ Cardiac Arrest/Post–Cardiac Arrest Care ☐ Megacode Practice

Debriefing Tool

ACLS Sample Scenario: Megacode Practice Learning Station

Action	Gather	Analyze	Summarize
	Student Observations (primary is Team Leader and Timer/Recorder)	**Done Well**	**Student-Led Summary**
• Assigns team roles and directs the team (effective team dynamics) • Directs the systematic approach • Directs team to administer 100% oxygen • Directs team to apply monitor leads • Directs IV or IO access • Directs appropriate defibrillation and drug treatment • Directs reassessment of patient in response to treatments • Summarizes specific treatments • Verbalizes indications for advanced airway if needed • Considers reversible causes • Directs post-cardiac arrest care	• Can you describe the events from your perspective? • How did you think your treatments went? • Can you review the events of the scenario? *(directed to the Timer/Recorder)* • What could you have improved? • What did the team do well?	• How were you able to [*insert action here*]? • Why do you think you were able to [*insert action here*]? • Tell me a little more about how you [*insert action here*].	• What are the main things you learned? • Can someone summarize the key points made? • What are the main take-home messages?
	Instructor Observations	**Needs Improvement**	**Instructor-Led Summary**
	• I noticed that [*insert action here*]. • I observed that [*insert action here*]. • I saw that [*insert action here*].	• Why do you think [*insert action here*] occurred? • How do you think [*insert action here*] could have been improved? • What was your thinking while [*insert action here*]? • What prevented you from [*insert action here*]?	• Let's summarize what we learned... • Here is what I think we learned... • The main take-home messages are...

Learning Objectives

- Apply the BLS, Primary, and Secondary Assessments sequence for a systematic evaluation of adult patients
- Perform prompt, high-quality BLS, including prioritizing early chest compressions and integrating early AED use
- Recognize respiratory arrest
- Perform early management of respiratory arrest
- Recognize bradyarrhythmias and tachyarrhythmias that may result in cardiac arrest or complicate resuscitation outcome
- Perform early management of bradyarrhythmias and tachyarrhythmias that may result in cardiac arrest or complicate resuscitation outcome
- Discuss early recognition and management of ACS, including appropriate disposition
- Discuss early recognition and management of stroke, including appropriate disposition
- Recognize cardiac arrest
- Perform early management of cardiac arrest until termination of resuscitation or transfer of care, including post-cardiac arrest care
- Evaluate resuscitative efforts during a cardiac arrest through continuous assessment of CPR quality, monitoring the patient's physiologic response and delivering real-time feedback to the team
- Model effective communication as a member or leader of a high-performance team
- Recognize the impact of team dynamics on overall team performance

General Debriefing Principles

- Use the table on the right to guide your debriefing.
- Debriefings are 10 minutes long (unless more time is needed).
- Address all objectives.
- Summarize take-home messages at the end of the debriefing.
- **Encourage** students to self-reflect, and engage all participants.
- **Avoid** mini-lectures, and prevent closed-ended questions from dominating the discussion.

Megacode Practice Learning Station Checklist: Case 49/52/57/60/62

Tachycardia → VF → PEA → PCAC

Student Name _____ Date of Test _____

Critical Performance Steps	Compression rate 100-120/min	Compression depth of ≥2 inches	Chest compression fraction >80%	Chest recoil (optional)	Ventilation (optional)	Check if done correctly
Team Leader						
Assigns team member roles						
Ensures high-quality CPR at all times	☐	☐	☐	☐	☐	
Ensures that team members communicate well						
Tachycardia Management						
Starts oxygen if needed, places monitor, starts IV						
Places monitor leads in proper position						
Recognizes unstable tachycardia						
Performs immediate synchronized cardioversion						
VF Management						
Recognizes VF						
Clears before analyze and shock						
Immediately resumes CPR after shocks						
Appropriate airway management						
Appropriate cycles of drug-rhythm check/shock-CPR						
Administers appropriate drug(s) and doses						
PEA Management						
Recognizes PEA						
Verbalizes potential reversible causes of PEA (H's and T's)						
Administers appropriate drug(s) and doses						
Immediately resumes CPR after rhythm and pulse checks						
Post-Cardiac Arrest Care						
Identifies ROSC						
Ensures BP and 12-lead ECG are performed, O₂ saturation is monitored, verbalizes need for endotracheal intubation and waveform capnography, and orders laboratory tests						
Considers targeted temperature management						

STOP TEST

Test Results	Circle **PASS** or **NR** to indicate pass or needs remediation:	PASS	NR

Instructor Initials _____ Instructor Number _____ Date _____

Learning Station Competency

☐ Bradycardia ☐ Tachycardia ☐ Cardiac Arrest/Post-Cardiac Arrest Care ☐ Megacode Practice

---

Case 57: Emergency Department Megacode Practice—Unstable Ventricular Tachycardia

(Unstable Tachycardia > VF > PEA > PCAC)

Scenario Rating: 2

Lead-in: You are an emergency department care provider. A man presents with chest pressure, shortness of breath, light-headedness, and palpitations.

Vital Signs

Heart rate: 130/min
Blood pressure: Unable to obtain
Respiratory rate: 24/min
SpO₂: 78% (poor waveform)

Temperature: 36.9°C
Weight: 80 kg
Age: 64 years

Initial Assessment

- The patient is in the acute care area of the emergency department.
- On initial assessment, he appears uncomfortable, pale, and diaphoretic.
- The carotid pulse is barely palpable.

What are your initial actions?

- His initial finger-stick glucose is 56 mg/dL (3.1 mmol/L).
- The rhythm on the monitor shows **VT**.

Instructor notes: The palpitations started abruptly approximately 30 minutes ago. There is no sensation of presyncope or dyspnea. He feels well other than his heart, which is racing. He had 1 hour of central chest discomfort that worsened with exertion before the palpitations began. There has been no preexisting illness. A review of systems is otherwise normal.

Instructor notes: The patient has a medical history of hypertension, and he is a former smoker. His medications are metoprolol 25 mg by mouth once daily, taken for years, and aspirin 81 mg by mouth once daily, taken for years. He has no allergies.

His lab data showed normal electrolytes and elevated creatine kinase and troponin I. His imaging **(provided if requested)** showed a normal chest x-ray. An ECG showed monomorphic VT.

Adult Tachycardia With a Pulse Algorithm (VT)

Instructor notes: The student should follow the Adult Tachycardia With a Pulse Algorithm. The teaching point for synchronized cardioversion is ensuring that the defibrillator/monitor is tracking the QRS and not the T waves before synchronized cardioversion.

If the monitor is tracking incorrectly, there is a danger in causing an R-on-T phenomenon. Change the leads to maximize the ratio of QRS to T-wave amplitude to address this problem.

Focus on good team communication, safe cardioversion, adequate monitoring, and IV access. The sedation technique for the cardioversion could be included.

Adult Cardiac Arrest Algorithm (VF)

Instructor notes: The patient should suddenly develop **VF**.

The student will follow the VF/pVT pathway of the Adult Cardiac Arrest Algorithm. Now, the student Team Leader will assign team functions and monitor for high-quality CPR.

The case should continue through safe defibrillation, administration of a vasopressor, and consideration of an antiarrhythmic drug.

Adult Cardiac Arrest Algorithm (PEA)

Instructor notes: The patient is now in PEA. The student continues to monitor high-quality CPR and follows the PEA pathway of the Adult Cardiac Arrest Algorithm.

Although the patient is likely in cardiogenic shock, the student should state a differential diagnosis of PEA.

Post-Cardiac Arrest Care Algorithm

Instructor notes: The team continues high-quality chest compressions, the patient has ROSC, and the team initiates the Post-Cardiac Arrest Care Algorithm.

Give specific attention to the likely cause of the patient's arrhythmia, including acute myocardial infarction.

Consider postarrest ventilation goals, hemodynamic goals, targeted temperature management, and urgent assessment for coronary angiogram.

Debriefing Tool

ACLS Sample Scenario: Megacode Practice Learning Station

Action	Gather		Analyze		Summarize	
	Student Observations (primary is Team Leader and Timer/Recorder)	**Instructor Observations**	**Done Well**	**Needs Improvement**	**Student-Led Summary**	**Instructor-Led Summary**
• Assigns team roles and directs the team (effective team dynamics) • Directs the systematic approach • Directs team to administer 100% oxygen • Directs team to apply monitor leads • Directs IV or IO access • Directs appropriate defibrillation and drug treatment • Directs reassessment of patient in response to treatments • Summarizes specific treatments • Verbalizes indications for advanced airway if needed • Considers reversible causes • Directs post-cardiac arrest care	• Can you describe the events from your perspective? • How did you think your treatments went? • Can you review the events of the scenario? (directed to the Timer/Recorder) • What could you have improved? • What did the team do well?	• I noticed that [insert action here]. • I observed that [insert action here]. • I saw that [insert action here].	• How were you able to [insert action here]? • Why do you think you were able to [insert action here]? • Tell me a little more about how you [insert action here].	• Why do you think [insert action here] occurred? • How do you think [insert action here] could have been improved? • What was your thinking while [insert action here]? • What prevented you from [insert action here]?	• What are the main things you learned? • Can someone summarize the key points made? • What are the main take-home messages?	• Let's summarize what we learned… • Here is what I think we learned… • The main take-home messages are…

Learning Objectives

- Apply the BLS, Primary, and Secondary Assessments sequence for a systematic evaluation of adult patients
- Perform prompt, high-quality BLS, including prioritizing early chest compressions and integrating early AED use
- Recognize respiratory arrest
- Perform early management of respiratory arrest
- Recognize bradyarrhythmias and tachyarrhythmias that may result in cardiac arrest or complicate resuscitation outcome
- Perform early management of bradyarrhythmias and tachyarrhythmias that may result in cardiac arrest or complicate resuscitation outcome
- Discuss early recognition and management of ACS, including appropriate disposition
- Discuss early recognition and management of stroke, including appropriate disposition
- Recognize cardiac arrest
- Perform early management of cardiac arrest until termination of resuscitation or transfer of care, including post-cardiac arrest care
- Evaluate resuscitative efforts during a cardiac arrest through continuous assessment of CPR quality, monitoring the patient's physiologic response and delivering real-time feedback to the team
- Model effective communication as a member or leader of a high-performance team
- Recognize the impact of team dynamics on overall team performance

General Debriefing Principles

- Use the table on the right to guide your debriefing.
- Debriefings are 10 minutes long (unless more time is needed).
- Address all objectives.
- Summarize take-home messages at the end of the debriefing.
- *Encourage* students to self-reflect, and engage all participants.
- *Avoid* mini-lectures, and prevent closed-ended questions from dominating the discussion.

Case 58: Emergency Department Megacode Practice— Unstable Ventricular Tachycardia

(Unstable Tachycardia > pVT > PEA > PCAC)

Scenario Rating: 2

Lead-in: You are an emergency department care provider. A man was smoking when he developed sudden-onset palpitations. Moments later, he experienced light-headedness and 2 syncopal episodes, each lasting seconds.

Vital Signs

Heart rate: 180/min
Blood pressure: 80/45 mm Hg
Respiratory rate: 24/min
SpO₂: 92%

Temperature: 37°C
Weight:
Age: 75 years

Initial Assessment

- He continues to feel palpitations in the emergency department.
- On questioning, he admits to drinking heavily for the previous 30 hours.
- During the interview, the patient becomes progressively more short of breath and light-headed.

What are your initial actions?

Adult Tachycardia With a Pulse Algorithm

Instructor notes: A rhythm strip shows **atrial fibrillation.**

Focus on safe synchronized cardioversion and a discussion about the approach to sedation and analgesia in this scenario.

After 2 failed synchronized cardioversions, the patient loses pulses and becomes apneic and unresponsive. The monitor shows **VT.**

Adult Cardiac Arrest Algorithm (pVT)

Instructor notes: Follow the pVT pathway of the Adult Cardiac Arrest Algorithm. Focus on safe defibrillation, high-quality compressions, and a consideration of differential diagnoses.

Adult Cardiac Arrest Algorithm (PEA)

Instructor notes: After the second defibrillation attempt, the patient's rhythm changes to a **wide-complex regular rhythm** (with P waves) at 70/min. The patient still has no pulses.

The student should follow the PEA pathway of the Adult Cardiac Arrest Algorithm. The student should focus on high-quality chest compressions and may consider an advanced airway and underlying causes, including pulmonary embolism and myocardial infarction hemorrhage, among other things.

Post–Cardiac Arrest Care Algorithm

Instructor notes: The team continues high-quality chest compressions, the patient has ROSC, and the team initiates the Post–Cardiac Arrest Care Algorithm.

Give specific attention to the likely cause of the patient's arrhythmia.

Consider postarrest ventilation goals, hemodynamic goals, targeted temperature management, and urgent assessment for coronary angiogram.

Megacode Practice Learning Station Checklist: Case 55/58

Tachycardia → Pulseless VT → PEA → PCAC

Student Name _____ Date of Test _____

Critical Performance Steps						Check if done correctly
Team Leader						
Assigns team member roles						
Ensures high-quality CPR at all times	Compression rate 100-120/min ☐	Compression depth of ≥2 inches ☐	Chest compression fraction >80% ☐	Chest recoil (optional) ☐	Ventilation (optional) ☐	
Ensures that team members communicate well						
Tachycardia Management						
Starts oxygen if needed, places monitor, starts IV						
Places monitor leads in proper position						
Recognizes unstable tachycardia						
Recognizes symptoms due to tachycardia						
Performs immediate synchronized cardioversion						
Pulseless VT Management						
Recognizes pulseless VT						
Clears before analyze and shock						
Immediately resumes CPR after shocks						
Appropriate airway management						
Appropriate cycles of drug-rhythm check/shock-CPR						
Administers appropriate drug(s) and doses						
PEA Management						
Recognizes PEA						
Verbalizes potential reversible causes of PEA (H's and T's)						
Administers appropriate drug(s) and doses						
Immediately resumes CPR after rhythm and pulse checks						
Post–Cardiac Arrest Care						
Identifies ROSC						
Ensures BP and 12-lead ECG are performed, O₂ saturation is monitored, verbalizes need for endotracheal intubation and waveform capnography, and orders laboratory tests						
Considers targeted temperature management						

STOP TEST

Test Results	Circle **PASS** or **NR** to indicate pass or needs remediation:	PASS	NR

Instructor Initials _____ Instructor Number _____ Date _____

Learning Station Competency
☐ Bradycardia ☐ Tachycardia ☐ Cardiac Arrest/Post–Cardiac Arrest Care ☐ Megacode Practice

Debriefing Tool

ACLS Sample Scenario: Megacode Practice Learning Station

Action	Gather	Analyze	Summarize
	Student Observations (primary is Team Leader and Timer/Recorder)	**Done Well**	**Student-Led Summary**
• Assigns team roles and directs the team (effective team dynamics)	• Can you describe the events from your perspective?	• How were you able to [insert action here]?	• What are the main things you learned?
• Directs the systematic approach	• How did you think your treatments went?	• Why do you think you were able to [insert action here]?	• Can someone summarize the key points made?
• Directs team to administer 100% oxygen	• Can you review the events of the scenario? (directed to the Timer/Recorder)	• Tell me a little more about how you [insert action here].	• What are the main take-home messages?
• Directs team to apply monitor leads	• What could you have improved?		
• Directs IV or IO access	• What did the team do well?		
• Directs appropriate defibrillation and drug treatment	**Instructor Observations**	**Needs Improvement**	**Instructor-Led Summary**
• Directs reassessment of patient in response to treatments	• I noticed that [insert action here].	• Why do you think [insert action here] occurred?	• Let's summarize what we learned…
• Summarizes specific treatments	• I observed that [insert action here].	• How do you think [insert action here] could have been improved?	• Here is what I think we learned…
• Verbalizes indications for advanced airway if needed	• I saw that [insert action here].	• What was your thinking while [insert action here]?	• The main take-home messages are…
• Considers reversible causes		• What prevented you from [insert action here]?	
• Directs post-cardiac arrest care			

Learning Objectives

- Apply the BLS, Primary, and Secondary Assessments sequence for a systematic evaluation of adult patients
- Perform prompt, high-quality BLS, including prioritizing early chest compressions and integrating early AED use
- Recognize respiratory arrest
- Perform early management of respiratory arrest
- Recognize bradyarrhythmias and tachyarrhythmias that may result in cardiac arrest or complicate resuscitation outcome
- Perform early management of bradyarrhythmias and tachyarrhythmias that may result in cardiac arrest or complicate resuscitation outcome
- Discuss early recognition and management of ACS, including appropriate disposition
- Discuss early recognition and management of stroke, including appropriate disposition
- Recognize cardiac arrest
- Perform early management of cardiac arrest until termination of resuscitation or transfer of care, including post–cardiac arrest care
- Evaluate resuscitative efforts during a cardiac arrest through continuous assessment of CPR quality, monitoring the patient's physiologic response and delivering real-time feedback to the team
- Model effective communication as a member or leader of a high-performance team
- Recognize the impact of team dynamics on overall team performance

General Debriefing Principles

- Use the table on the right to guide your debriefing.
- Debriefings are 10 minutes long (unless more time is needed).
- Address all objectives.
- Summarize take-home messages at the end of the debriefing.
- *Encourage* students to self-reflect, and engage all participants.
- *Avoid* mini-lectures, and prevent closed-ended questions from dominating the discussion.

Case 59: Emergency Department Megacode Practice—Unstable Bradycardia

(Unstable Bradycardia > VF > Asystole > PCAC)

Scenario Rating: 2

Lead-in: EMS is called because a man with diabetes developed sudden-onset chest discomfort and diaphoresis.

Vital Signs
Heart rate: 42/min
Blood pressure: 110/70 mm Hg
Respiratory rate:
SpO$_2$:
Temperature:
Weight:
Age: 55 years

Initial Assessment

- On EMS arrival, the patient is sitting on a bench.
- He has 8/10 chest pain and his shirt is drenched with sweat.
- His lungs are clear to auscultation.
- A 12-lead ECG is performed and shows ST elevation in the inferior and ST depression in the anterior precordial leads.
- EMS transports the patient to your hospital and places him in bed 3.

What are your initial actions?

Adult Bradycardia Algorithm

Instructor notes: The patient is placed on a cardiac monitor. He chewed 325 mg of aspirin on scene. His blood pressure is 70 mm Hg systolic, and his monitor **(show)** reveals bradycardia at 42/min with AV dissociation and evidence of complete heart block **(third-degree AV block)**.

What do you do next?

Adult Cardiac Arrest Algorithm (VF)

Instructor notes: As you are drawing up atropine, the patient becomes unresponsive. You look at the monitor **(show)**, and it reveals **VF**; prompt defibrillation is performed. The patient returns to sinus rhythm and is responsive, alert, and oriented.

What are your next actions?

Adult Cardiac Arrest Algorithm (Asystole)

Instructor notes: He has another arrest **(VF)**. After defibrillation, CPR is initiated; after 2 minutes of CPR, the monitor reveals **asystole**.

What do you do next?

Instructor notes: After giving epinephrine, CPR is continued; there is ROSC.

Post-Cardiac Arrest Care Algorithm

Instructor notes: The patient is comatose and unresponsive.

He is intubated, and ventilation is initiated. Follow the Post-Cardiac Arrest Care Algorithm.

Megacode Practice Learning Station Checklist: Case 56/59

Bradycardia → VF → Asystole → PCAC

Student Name _____ Date of Test _____

Critical Performance Steps						Check if done correctly
Team Leader						
Assigns team member roles						
Ensures high-quality CPR at all times	Compression rate 100–120/min ☐	Compression depth of ≥2 inches ☐	Chest compression fraction >80% ☐	Chest recoil (optional) ☐	Ventilation (optional) ☐	
Ensures that team members communicate well						
Bradycardia Management						
Starts oxygen if needed, places monitor, starts IV						
Places monitor leads in proper position						
Recognizes symptomatic bradycardia						
Administers correct dose of atropine						
Prepares for second-line treatment						
VF Management						
Recognizes VF						
Clears before analyze and shock						
Immediately resumes CPR after shocks						
Appropriate airway management						
Appropriate cycles of drug-rhythm check/shock-CPR						
Administers appropriate drug(s) and doses						
Asystole Management						
Recognizes asystole						
Verbalizes potential reversible causes of asystole (H's and T's)						
Administers appropriate drug(s) and doses						
Immediately resumes CPR after rhythm and pulse checks						
Post-Cardiac Arrest Care						
Identifies ROSC						
Ensures BP and 12-lead ECG are performed, O$_2$ saturation is monitored, verbalizes need for endotracheal intubation and waveform capnography, and orders laboratory tests						
Considers targeted temperature management						

STOP TEST

Test Results	Circle **PASS** or **NR** to indicate pass or needs remediation:	PASS	NR

Instructor Initials _____ Instructor Number _____ Date _____

Learning Station Competency
☐ Bradycardia ☐ Tachycardia ☐ Cardiac Arrest/Post-Cardiac Arrest Care ☐ Megacode Practice

Debriefing Tool

ACLS Sample Scenario: Megacode Practice Learning Station

Action	Gather	Analyze	Summarize
	Student Observations (primary is Team Leader and Timer/Recorder)	**Done Well**	**Student-Led Summary**
• Assigns team roles and directs the team (effective team dynamics)	• Can you describe the events from your perspective?	• How were you able to [insert action here]?	• What are the main things you learned?
• Directs the systematic approach	• How did you think your treatments went?	• Why do you think you were able to [insert action here]?	• Can someone summarize the key points made?
• Directs team to administer 100% oxygen	• Can you review the events of the scenario? (directed to the Timer/Recorder)	• Tell me a little more about how you [insert action here].	• What are the main take-home messages?
• Directs team to apply monitor leads	• What could you have improved?		
• Directs IV or IO access	• What did the team do well?		
• Directs appropriate defibrillation and drug treatment			
• Directs reassessment of patient in response to treatments			
• Summarizes specific treatments	**Instructor Observations**	**Needs Improvement**	**Instructor-Led Summary**
• Verbalizes indications for advanced airway if needed	• I noticed that [insert action here].	• Why do you think [insert action here] occurred?	• Let's summarize what we learned…
• Considers reversible causes	• I observed that [insert action here].	• How do you think [insert action here] could have been improved?	• Here is what I think we learned…
• Directs post–cardiac arrest care	• I saw that [insert action here].	• What was your thinking while [insert action here]?	• The main take-home messages are…
		• What prevented you from [insert action here]?	

Learning Objectives

• Apply the BLS, Primary, and Secondary Assessments sequence for a systematic evaluation of adult patients

• Perform prompt, high-quality BLS, including prioritizing early chest compressions and integrating early AED use

• Recognize respiratory arrest

• Perform early management of respiratory arrest

• Recognize bradyarrhythmias and tachyarrhythmias that may result in cardiac arrest or complicate resuscitation outcome

• Perform early management of bradyarrhythmias and tachyarrhythmias that may result in cardiac arrest or complicate resuscitation outcome

• Discuss early recognition and management of ACS, including appropriate disposition

• Discuss early recognition and management of stroke, including appropriate disposition

• Recognize cardiac arrest

• Perform early management of cardiac arrest until termination of resuscitation or transfer of care, including post–cardiac arrest care

• Evaluate resuscitative efforts during a cardiac arrest through continuous assessment of CPR quality, monitoring the patient's physiologic response and delivering real-time feedback to the team

• Model effective communication as a member or leader of a high-performance team

• Recognize the impact of team dynamics on overall team performance

General Debriefing Principles

• Use the table on the right to guide your debriefing.

• Debriefings are 10 minutes long (unless more time is needed).

• Address all objectives.

• Summarize take-home messages at the end of the debriefing.

• *Encourage* students to self-reflect, and engage all participants.

• *Avoid* mini-lectures, and prevent closed-ended questions from dominating the discussion.

Megacode Practice Learning Station Checklist: Case 49/52/57/60/62
Tachycardia → VF → PEA → PCAC

Student Name _____   Date of Test _____

Critical Performance Steps						Check if done correctly
Team Leader						
Assigns team member roles						
Ensures high-quality CPR at all times	Compression rate 100–120/min ☐	Compression depth of ≥2 inches ☐	Chest compression fraction >80% ☐	Chest recoil (optional) ☐	Ventilation (optional) ☐	
Ensures that team members communicate well						
Tachycardia Management						
Starts oxygen if needed, places monitor, starts IV						
Places monitor leads in proper position						
Recognizes unstable tachycardia						
Performs immediate synchronized cardioversion						
VF Management						
Recognizes VF						
Clears before analyze and shock						
Immediately resumes CPR after shocks						
Appropriate airway management						
Appropriate cycles of drug–rhythm check/shock–CPR						
Administers appropriate drug(s) and doses						
PEA Management						
Recognizes PEA						
Verbalizes potential reversible causes of PEA (H's and T's)						
Administers appropriate drug(s) and doses						
Immediately resumes CPR after rhythm and pulse checks						
Post–Cardiac Arrest Care						
Identifies ROSC						
Ensures BP and 12-lead ECG are performed, O₂ saturation is monitored, verbalizes need for endotracheal intubation and waveform capnography, and orders laboratory tests						
Considers targeted temperature management						

STOP TEST

Test Results   Circle **PASS** or **NR** to indicate pass or needs remediation: | **PASS** | **NR** |

Instructor Initials _____   Instructor Number _____   Date _____

Learning Station Competency
☐ Bradycardia ☐ Tachycardia ☐ Cardiac Arrest/Post–Cardiac Arrest Care ☐ Megacode Practice

---

Case 60: In-Hospital Megacode Practice—Stable/Unstable Tachycardia (Stable/Unstable Tachycardia > VF > PEA > PCAC)

Scenario Rating: 3

Lead-in: You are a medical emergency team member called to urgently assess a woman admitted to the medical floor with pneumonia. Overnight, she was becoming progressively short of breath with increased work of breathing. This morning, the nursing staff found her obtunded in extreme respiratory distress.

Vital Signs
Heart rate: 138/min, normal sinus rhythm
Blood pressure: 92/45 mm Hg
Respiratory rate: 20/min
SpO₂: 92%

Temperature: 50 kg
Weight: 50 kg
Age: 81 years

Initial Assessment
- The patient was brought to the hospital by EMS for an altered level of consciousness and shortness of breath.
- She had been feeling unwell for approximately a week with a productive cough.
- She was admitted from the emergency department with a diagnosis of pneumonia and started on antibiotics.
- Despite this, her work of breathing has increased overnight, and this morning, her Glasgow Coma Scale score has decreased.

What are your initial actions?
- She is unable to communicate with you because of her level of consciousness.
- She is in severe respiratory distress with accessory muscle use and labored breathing.
- She also displays paradoxical respirations.
- She is on 100% oxygen by nonrebreathing mask.
- Her medical history includes hysterectomy, appendectomy, and hypothyroidism.
- Her medications are levothyroxine and levofloxacin.
- She has no allergies.
- Her blood sugar is 59 mg/dL (3.3 mmol/L).
- She has no labs available, but a chest x-ray shows pneumonia, and an ECG shows **sinus tachycardia.**

Adult Tachycardia With a Pulse Algorithm
Instructor notes: During the interview and initial assessment, her level of consciousness continues to decrease, and her respiratory effort slowly decreases to zero. She becomes apneic, and her hypoxia worsens, with SpO₂ into the 60s. Her tachycardia increases to 160/min. She maintains pulses, and her blood pressure drops to 82/42 mm Hg.

What are your next actions?

Adult Cardiac Arrest Algorithm (VF)
Instructor notes: As the student manages the respiratory arrest (either during bag-mask ventilation or after successful intubation), the patient develops **VF** and loses her pulse. CPR is initiated, and pads for defibrillation are placed. The student should defibrillate early. The student should verify the position of the endotracheal tube, if placed, or remove it if it cannot be confirmed (bag-mask device).
The VF is resistant to multiple defibrillations, epinephrine, and antiarrhythmic medications. Focus on high-quality chest compressions, minimizing hands-off time, safe defibrillation technique, and consideration of reversible causes.

Adult Cardiac Arrest Algorithm (PEA)
Instructor notes: Despite adequate management of VF, the patient will develop PEA.
The focus of the team should be on high-quality CPR, ongoing epinephrine as indicated, and a verbalization of the differential diagnosis beyond sepsis.

Post–Cardiac Arrest Care Algorithm
Instructor notes: After 2 rounds of CPR and drugs, the patient will regain pulses. The student will be expected to reassess vital signs and initiate the Post–Cardiac Arrest Care Algorithm.
Discussion points for the advanced learner may include indications and contraindications for targeted temperature management in this patient with sepsis, blood gas management and targets, and general sepsis management (eg, blood pressure and perfusion goals).

Debriefing Tool

ACLS Sample Scenario: Megacode Practice Learning Station

Action	Gather	Analyze	Summarize
	Student Observations	**Done Well**	**Student-Led Summary**
• Assigns team roles and directs the team (effective team dynamics) • Directs the systematic approach • Directs team to administer 100% oxygen • Directs team to apply monitor leads • Directs IV or IO access • Directs appropriate defibrillation and drug treatment • Directs reassessment of patient in response to treatments • Summarizes specific treatments • Verbalizes indications for advanced airway if needed • Considers reversible causes • Directs post–cardiac arrest care	(primary is Team Leader and Timer/ Recorder) • Can you describe the events from your perspective? • How did you think your treatments went? • Can you review the events of the scenario? *(directed to the Timer/Recorder)* • What could you have improved? • What did the team do well?	• How were you able to [insert action here]? • Why do you think you were able to [insert action here]? • Tell me a little more about how you [insert action here].	• What are the main things you learned? • Can someone summarize the key points made? • What are the main take-home messages?
	Instructor Observations	**Needs Improvement**	**Instructor-Led Summary**
	• I noticed that [insert action here]. • I observed that [insert action here]. • I saw that [insert action here].	• Why do you think [insert action here] occurred? • How do you think [insert action here] could have been improved? • What was your thinking while [insert action here]? • What prevented you from [insert action here]?	• Let's summarize what we learned… • Here is what I think we learned… • The main take-home messages are…

Learning Objectives

- Apply the BLS, Primary, and Secondary Assessments sequence for a systematic evaluation of adult patients
- Perform prompt, high-quality BLS, including prioritizing early chest compressions and integrating early AED use
- Recognize respiratory arrest
- Perform early management of respiratory arrest
- Recognize bradyarrhythmias and tachyarrhythmias that may result in cardiac arrest or complicate resuscitation outcome
- Perform early management of bradyarrhythmias and tachyarrhythmias that may result in cardiac arrest or complicate resuscitation outcome
- Discuss early recognition and management of ACS, including appropriate disposition
- Discuss early recognition and management of stroke, including appropriate disposition
- Recognize cardiac arrest
- Perform early management of cardiac arrest until termination of resuscitation or transfer of care, including post–cardiac arrest care
- Evaluate resuscitative efforts during a cardiac arrest through continuous assessment of CPR quality, monitoring the patient's physiologic response and delivering real-time feedback to the team
- Model effective communication as a member or leader of a high-performance team
- Recognize the impact of team dynamics on overall team performance

General Debriefing Principles

- Use the table on the right to guide your debriefing.
- Debriefings are 10 minutes long (unless more time is needed).
- Address all objectives.
- Summarize take-home messages at the end of the debriefing.
- *Encourage* students to self-reflect, and engage all participants.
- *Avoid* mini-lectures, and prevent closed-ended questions from dominating the discussion.

Megacode Practice Learning Station Checklist: Case 61

Tachycardia → VF → PEA → PCAC

Student Name _____ Date of Test _____

Critical Performance Steps						Check if done correctly
Team Leader						
Assigns team member roles						
Ensures high-quality CPR at all times	Compression rate 100-120/min ☐	Compression depth of ≥2 inches ☐	Chest compression fraction >80% ☐	Chest recoil (optional) ☐	Ventilation (optional) ☐	
Ensures that team members communicate well						
Tachycardia Management						
Starts oxygen if needed, places monitor, starts IV						
Places monitor leads in proper position						
Recognizes unstable tachycardia						
Recognizes symptoms due to gunshot wound						
VF Management						
Recognizes VF						
Clears before analyze and shock						
Immediately resumes CPR after shocks						
Appropriate airway management						
Appropriate cycles of drug-rhythm check/shock-CPR						
Administers appropriate drug(s) and doses						
PEA Management						
Recognizes PEA						
Verbalizes potential reversible causes of PEA (H's and T's)						
Administers appropriate drug(s) and doses						
Immediately resumes CPR after rhythm and pulse checks						
Post-Cardiac Arrest Care						
Identifies ROSC						
Ensures BP and 12-lead ECG are performed, O_2 saturation is monitored, verbalizes need for endotracheal intubation and waveform capnography, and orders laboratory tests						
Considers targeted temperature management						

STOP TEST

Test Results	Circle **PASS** or **NR** to indicate pass or needs remediation:	**PASS**	**NR**

Instructor Initials _____ Instructor Number _____ Date _____

Learning Station Competency
☐ Bradycardia ☐ Tachycardia ☐ Cardiac Arrest/Post-Cardiac Arrest Care ☐ Megacode Practice

---

Case 61: In-Hospital Intermediate Medical-Surgical Unit Megacode Practice—Stable/Unstable Tachycardia

(Stable/Unstable Tachycardia > VF > PEA > PCAC)

Scenario Rating: 3

Lead-in: You are a healthcare provider on an intermediate medical-surgical unit, checking on your patients, when you hear an overhead page (coded) that an intruder is in the hospital. One of your patients was involved in a bar fight and sustained several life-threatening injuries. As the message is delivered, you hear him screaming, "I'm dying— I've been shot!" and you see an unfamiliar man run out of the unit.

Vital Signs
Heart rate: 130/min
Blood pressure: 90/60 mm Hg
Respiratory rate: 40/min
SpO₂:

Temperature:
Weight:
Age: 22 years

Initial Assessment

- While you assess your patient, replacing his nonrebreathing mask and checking IV patency, you notice a chest wound at his left lower rib cage.

What are your initial actions?

Instructor notes: This patient has high potential to experience a respiratory arrest. The focus of this case initially is tachycardia, tachypnea, and hypotension.

Because you know the history of the patient, stabilizing vital signs and the open wound and calming your patient are priorities. You should continue to monitor narrow, rapid cardiac rhythm, increased respiratory rate, and hypotension.

Adult Tachycardia With a Pulse Algorithm

Instructor notes: Your patient most likely has a sucking chest wound, which can impair breathing due to interruption in the lungs, the diaphragm, and/or the chest wall.

Because your patient has a large defect in his chest wall, he will need a chest tube and, most likely, surgery. So, his **tachycardia** could be caused by the impaired lung integrity or loss of blood from the gunshot wound.

You should be aware of signs of distress, such as continued dyspnea, chest pain, and decreased breath sounds on the side of the injury. If these signs are not acknowledged, your patient will have a respiratory arrest.

Adult Cardiac Arrest Algorithm (VF)

Instructor notes: Shortly after your patient experiences respiratory arrest and you begin ventilation, the patient goes into **VF**. Initiate high-quality CPR and prepare to defibrillate.

Adult Cardiac Arrest Algorithm (PEA)

Instructor notes: Despite adequate management of VF, the patient remains in cardiac arrest.

Options to consider:
- Indication for an emergency thoracotomy in the emergency department or on a surgical floor
- High-quality CPR, ongoing epinephrine as indicated, and a verbalization of the differential diagnosis while preparing to move to surgery

After the second shock and continued CPR, the rhythm changes to a **wide-complex tachycardia**. There is no pulse.

Post-Cardiac Arrest Care Algorithm

Instructor notes: After another round of CPR and medications, the patient regains a pulse. The student will be expected to reassess vital signs and initiate the Post-Cardiac Arrest Care Algorithm.

Debriefing Tool

ACLS Sample Scenario: Megacode Practice Learning Station

Learning Objectives

- Apply the BLS, Primary, and Secondary Assessments sequence for a systematic evaluation of adult patients
- Perform prompt, high-quality BLS, including prioritizing early chest compressions and integrating early AED use
- Recognize respiratory arrest
- Perform early management of respiratory arrest
- Recognize bradyarrhythmias and tachyarrhythmias that may result in cardiac arrest or complicate resuscitation outcome
- Perform early management of bradyarrhythmias and tachyarrhythmias that may result in cardiac arrest or complicate resuscitation outcome
- Discuss early recognition and management of ACS, including appropriate disposition
- Discuss early recognition and management of stroke, including appropriate disposition
- Recognize cardiac arrest
- Perform early management of cardiac arrest until termination of resuscitation or transfer of care, including post–cardiac arrest care
- Evaluate resuscitative efforts during a cardiac arrest through continuous assessment of CPR quality, monitoring the patient's physiologic response and delivering real-time feedback to the team
- Model effective communication as a member or leader of a high-performance team
- Recognize the impact of team dynamics on overall team performance

General Debriefing Principles

- Use the table on the right to guide your debriefing.
- Debriefings are 10 minutes long (unless more time is needed).
- Address all objectives.
- Summarize take-home messages at the end of the debriefing.
- *Encourage* students to self-reflect, and engage all participants.
- *Avoid* mini-lectures, and prevent closed-ended questions from dominating the discussion.

Action	Gather	Analyze	Summarize
• Assigns team roles and directs the team (effective team dynamics) • Directs the systematic approach • Directs team to administer 100% oxygen • Directs team to apply monitor leads • Directs IV or IO access • Directs appropriate defibrillation and drug treatment • Directs reassessment of patient in response to treatments • Summarizes specific treatments • Verbalizes indications for advanced airway if needed • Considers reversible causes • Directs post–cardiac arrest care	**Student Observations** (primary is Team Leader and Timer/Recorder) • Can you describe the events from your perspective? • How did you think your treatments went? • Can you review the events of the scenario? *(directed to the Timer/Recorder)* • What could you have improved? • What did the team do well?	**Done Well** • How were you able to *[insert action here]*? • Why do you think you were able to *[insert action here]*? • Tell me a little more about how you *[insert action here]*.	**Student-Led Summary** • What are the main things you learned? • Can someone summarize the key points made? • What are the main take-home messages?
	Instructor Observations • I noticed that *[insert action here]*. • I observed that *[insert action here]*. • I saw that *[insert action here]*.	**Needs Improvement** • Why do you think *[insert action here]* occurred? • How do you think *[insert action here]* could have been improved? • What was your thinking while *[insert action here]*? • What prevented you from *[insert action here]*?	**Instructor-Led Summary** • Let's summarize what we learned… • Here is what I think we learned… • The main take-home messages are…

Megacode Practice Learning Station Checklist: Case 49/52/57/60/62
Tachycardia → VF → PEA → PCAC

Student Name _____ Date of Test _____

Critical Performance Steps					Check if done correctly
Team Leader					
Assigns team member roles					
Ensures high-quality CPR at all times	Compression rate 100-120/min ☐	Compression depth of ≥2 inches ☐	Chest compression fraction >80% ☐	Chest recoil (optional) ☐ Ventilation (optional) ☐	
Ensures that team members communicate well					
Tachycardia Management					
Starts oxygen if needed, places monitor, starts IV					
Places monitor leads in proper position					
Recognizes unstable tachycardia					
Performs immediate synchronized cardioversion					
VF Management					
Recognizes VF					
Clears before analyze and shock					
Immediately resumes CPR after shocks					
Appropriate airway management					
Appropriate cycles of drug–rhythm check/shock–CPR					
Administers appropriate drug(s) and doses					
PEA Management					
Recognizes PEA					
Verbalizes potential reversible causes of PEA (H's and T's)					
Administers appropriate drug(s) and doses					
Immediately resumes CPR after rhythm and pulse checks					
Post–Cardiac Arrest Care					
Identifies ROSC					
Ensures BP and 12-lead ECG are performed, O₂ saturation is monitored, verbalizes need for endotracheal intubation and waveform capnography, and orders laboratory tests					
Considers targeted temperature management					

STOP TEST

Test Results	Circle **PASS** or **NR** to indicate pass or needs remediation:	**PASS**	**NR**

Instructor Initials _____ Instructor Number _____ Date _____

Learning Station Competency
☐ Bradycardia ☐ Tachycardia ☐ Cardiac Arrest/Post–Cardiac Arrest Care ☐ Megacode Practice

---

Case 62: In-Hospital Megacode Practice—
Unstable Ventricular Tachycardia
(Unstable Tachycardia > VF > PEA > PCAC)

Scenario Rating: 1

Lead-in: You are a healthcare provider caring for a man awaiting surgery for a small bowel obstruction. He signals with his call light and says that he is experiencing increasing shortness of breath, anxiety, and a feeling of impending doom.

Vital Signs
Heart rate: 152/min
Blood pressure: 90/52 mm Hg
Respiratory rate: 24/min
SpO₂: 93%

Temperature:
Weight:
Age: 71 years

Initial Assessment

What are your initial actions?

- Upon assessment, you notice the portable telemetry monitor shows a wide, monomorphic, rapid rhythm, which you identify as **VT**.
- He begins to experience diaphoresis, increasing shortness of breath, and apprehension.

Adult Tachycardia With a Pulse Algorithm

Instructor notes: The student should realize that the patient is in unstable VT. Following the Adult Tachycardia With a Pulse Algorithm, a critical action is recognizing the arrhythmia and its need for immediate treatment.

The student should also recognize that the patient is symptomatic and prepare for immediate cardioversion. Consideration of drug therapy should not delay cardioversion.

Adult Cardiac Arrest Algorithm (VF)

Instructor notes: The patient suddenly develops **VF**. The student will follow the VF/pVT pathway of the Adult Cardiac Arrest Algorithm.

A Team Leader designates team functions and monitors for high-quality CPR. The case should continue through safe defibrillation, administration of epinephrine, and consideration of an antiarrhythmic drug.

Adult Cardiac Arrest Algorithm (PEA)

Instructor notes: The situation continues, and the patient is now in PEA. The team should continuously monitor high-quality CPR and follow the PEA pathway of the Adult Cardiac Arrest Algorithm.

A likely occurrence is that the patient is in cardiogenic shock, so the student should be able to state and discuss the differentiating diagnoses associated with PEA.

Post–Cardiac Arrest Care Algorithm

Instructor notes: As a member of the resuscitation team, the student continues high-quality chest compressions.

The patient has ROSC, and the student should initiate the Post-Cardiac Arrest Care Algorithm.

Debriefing Tool

ACLS Sample Scenario: Megacode Practice Learning Station

Action	Gather	Analyze	Summarize
	Student Observations (primary is Team Leader and Timer/Recorder)	**Done Well**	**Student-Led Summary**
• Assigns team roles and directs the team (effective team dynamics) • Directs the systematic approach • Directs team to administer 100% oxygen • Directs team to apply monitor leads • Directs IV or IO access • Directs appropriate defibrillation and drug treatment • Directs reassessment of patient in response to treatments • Summarizes specific treatments • Verbalizes indications for advanced airway if needed • Considers reversible causes • Directs post–cardiac arrest care	• Can you describe the events from your perspective? • How did you think your treatments went? • Can you review the events of the scenario? *(directed to the Timer/Recorder)* • What could you have improved? • What did the team do well?	• How were you able to *[insert action here]*? • Why do you think you were able to *[insert action here]*? • Tell me a little more about how you *[insert action here]*.	• What are the main things you learned? • Can someone summarize the key points made? • What are the main take-home messages?
	Instructor Observations	**Needs Improvement**	**Instructor-Led Summary**
	• I noticed that *[insert action here]*. • I observed that *[insert action here]*. • I saw that *[insert action here]*.	• Why do you think *[insert action here]* occurred? • How do you think *[insert action here]* could have been improved? • What was your thinking while *[insert action here]*? • What prevented you from *[insert action here]*?	• Let's summarize what we learned… • Here is what I think we learned… • The main take-home messages are…

Learning Objectives

- Apply the BLS, Primary, and Secondary Assessments sequence for a systematic evaluation of adult patients
- Perform prompt, high-quality BLS, including prioritizing early chest compressions and integrating early AED use
- Recognize respiratory arrest
- Perform early management of respiratory arrest
- Recognize bradyarrhythmias and tachyarrhythmias that may result in cardiac arrest or complicate resuscitation outcome
- Perform early management of bradyarrhythmias and tachyarrhythmias that may result in cardiac arrest or complicate resuscitation outcome
- Discuss early recognition and management of ACS, including appropriate disposition
- Discuss early recognition and management of stroke, including appropriate disposition
- Recognize cardiac arrest
- Perform early management of cardiac arrest until termination of resuscitation or transfer of care, including post–cardiac arrest care
- Evaluate resuscitative efforts during a cardiac arrest through continuous assessment of CPR quality, monitoring the patient's physiologic response and delivering real-time feedback to the team
- Model effective communication as a member or leader of a high-performance team
- Recognize the impact of team dynamics on overall team performance

General Debriefing Principles

- Use the table on the right to guide your debriefing.
- Debriefings are 10 minutes long (unless more time is needed).
- Address all objectives.
- Summarize take-home messages at the end of the debriefing.
- *Encourage* students to self-reflect, and engage all participants.
- *Avoid* mini-lectures, and prevent closed-ended questions from dominating the discussion.

Megacode Testing Checklist: Scenarios 1/3/8
Bradycardia → Pulseless VT → PEA → PCAC

Student Name _____ Date of Test _____

Critical Performance Steps						Check if done correctly
Team Leader						
Assigns team member roles						
Ensures high-quality CPR at all times	Compression rate 100–120/min ☐	Compression depth of ≥2 inches ☐	Chest compression fraction >80% ☐	Chest recoil (optional) ☐	Ventilation (optional) ☐	
Ensures that team members communicate well						
Bradycardia Management						
Starts oxygen if needed, places monitor, starts IV						
Places monitor leads in proper position						
Recognizes symptomatic bradycardia						
Administers correct dose of atropine						
Prepares for second-line treatment						
Pulseless VT Management						
Recognizes pVT						
Clears before analyze and shock						
Immediately resumes CPR after shocks						
Appropriate airway management						
Appropriate cycles of drug–rhythm check/shock–CPR						
Administers appropriate drug(s) and doses						
PEA Management						
Recognizes PEA						
Verbalizes potential reversible causes of PEA (H's and T's)						
Administers appropriate drug(s) and doses						
Immediately resumes CPR after rhythm checks						
Post–Cardiac Arrest Care						
Identifies ROSC						
Ensures BP and 12-lead ECG are performed, O₂ saturation is monitored, verbalizes need for endotracheal intubation and waveform capnography, and orders laboratory tests						
Considers targeted temperature management						

STOP TEST

Test Results	Circle **PASS** or **NR** to indicate pass or needs remediation:	**PASS**	**NR**

Instructor Initials _____ Instructor Number _____ Date _____

Learning Station Competency
☐ Bradycardia ☐ Tachycardia ☐ Cardiac Arrest/Post–Cardiac Arrest Care ☐ Megacode Practice

---

Megacode 1— Out-of-Hospital Unstable Bradycardia
(Unstable Bradycardia > pVT > PEA > PCAC)

Lead-in: You are a paramedic treating a man who had a syncopal episode.

Vital Signs
Heart rate:
Blood pressure: 78/42 mm Hg
Respiratory rate:
SpO₂:
Temperature:
Weight:
Age: 62 years

Initial Assessment
- The patient is conscious and alert.

What are your initial actions?
- His skin is pale, and he is diaphoretic.
- The patient is not following commands.
- There is no radial pulse, but the carotid pulse is weak and slow.

Adult Bradycardia Algorithm
Instructor notes: The ECG monitor shows a **sinus bradycardia** with occasional PVC.

The student should follow the Adult Bradycardia Algorithm and be prepared to administer a single dose of atropine while preparing for transcutaneous pacing.

Adult Cardiac Arrest Algorithm (pVT)
Instructor notes: With the introduction of the pacing impulse, the ECG monitor displays VT. There is no pulse.

The student should immediately discontinue pacing and defibrillate the patient. The student will follow the VF/pVT pathway of the Adult Cardiac Arrest Algorithm.

The student should assign team functions and monitor for high-quality CPR. The case should continue through safe defibrillation and administration of epinephrine and amiodarone.

Adult Cardiac Arrest Algorithm (PEA)
Instructor notes: After the third shock, the patient develops an **organized rhythm that is slow.** There is no pulse. The patient is now in PEA.

The student continues to monitor high-quality CPR and follows the PEA pathway of the Adult Cardiac Arrest Algorithm.

The student should consider reversible causes.

Post–Cardiac Arrest Care Algorithm
Instructor notes: After ensuring effective ventilation, the student can now detect a carotid pulse. The patient has ROSC.

The student should initiate the Post-Cardiac Arrest Care Algorithm.

Megacode Testing Checklist: Scenarios 2/5
Bradycardia → VF → Asystole → PCAC

Student Name _____ Date of Test _____

Critical Performance Steps						Check if done correctly
Team Leader						
Assigns team member roles						
Ensures high-quality CPR at all times	Compression rate 100-120/min ☐	Compression depth ≥2 inches ☐	Chest compression fraction >80% ☐	Chest recoil (optional) ☐	Ventilation (optional) ☐	
Ensures that team members communicate well						
Bradycardia Management						
Starts oxygen if needed, places monitor, starts IV						
Places monitor leads in proper position						
Recognizes symptomatic bradycardia						
Administers correct dose of atropine						
Prepares for second-line treatment						
VF Management						
Recognizes VF						
Clears before analyze and shock						
Immediately resumes CPR after shocks						
Appropriate airway management						
Appropriate cycles of drug-rhythm check/shock-CPR						
Administers appropriate drug(s) and doses						
Asystole Management						
Recognizes asystole						
Verbalizes potential reversible causes of asystole (H's and T's)						
Administers appropriate drug(s) and doses						
Immediately resumes CPR after rhythm checks						
Post-Cardiac Arrest Care						
Identifies ROSC						
Ensures BP and 12-lead ECG are performed, O₂ saturation is monitored, verbalizes need for endotracheal intubation and waveform capnography, and orders laboratory tests						
Considers targeted temperature management						

STOP TEST

Test Results	Circle **PASS** or **NR** to indicate pass or needs remediation:	**PASS**	**NR**

Instructor Initials _____ Instructor Number _____ Date _____

Learning Station Competency
☐ Bradycardia ☐ Tachycardia ☐ Cardiac Arrest/Post–Cardiac Arrest Care ☐ Megacode Practice

---

Megacode 2—Out-of-Hospital Unstable Bradycardia
(Unstable Bradycardia > VF > Asystole > PCAC)

Lead-in: You are called to a restaurant for a man who suddenly became unresponsive, vomited, and then stopped breathing. You have a 4-minute response to the scene in your ALS ambulance.

Vital Signs
Heart rate: 44/min and very strong
Blood pressure: 84/50 mm Hg
Respiratory rate: 3/min
SpO₂:
Temperature:
Weight:
Age:

Initial Assessment

- You arrive at the scene to find 3 firefighters assisting the patient.
- One is maintaining an open airway, another is suctioning the patient, and the third is getting vital signs.
- Witnesses state that the patient had a normal day but seemed irritated.

Adult Bradycardia Algorithm

Instructor notes: The patient is in **sinus bradycardia** when the limb leads are applied, and the 12-lead ECG is not suspicious for injury or ischemia.

An IV is being initiated when the patient has a 5-second episode of grand mal seizures and then remains unresponsive. Bag-mask ventilation is initiated with oxygen. Shortly after that, the patient has no respirations and no pulse. The monitor shows **VF**.

Adult Cardiac Arrest Algorithm (VF)

Instructor notes: Defibrillation is attempted, and then CPR is provided for 2 minutes. During this time, his wife says that he is normally healthy and takes only vitamin supplements but that he's been under extreme stress at work lately.

After the first 2 minutes of CPR, the rhythm is still VF. Another shock is given, followed by more CPR. Epinephrine is given, and an advanced airway is placed, with an ETCO₂ reading of 22 mm Hg noted. Two minutes later, the rhythm is asystole, confirmed in 2 leads.

Adult Cardiac Arrest Algorithm (Asystole)

Instructor notes: CPR continues, and treatable causes are considered.

After 2 minutes of CPR, the monitor shows a borderline wide–complex organized rhythm with a rate of 56/min, and there are pulses present.

Post–Cardiac Arrest Care Algorithm

Instructor notes: Blood pressure is 180/108 mm Hg. The patient is still apneic with a capnography reading of 50 mm Hg.

A finger-stick glucose reading (**if asked for by Team Leader**) is 187 mg/dL (10.4 mmol/L), and he remains unresponsive.

For transport considerations, the nearest emergency department is 4 minutes from the scene, the nearest comprehensive stroke center is 12 minutes from the scene, and a cardiac arrest receiving center is 16 minutes from the scene.

Megacode Testing Checklist: Scenarios 1/3/8
Bradycardia → Pulseless VT → PEA → PCAC

Student Name _____ Date of Test _____

Critical Performance Steps	Check if done correctly
Team Leader	
Assigns team member roles	
Ensures high-quality CPR at all times	Compression rate 100-120/min ☐ · Compression depth of ≥2 inches ☐ · Chest compression fraction >80% ☐ · Chest recoil (optional) ☐ · Ventilation (optional) ☐
Ensures that team members communicate well	
Bradycardia Management	
Starts oxygen if needed, places monitor, starts IV	
Places monitor leads in proper position	
Recognizes symptomatic bradycardia	
Administers correct dose of atropine	
Prepares for second-line treatment	
Pulseless VT Management	
Recognizes pVT	
Clears before analyze and shock	
Immediately resumes CPR after shocks	
Appropriate airway management	
Appropriate cycles of drug–rhythm check/shock–CPR	
Administers appropriate drug(s) and doses	
PEA Management	
Recognizes PEA	
Verbalizes potential reversible causes of PEA (H's and T's)	
Administers appropriate drug(s) and doses	
Immediately resumes CPR after rhythm checks	
Post–Cardiac Arrest Care	
Identifies ROSC	
Ensures BP and 12-lead ECG are performed, O_2 saturation is monitored, verbalizes need for endotracheal intubation and waveform capnography, and orders laboratory tests	
Considers targeted temperature management	

STOP TEST

Test Results	Circle **PASS** or **NR** to indicate pass or needs remediation:	PASS	NR

Instructor Initials _____ Instructor Number _____ Date _____

Learning Station Competency
☐ Bradycardia ☐ Tachycardia ☐ Cardiac Arrest/Post–Cardiac Arrest Care ☐ Megacode Practice

---

Megacode 3—Out-of-Hospital Unstable Bradycardia
(Unstable Bradycardia > pVT > PEA > PCAC)

Lead-in: Your ALS ambulance is dispatched to help an elderly man having chest pain. A BLS engine is also responding. You arrive to find the firefighters placing a nonrebreathing oxygen mask on the patient.

Vital Signs
Heart rate: **Temperature:**
Blood pressure: 86/48 mm Hg by Doppler   **Weight:**
Respiratory rate: 18/min and nonlabored   **Age:**
SpO₂:

Initial Assessment
- The patient is sitting with his back against a wall, alert and talking with firefighters.
- He says his chest feels heavy and he might need to vomit; this started abruptly while he waited in line at the bank.
- He has had cardiac problems in the past, and he received a heart transplant 2 years ago.

What are your initial actions?

Instructor notes: His pulse is slow and weak, and he is grossly diaphoretic and pale and gray. The monitor displays a **third-degree AV block** with wider QRS complexes and a rate of 32/min.

He takes multiple medications, but they are at his home. He is allergic to sulfa. The 12-lead ECG is suspicious for injury in leads II, III, and aVF, and lead V_4R is flat.

Adult Bradycardia Algorithm

Instructor notes: If students try to give atropine, it will have no effect because of heart denervation.

The transcutaneous pacemaker is applied, but before it acquires capture, the patient becomes unresponsive, the rhythm changes to **VT**, and he becomes apneic. There is no pulse.

Adult Cardiac Arrest Algorithm (pVT)

Instructor notes: Defibrillation is attempted, and then high-quality CPR is given for 2 minutes, during which peripheral IVs are established in each arm. After 2 minutes, the rhythm is still VT.

Defibrillation is attempted again, with CPR and epinephrine administered.

Bag-mask ventilation is performed without difficulty, so an advanced airway isn't necessary unless the Team Leader feels it's indicated.

After 2 minutes, the rhythm is **sinus bradycardia** with marginally wide QRS complexes. A pulse is not present.

Adult Cardiac Arrest Algorithm (PEA)

Instructor notes: CPR is continued, an advanced airway is now placed, and capnography is connected, with a reading of 22 mm Hg.

After 2 minutes of CPR, the rhythm is nearly the same, and the QRS complexes aren't as wide, but the rate is the same.

A carotid pulse is present, but a radial pulse can't be felt. The ETCO₂ reading is now 48 mm Hg.

Post–Cardiac Care Algorithm

Instructor notes: The patient will bat his eyes to loud voices, and he begins breathing at 8 breaths per minute. His blood pressure by Doppler is 68/40 mm Hg.

The Team Leader should consider dopamine infusion for blood pressure support and/or epinephrine infusion to support perfusion.

The closest emergency department is 3 minutes from the scene, and a STEMI receiving center is 12 minutes from the scene.

Megacode 4—Out-of-Hospital Unstable Ventricular Tachycardia (Unstable Tachycardia > VF > PEA > PCAC)

Lead-in: Your ALS ambulance is dispatched to a car that has pulled to the side of the highway. The caller was driving the patient to an appointment, but she was sick and needed to stop. She reports shortness of breath and weakness.

Vital Signs
Heart rate: 150/min
Blood pressure: 84/54 mm Hg
Respiratory rate: 20/min with mildly labored breathing
SpO$_2$: 94% on 15 L/min of oxygen

Temperature:
Weight:
Age: 65 years

Initial Assessment

- Your unit arrives to the scene to find the patient in the passenger seat of an SUV, awake and talking in 2- to 3-word sentences.
- Her lungs have fine crackles in both bases.
- There are palpable carotid and radial pulses.

What are your initial actions?

Adult Tachycardia With a Pulse Algorithm

Instructor notes: The student's partner attaches the cardiac monitor, and the initial rhythm is **monomorphic wide-complex tachycardia.**

Due to the overall patient condition, the Team Leader should consider cardioversion. A peripheral IV is attempted without success. Cardioversion is performed without a change in condition.

While the student prepares to increase the energy to cardiovert again, the patient's head slumps, and she stops breathing. The monitor now shows **VF.**

Adult Cardiac Arrest Algorithm (VF)

Instructor notes: The patient is rapidly moved from the car to the stretcher. CPR is initiated, defibrillation is quickly delivered, and CPR is continued.

The stretcher (with CPR in progress) is moved to the ambulance to access equipment. During CPR, an IO access is achieved, and bag-mask ventilation is performed with mild difficulty.

After 2 minutes, the rhythm is still VF, defibrillation is performed, and CPR continues. Epinephrine is given, and an advanced airway is placed, with a capnography reading of 25 mm Hg.

After 2 minutes, the rhythm is an **organized wide-complex rhythm** at a rate of 70/min, but no pulses are present.

Adult Cardiac Arrest Algorithm (PEA)

Instructor notes: CPR is continued, and capnography readings continue to hover between 22 and 27 mm Hg during CPR.

Treatable causes are considered, and the person driving the vehicle states, "I was taking her to dialysis because she missed her appointment 2 days ago."

Calcium chloride or gluconate and sodium bicarbonate should be considered for this patient to offset hyperkalemia.

After this, at the next rhythm check, the monitor shows a **marginally wide-complex rhythm,** with severely peaked T waves, and a rate of 100/min. The patient now has a pulse at the carotid.

Post-Cardiac Arrest Care Algorithm

Instructor notes: The patient is starting to have spontaneous respirations (disorganized) with a capnography reading of 60 mm Hg and SpO$_2$ of 100% with oxygen. Her blood pressure is 94/56 mm Hg. A finger-stick glucose reading of 330 mg/dL (18.3 mmol/L) is obtained.

The nearest emergency department is 7 minutes away; a tertiary care center is 14 minutes away.

Megacode Testing Checklist: Scenarios 4/7/10
Tachycardia → VF → PEA → PCAC

Student Name _____   Date of Test _____

Critical Performance Steps					Check if done correctly
Team Leader					
Assigns team member roles					
Ensures high-quality CPR at all times	Compression rate 100-120/min ☐	Compression depth of ≥2 inches ☐	Chest compression fraction >80% ☐	Chest recoil (optional) ☐ Ventilation (optional) ☐	
Ensures that team members communicate well					
Tachycardia Management					
Starts oxygen if needed, places monitor, starts IV					
Places monitor leads in proper position					
Recognizes unstable tachycardia					
Recognizes symptoms due to tachycardia					
Performs immediate synchronized cardioversion					
VF Management					
Recognizes VF					
Clears before analyze and shock					
Immediately resumes CPR after shocks					
Appropriate airway management					
Appropriate cycles of drug-rhythm check/shock-CPR					
Administers appropriate drug(s) and doses					
PEA Management					
Recognizes PEA					
Verbalizes potential reversible causes of PEA (H's and T's)					
Administers appropriate drug(s) and doses					
Immediately resumes CPR after rhythm checks					
Post-Cardiac Arrest Care					
Identifies ROSC					
Ensures BP and 12-lead ECG are performed, O$_2$ saturation is monitored, verbalizes need for endotracheal intubation and waveform capnography, and orders laboratory tests					
Considers targeted temperature management					

STOP TEST

Test Results	Circle **PASS** or **NR** to indicate pass or needs remediation:	**PASS**	**NR**

Instructor Initials _____   Instructor Number _____   Date _____

Learning Station Competency
☐ Bradycardia ☐ Tachycardia ☐ Cardiac Arrest/Post–Cardiac Arrest Care ☐ Megacode Practice

Megacode Testing Checklist: Scenarios 2/5

Bradycardia → VF → Asystole → PCAC

Student Name _____ Date of Test _____

	Critical Performance Steps						Check if done correctly
Team Leader							
Assigns team member roles							
	Compression rate 100–120/min	Compression depth of ≥2 inches	Chest compression fraction >80%	Chest recoil (optional)	Ventilation (optional)		
Ensures high-quality CPR at all times	☐	☐	☐	☐	☐		
Ensures that team members communicate well							
Bradycardia Management							
Starts oxygen if needed, places monitor, starts IV							
Places monitor leads in proper position							
Recognizes symptomatic bradycardia							
Administers correct dose of atropine							
Prepares for second-line treatment							
VF Management							
Recognizes VF							
Clears before analyze and shock							
Immediately resumes CPR after shocks							
Appropriate airway management							
Appropriate cycles of drug–rhythm check/shock–CPR							
Administers appropriate drug(s) and doses							
Asystole Management							
Recognizes asystole							
Verbalizes potential reversible causes of asystole (H's and T's)							
Administers appropriate drug(s) and doses							
Immediately resumes CPR after rhythm checks							
Post–Cardiac Arrest Care							
Identifies ROSC							
Ensures BP and 12-lead ECG are performed, O₂ saturation is monitored, verbalizes need for endotracheal intubation and waveform capnography, and orders laboratory tests							
Considers targeted temperature management							

STOP TEST

Test Results Circle **PASS** or **NR** to indicate pass or needs remediation: | **PASS** | **NR** |

Instructor Initials _____ Instructor Number _____ Date _____

Learning Station Competency
☐ Bradycardia ☐ Tachycardia ☐ Cardiac Arrest/Post–Cardiac Arrest Care ☐ Megacode Practice

---

Megacode 5—Emergency Department Unstable Bradycardia (Unstable Bradycardia > VF > Asystole > PCAC)

Lead-in: You are working in the emergency department when paramedics bring in a drowsy man. They are concerned about a drug overdose.

Vital Signs
Heart rate:
Blood pressure:
Respiratory rate:
SpO₂:

Temperature:
Weight:
Age: 28 years

Initial Assessment

- Paramedics say that the patient has a history of depression and also takes diltiazem for an unknown reason.
- A family member on scene said that the patient has had a very low mood lately and threatened suicide earlier in the day.
- An empty bottle of diltiazem was found beside the patient when the paramedics arrived.

What are your initial actions?

- Assessing the patient on the paramedic stretcher, you find the patient very drowsy and slurring his words.
- You cannot get any useful information from the patient on his history.

Adult Bradycardia Algorithm

Instructor notes: His vital signs include heart rate 30/min, respiratory rate 16/min, blood pressure 80/48 mm Hg, SpO₂ 98% on 3 L by nasal prongs, temperature 36.5°C, and blood glucose 195 mg/dL (10.8 mmol/L).

A rhythm strip shows **wide QRS ventricular escape rhythm** at 30, with a long QT. His heart rate continues to drop, and then the patient suddenly becomes unresponsive and loses his pulse. The monitor shows **VF.**

Adult Cardiac Arrest Algorithm (VF)

Instructor notes: Students should follow the VF pathway of the Adult Cardiac Arrest Algorithm.

Advanced students may consider discussing intravenous lipid emulsion therapy and extracorporeal CPR.

Adult Cardiac Arrest Algorithm (Asystole)

Instructor notes: After the second shock, the patient's rhythm changes to asystole. The student should follow the asystole pathway of the Adult Cardiac Arrest Algorithm with special attention given to high-quality CPR and good team communication.

Post–Cardiac Arrest Care Algorithm

Instructor notes: After several rounds of CPR and ACLS, the patient has ROSC. The rhythm on the monitor is a ventricular escape bradycardia with hypotension.

The student should consider the toxicological aspects of the case as well as the differential diagnosis.

A discussion around the treatment of calcium channel blocker overdose and available treatment options may be included for advanced learners.

Megacode Testing Checklist: Scenarios 6/11
Bradycardia → VF → PEA → PCAC

Student Name _____ Date of Test _____

Critical Performance Steps						Check if done correctly
Team Leader						
Assigns team member roles						
Ensures high-quality CPR at all times	Compression rate 100–120/min ☐	Compression depth of ≥2 inches ☐	Chest compression fraction >80% ☐	Chest recoil (optional) ☐	Ventilation (optional) ☐	
Ensures that team members communicate well						
Bradycardia Management						
Starts oxygen if needed, places monitor, starts IV						
Places monitor leads in proper position						
Recognizes symptomatic bradycardia						
Administers correct dose of atropine						
Prepares for second-line treatment						
VF Management						
Recognizes VF						
Clears before analyze and shock						
Immediately resumes CPR after shocks						
Appropriate airway management						
Appropriate cycles of drug–rhythm check/shock–CPR						
Administers appropriate drug(s) and doses						
PEA Management						
Recognizes PEA						
Verbalizes potential reversible causes of PEA (H's and T's)						
Administers appropriate drug(s) and doses						
Immediately resumes CPR after rhythm checks						
Post–Cardiac Arrest Care						
Identifies ROSC						
Ensures BP and 12-lead ECG are performed, O₂ saturation is monitored, verbalizes need for endotracheal intubation and waveform capnography, and orders laboratory tests						
Considers targeted temperature management						

STOP TEST

Test Results	Circle **PASS** or **NR** to indicate pass or needs remediation:	PASS	NR

Instructor Initials _____ Instructor Number _____ Date _____

Learning Station Competency
☐ Bradycardia ☐ Tachycardia ☐ Cardiac Arrest/Post–Cardiac Arrest Care ☐ Megacode Practice

---

Megacode 6—In-Hospital Unstable Bradycardia
(Unstable Bradycardia > VF > PEA > PCAC)

Lead-in: A man admitted to the hospital with pneumonia has chest pain on the second day of his hospital course. You are called to evaluate him.

Vital Signs
Heart rate: Temperature:
Blood pressure: Weight:
Respiratory rate: Age: 58 years
SpO₂:

Initial Assessment

What are your initial actions?

Adult Bradycardia Algorithm

Instructor notes: The patient's vital signs are heart rate 35/min, respiratory rate 18/min, and blood pressure 88/49 mm Hg.

The monitor shows a **third-degree heart block**. The initial dose of atropine will not have much effect, and pacing should be initiated.

With pacing, the patient's blood pressure will also improve such that the patient can now go to the cardiac cath lab.

Adult Cardiac Arrest Algorithm (VF)

Instructor notes: Just after completing cardiac catheterization (with findings of 100% right coronary artery occlusion), the patient will develop VF.

The patient will be refractory to at least 3 shocks, thus allowing the student to progress through the algorithm. Chest compressions should be initiated with high-quality CPR and the airway managed initially with bag-mask ventilation and, ultimately, probably intubation and epinephrine/amiodarone.

Errors would be to provide epinephrine before at least 2 shocks. After the third shock, the patient will go into a **sinus tachycardia** with no pulse (PEA).

Of note, if the student chose to relook at the coronary arteries, this would be an appropriate step and they would be patent (ie, the underlying cause could be arterial reocclusion, but this advanced reasoning is beyond the expectations of the scenario).

Adult Cardiac Arrest Algorithm (PEA)

Instructor notes: The patient is now in PEA. The student continues to monitor high-quality CPR, and epinephrine should be provided.

After a dose of epinephrine, the student will notice that the continuous ETCO₂ rises to 40 mm Hg. The student should recognize that ROSC is likely and stop CPR, even if the full 2 minutes is not performed, because the ETCO₂ is indicating ROSC (a good opportunity for this teaching point).

Underlying causes during this event that could be considered include cardiac tamponade, and, if an ultrasound is performed, there would be no fluid present.

Post–Cardiac Arrest Care Algorithm

Instructor notes: After the student recognizes ROSC (ETCO₂ rises to 40 mm Hg) and checks a pulse, the patient will be found to be hemodynamically unstable, with heart rate 110/min and blood pressure 70/30 mm Hg.

The student should ask for the vital signs, not state them. The patient should receive a fluid bolus, and a vasopressor infusion should be initiated (blood pressure will not improve with fluids alone).

The patient will not follow commands and is a candidate for targeted temperature management.

Megacode 7—In-Hospital Unstable Ventricular Tachycardia (Unstable Tachycardia > VF > PEA > PCAC)

Lead-in: You are a healthcare provider caring for a patient who was admitted for chest pain, and you to rule out myocardial infarction. He was diagnosed with stable angina 10 years ago, but over the past few months, his pain has been increasing in duration and intensity.

Vital Signs
Heart rate: 82/min
Blood pressure: 124/74 mm Hg
Respiratory rate: 16/min
SpO₂: 98%

Temperature:
Weight:
Age:

Initial Assessment
What are your initial actions?

Instructor notes: At the change of shift, the patient denied chest pain. The student leaves the room and is soon called back by the patient's son.

The student enters the room and assesses that the patient is clutching his chest, stating he has chest pain, and displaying diaphoresis. His vital signs are now heart rate 160/min, respiratory rate 22/min, blood pressure 156/92 mm Hg, and SpO₂ 93%.

His bedside monitor shows a **monomorphic, wide, and rapid rhythm,** which is different from previously recorded rhythms. The patient may have an acute coronary syndrome. Because of the patient's history, the student will initially focus on the tachycardia rhythm.

The student will question the patient on his current symptoms and ensure IV line patency and cardiac monitoring. Nitroglycerin may be initiated as long as the blood pressure is greater than 90 mm Hg systolic and the patient continues to have chest pain. Administration of aspirin is appropriate as long as the patient is responsive.

Adult Tachycardia With a Pulse Algorithm

Instructor notes: The symptoms of the patient's tachycardia require management and treatment. The student can differentiate that the patient is in VT and is symptomatic. The treatment for this is immediate cardioversion, and drug therapy should not delay the cardioversion.

Adult Cardiac Arrest Algorithm (VF)

Instructor notes: Upon delivery of the cardioversion shock, the patient develops a different rhythm, which is identified as **VF.** Now, the student will follow the VF/pVT pathway of the Adult Cardiac Arrest Algorithm.

The Team Leader assigns team functions and monitors for high-quality CPR. The case continues through safe defibrillation, administering a vasopressor, and considering an antiarrhythmic drug.

Adult Cardiac Arrest Algorithm (PEA)

Instructor notes: Despite the student's actions, the patient is now showing **second-degree AV block** on the monitor with no pulse (PEA).

The Team Leader should continue to monitor high-quality CPR and follow the PEA pathway of the Adult Cardiac Arrest Algorithm.

The patient may be in cardiogenic shock, so the student must be able to differentiate and discuss potential causes of PEA.

Post–Cardiac Arrest Care Algorithm

Instructor notes: The team continues high-quality chest compressions, and the patient has ROSC. At this point, you should initiate the Post–Cardiac Arrest Care Algorithm.

Megacode Testing Checklist: Scenarios 4/7/10
Tachycardia → VF → PEA → PCAC

Student Name _____ Date of Test _____

Critical Performance Steps	Compression rate 100-120/min	Compression depth of ≥2 inches	Chest compression fraction >80%	Chest recoil (optional)	Ventilation (optional)	Check if done correctly
Team Leader						
Assigns team member roles						
Ensures high-quality CPR at all times	☐	☐	☐	☐	☐	
Ensures that team members communicate well						
Tachycardia Management						
Starts oxygen if needed, places monitor, starts IV						
Places monitor leads in proper position						
Recognizes unstable tachycardia						
Recognizes symptoms due to tachycardia						
Performs immediate synchronized cardioversion						
VF Management						
Recognizes VF						
Clears before analyze and shock						
Immediately resumes CPR after shocks						
Appropriate airway management						
Appropriate cycles of drug-rhythm check/shock–CPR						
Administers appropriate drug(s) and doses						
PEA Management						
Recognizes PEA						
Verbalizes potential reversible causes of PEA (H's and T's)						
Administers appropriate drug(s) and doses						
Immediately resumes CPR after rhythm checks						
Post–Cardiac Arrest Care						
Identifies ROSC						
Ensures BP and 12-lead ECG are performed, O₂ saturation is monitored, verbalizes need for endotracheal intubation and waveform capnography, and orders laboratory tests						
Considers targeted temperature management						

STOP TEST

Test Results	Circle **PASS** or **NR** to indicate pass or needs remediation:	**PASS**	**NR**

Instructor Initials _____ Instructor Number _____ Date _____

Learning Station Competency
☐ Bradycardia ☐ Tachycardia ☐ Cardiac Arrest/Post–Cardiac Arrest Care ☐ Megacode Practice

Megacode 8—In-Hospital Unstable Bradycardia
(Unstable Bradycardia > pVT > PEA > PCAC)

Lead-in: A man who was admitted to the hospital with palpitations now reports chest discomfort, and you are called to evaluate him.

Vital Signs
Heart rate: 50/min
Blood pressure: 150/70 mm Hg
Respiratory rate: 24/min
SpO₂: 90% on room air
Temperature:
Weight:
Age: 72 years

Initial Assessment
What are your initial actions?
- A 12-lead ECG reveals an acute inferior STEMI.

Adult Bradycardia Algorithm
Instructor notes: The patient has a STEMI, bradycardia, and hypoxia. The patient should be placed on supplemental oxygen because of the hypoxia, the cath lab should be activated, and aspirin should be given.

The patient's heart rate is 50/min and the monitor shows **sinus bradycardia**. Because the blood pressure is stable, no intervention is necessary.

If the student chooses to give atropine, the side effects of this drug in acute myocardial infarction (when not clinically indicated) can be discussed.

Other interventions, such as anticoagulation, could be considered while preparing for the cath lab, although nitroglycerin should be avoided because of the inferior myocardial infarction.

Adult Cardiac Arrest Algorithm (pVT)
Instructor notes: While waiting to go to the cath lab, the patient becomes unresponsive, is pulseless, and has **VT** on the monitor.

One correct action would be immediate defibrillation (one could also have done precordial thump as a witnessed event) simultaneously with good CPR.

VT will persist despite a defibrillation attempt, and the patient will need high-quality CPR, bag-mask ventilation with or without intubation, and reevaluation of the rhythm after 2 minutes of CPR.

After a second defibrillation attempt, the patient's rhythm will change to PEA.

Adult Cardiac Arrest Algorithm (PEA)
Instructor notes: After epinephrine is given for PEA, the rhythm will go **back to VF.**

After another defibrillation attempt, the ETCO₂ will rise to 40 mm Hg after about 1 minute of CPR.

The student should recognize that ROSC is obtained, and CPR should be stopped rather than continue for an additional minute.

Post–Cardiac Arrest Care Algorithm
Instructor notes: After ROSC, the patient should have his vital signs checked (heart rate 108/min, blood pressure 80/60 mm Hg, SpO₂ 95%).

He should be given a fluid bolus for hypotension and rapidly transported to the cath lab for revascularization.

He is unresponsive, so plans can be made to initiate targeted temperature management, ideally simultaneously with revascularization in the cath lab.

Megacode Testing Checklist: Scenarios 1/3/8
Bradycardia → Pulseless VT → PEA → PCAC

Student Name _____ Date of Test _____

Critical Performance Steps	Check if done correctly
Team Leader	
Assigns team member roles	

	Compression rate 100-120/min	Compression depth of ≥2 inches	Chest compression fraction >80%	Chest recoil (optional)	Ventilation (optional)
Ensures high-quality CPR at all times	☐	☐	☐	☐	☐

Critical Performance Steps	Check if done correctly
Ensures that team members communicate well	
Bradycardia Management	
Starts oxygen if needed, places monitor, starts IV	
Places monitor leads in proper position	
Recognizes symptomatic bradycardia	
Administers correct dose of atropine	
Prepares for second-line treatment	
Pulseless VT Management	
Recognizes pVT	
Clears before analyze and shock	
Immediately resumes CPR after shocks	
Appropriate airway management	
Appropriate cycles of drug–rhythm check/shock–CPR	
Administers appropriate drug(s) and doses	
PEA Management	
Recognizes PEA	
Verbalizes potential reversible causes of PEA (H's and T's)	
Administers appropriate drug(s) and doses	
Immediately resumes CPR after rhythm checks	
Post–Cardiac Arrest Care	
Identifies ROSC	
Ensures BP and 12-lead ECG are performed, O₂ saturation is monitored, verbalizes need for endotracheal intubation and waveform capnography, and orders laboratory tests	
Considers targeted temperature management	

STOP TEST

Test Results	Circle **PASS** or **NR** to indicate pass or needs remediation:	**PASS**	**NR**

Instructor Initials _____ Instructor Number _____ Date _____

Learning Station Competency
☐ Bradycardia ☐ Tachycardia ☐ Cardiac Arrest/Post–Cardiac Arrest Care ☐ Megacode Practice

Megacode Testing Checklist: Scenario 9
Tachycardia → PEA → VF → PCAC

Student Name _____ Date of Test _____

Critical Performance Steps	Compression rate 100-120/min	Compression depth of ≥2 inches	Chest compression fraction >80%	Chest recoil (optional)	Ventilation (optional)	Check if done correctly
Team Leader						
Assigns team member roles						
Ensures high-quality CPR at all times	☐	☐	☐	☐	☐	
Ensures that team members communicate well						
Tachycardia Management						
Starts oxygen if needed, places monitor, starts IV						
Places monitor leads in proper position						
Recognizes tachycardia (specific diagnosis)						
Recognizes no symptoms due to tachycardia						
Considers appropriate initial drug therapy						
PEA Management						
Recognizes PEA						
Verbalizes potential reversible causes of PEA (H's and T's)						
Administers appropriate drug(s) and doses						
Immediately resumes CPR after rhythm check and pulse checks						
VF Management						
Recognizes VF						
Clears before analyze and shock						
Immediately resumes CPR after shocks						
Appropriate airway management						
Appropriate cycles of drug-rhythm check/shock-CPR						
Administers appropriate drug(s) and doses						
Post-Cardiac Arrest Care						
Identifies ROSC						
Ensures BP and 12-lead ECG are performed, O₂ saturation is monitored, verbalizes need for endotracheal intubation and waveform capnography, and orders laboratory tests						
Considers targeted temperature management						

STOP TEST

Test Results	Circle **PASS** or **NR** to indicate pass or needs remediation:	PASS	NR

Instructor Initials _____ Instructor Number _____ Date _____

Learning Station Competency
☐ Bradycardia ☐ Tachycardia ☐ Cardiac Arrest/Post-Cardiac Arrest Care ☐ Megacode Practice

---

Megacode 9—In-Hospital Stable Tachycardia (SVT)
(Stable Tachycardia > PEA > VF > PCAC)

Lead-in: A woman with a history of lupus and asthma was admitted with pneumonia. She is doing well initially but develops tachycardia while receiving albuterol for ongoing wheezing.

Vital Signs
Heart rate: 160/min, and the monitor shows SVT
Blood pressure: 140/70 mm Hg
Respiratory rate:
SpO₂:

Temperature:
Weight:
Age: 42 years

Initial Assessment
What are your initial actions?

Adult Tachycardia With a Pulse Algorithm

Instructor notes: If the student gives adenosine in this scenario, the rhythm will change from SVT to sinus, but the patient will progress to severe respiratory distress with marked wheezing. Adenosine is relatively contraindicated in asthma exacerbation because of the effects on the adenosine receptors, and it will worsen the underlying asthma exacerbation, leading to respiratory distress. If the student recognizes this and chooses an alternative for SVT, that should be positively noted, but for the scenario, the patient will progress to respiratory failure anyway.

The patient is in profound respiratory distress with wheezing and will be refractory to any attempts at albuterol. The patient will clearly either need immediate intubation or her condition will progress to complete respiratory failure requiring bag-mask ventilation. After intubation, the patient's condition will progress to PEA. The student should recognize this by evaluating for pulse and blood pressure after the intubation. Also, the PEA theoretically could be caused or contributed to by excessive ventilation (ie, auto-PEEP) immediately after intubation.

Adult Cardiac Arrest Algorithm (PEA)

Instructor notes: The patient is in PEA after intubation with contributions from auto-PEEP given the severe asthma. The ventilation rate should be low, and the student should consider disconnecting the bag to allow full exhalation.

After the student attends to the ventilation rate and provision of epinephrine, the patient will have a rhythm change to **VF**.

Adult Cardiac Arrest Algorithm (VF)

Instructor notes: The patient is in VF, and immediate defibrillation is required. After attempting defibrillation, chest compressions can be initiated. After about 1 minute of chest compressions, ETCO₂ will rise from 12 mm Hg to 38 mm Hg.

The student should recognize ROSC, discontinue CPR, confirm pulse and blood pressure, and move to the Post-Cardiac Arrest Care Algorithm.

Post-Cardiac Arrest Care Algorithm

Instructor notes: After ROSC, the patient will have substantial auto-PEEP, and one immediate strategy will need to be avoiding excessive ventilation. The blood pressure will be relatively low (89/70 mm Hg) but responsive to fluids, and vasopressors are not necessarily needed, although they could be prepared in case the patient's condition worsens.

Because the causes of arrest are pneumonia and asthma, there should not be consideration for cardiac catheterization (if performed, a 12-lead ECG will show sinus tachycardia at rate of 110/min but otherwise normal).

The patient will not be following commands and thus would be a candidate for targeted temperature management. Oxygenation will be marginal, so the principle of avoiding hypoxia (as opposed to hyperoxia) will be in play.

Megacode 10—In-Hospital Unstable Ventricular Tachycardia (Unstable Tachycardia > VF > PEA > PCAC)

Lead-in: You are working in the cardiac care unit of your hospital. A woman who underwent PCI 3 hours ago is reporting heavy central chest pressure and nausea.

Vital Signs
Heart rate: 130/min
Blood pressure: 72/40 mm Hg
Respiratory rate: 20/min
SpO₂:

Temperature: 37°C
Weight:
Age: 51 years

Initial Assessment
What are your initial actions?

- On initial assessment, the patient reports feeling light-headed and nauseated, with severe central crushing chest pain.
- She appears drowsy, pale, and diaphoretic. The SpO₂ monitor is not showing a waveform and giving no reading.
- The rhythm strip shows a **regular wide-complex tachycardia** at 130/min.

Adult Tachycardia With a Pulse Algorithm

Instructor notes: A 12-lead ECG shows **VT** at 130/min. A previous ECG done before the procedure shows a normal sinus tachycardia with narrow complex.

The goals of this section will be for the student to recognize unstable VT and follow the algorithm, assess ABCs, provide supplemental O₂ ensure adequate IV access, discuss the pros and cons of analgesia and sedation, demonstrate safe synchronized cardioversion, and consider treatment for acute ischemia and acute coronary syndromes in this setting.

Adult Cardiac Arrest Algorithm (VF)

Instructor notes: After 2 failed synchronized cardioversions, the patient loses pulses and becomes apneic and unresponsive. The monitor shows **VF.**

Focus on safe defibrillation, high-quality compressions, and a consideration of differential diagnoses.

Adult Cardiac Arrest Algorithm (PEA)

Instructor notes: After the second defibrillation attempt, the patient's rhythm changes to a **wide-complex regular rhythm** (with P waves) at 70/min. The patient still has no pulses.

The student should follow the PEA pathway of the Adult Cardiac Arrest Algorithm. Students should focus on high-quality chest compressions and may consider advanced airway and underlying causes, including pulmonary embolism and myocardial infarction hemorrhage, among other things.

Post-Cardiac Arrest Care Algorithm

Instructor notes: The team continues high-quality chest compressions, the patient has ROSC, and the team initiates the Post-Cardiac Arrest Care Algorithm.

The students may consider myocardial ischemia and involvement of the interventional cardiologist (question acute stent obstruction).

If the patient cannot follow commands, targeted temperature management should be started.

Megacode Testing Checklist: Scenarios 4/7/10 Tachycardia → VF → PEA → PCAC

Student Name _____ Date of Test _____

Critical Performance Steps	Compression rate 100–120/min	Compression depth of ≥2 inches	Chest compression fraction >80%	Chest recoil (optional)	Ventilation (optional)	Check if done correctly
Team Leader						
Assigns team member roles						
Ensures high-quality CPR at all times	☐	☐	☐	☐	☐	
Ensures that team members communicate well						
Tachycardia Management						
Starts oxygen if needed, places monitor, starts IV						
Places monitor leads in proper position						
Recognizes unstable tachycardia						
Recognizes symptoms due to tachycardia						
Performs immediate synchronized cardioversion						
VF Management						
Recognizes VF						
Clears before analyze and shock						
Immediately resumes CPR after shocks						
Appropriate airway management						
Appropriate cycles of drug-rhythm check/shock-CPR						
Administers appropriate drug(s) and doses						
PEA Management						
Recognizes PEA						
Verbalizes potential reversible causes of PEA (H's and T's)						
Administers appropriate drug(s) and doses						
Immediately resumes CPR after rhythm checks						
Post-Cardiac Arrest Care						
Identifies ROSC						
Ensures BP and 12-lead ECG are performed, O₂ saturation is monitored, verbalizes need for endotracheal intubation and waveform capnography, and orders laboratory tests						
Considers targeted temperature management						

STOP TEST

Test Results	Circle **PASS** or **NR** to indicate pass or needs remediation:	**PASS**	**NR**

Instructor Initials _____ Instructor Number _____ Date _____

Learning Station Competency
☐ Bradycardia ☐ Tachycardia ☐ Cardiac Arrest/Post–Cardiac Arrest Care ☐ Megacode Practice

Megacode Testing Checklist: Scenarios 6/11
Bradycardia → VF → PEA → PCAC

Student Name _____ Date of Test _____

Critical Performance Steps	Compression rate 100–120/min	Compression depth of ≥2 inches	Chest compression fraction >80%	Chest recoil (optional)	Ventilation (optional)	Check if done correctly
Team Leader						
Assigns team member roles						
Ensures high-quality CPR at all times	☐	☐	☐	☐	☐	
Ensures that team members communicate well						
Bradycardia Management						
Starts oxygen if needed, places monitor, starts IV						
Places monitor leads in proper position						
Recognizes symptomatic bradycardia						
Administers correct dose of atropine						
Prepares for second-line treatment						
VF Management						
Recognizes VF						
Clears before analyze and shock						
Immediately resumes CPR after shocks						
Appropriate airway management						
Appropriate cycles of drug–rhythm check/shock–CPR						
Administers appropriate drug(s) and doses						
PEA Management						
Recognizes PEA						
Verbalizes potential reversible causes of PEA (H's and T's)						
Administers appropriate drug(s) and doses						
Immediately resumes CPR after rhythm checks						
Post-Cardiac Arrest Care						
Identifies ROSC						
Ensures BP and 12-lead ECG are performed, O₂ saturation is monitored, verbalizes need for endotracheal intubation and waveform capnography, and orders laboratory tests						
Considers targeted temperature management						

STOP TEST

Test Results	Circle **PASS** or **NR** to indicate pass or needs remediation:	PASS	NR

Instructor Initials _____ Instructor Number _____ Date _____

Learning Station Competency
☐ Bradycardia ☐ Tachycardia ☐ Cardiac Arrest/Post–Cardiac Arrest Care ☐ Megacode Practice

---

Megacode 11—In-Hospital Colonoscopy Suite Unstable Bradycardia
(Unstable Bradycardia > VF > PEA > PCAC)

Lead-in: A patient is undergoing his initial colon screening. Fifteen minutes into the procedure, under conscious sedation, the patient's respiratory rate drops to 4 and ETCO₂ is 55 mm Hg.

Vital Signs
Heart rate:
Blood pressure:
Respiratory rate:
SpO₂:
Temperature:
Weight:
Age: 51 years

Initial Assessment
What are your initial actions?

- This healthy man with a family history of colon cancer (maternal grandfather and uncle) is undergoing an initial screening colonoscopy.
- He has no significant past medical history except daily alcohol use (3 to 4 drinks per day).
- The patient had received a combination of fentanyl and midazolam for conscious sedation.
- It is noted that as the ETCO₂ rises, the patient becomes less arousable and then apneic.
- The Code Team is activated.

What are the next steps?

Instructor notes: IV reversal agents are ordered. Bag-mask ventilation is initiated. His vital signs are heart rate 30/min, respiratory rate 3/min, blood pressure 70/P mm Hg, and SpO₂ 82% on 4 L/min via nasal cannula.

Students should recognize the impending respiratory failure and consider reversal agents. The patient is placed on 100% oxygen, and flumazenil and naloxone are provided with improved oxygen saturations, but there is no change in respiratory rate. A supraglottic airway is placed.

Adult Bradycardia Algorithm
Instructor notes: The patient's respiratory status has been stabilized. The student should note the abnormal heart rate and hypotension. The bradycardia is **slow and narrow complex** without ST changes. The patient is unstable and given IV atropine (0.5 mg) twice without change in heart rate or blood pressure.

While the dopamine infusion is being prepared, the patient becomes unresponsive.

What is the next action?

Adult Cardiac Arrest Algorithm (VF)
Instructor notes: The monitor demonstrates **VF**.

What is the action?

Instructor notes: The patient has no pulse. CPR is started. The VF/pVT pathway should be followed. Shocks are delivered. Epinephrine and amiodarone are given.

An advanced airway is placed. A rhythm check shows SVT. No pulse or spontaneous respirations are confirmed.

Adult Cardiac Arrest Algorithm (PEA)
Instructor notes: CPR is continued. Bag-mask ventilation at 100% is continued. A second dose of epinephrine is given with no change in condition.

During the rhythm check, the monitor reveals a **narrow-complex tachycardia** and no pulse. The PEA pathway of the Adult Cardiac Arrest Algorithm is followed.

Post-Cardiac Arrest Care Algorithm
Instructor notes: The team continues high-quality chest compressions, the patient has ROSC, and the team initiates the Post–Cardiac Arrest Care Algorithm.

Megacode 12—In-Hospital Surgical Waiting Room Unstable Bradycardia → VF → Asystole/PEA > PCAC)

Lead-in: A woman sits in the surgical waiting room, awaiting news about her husband's surgery, when she suddenly becomes light-headed and dizzy and nearly passes out.

Vital Signs
Heart rate:
Blood pressure:
Respiratory rate:
SpO₂:

Temperature:
Weight:
Age: 67 years

Initial Assessment

- The patient has a past medical history of breast cancer (in remission) and diabetes.
- She is lying on the floor.
- You respond as a member of the medical emergency team that was activated.

What are your initial steps?

Instructor notes: She admits that she forgot to eat breakfast today. The rest of the team arrives. Her vital signs are heart rate 28/min, respiratory rate 18/min, blood pressure 68/P mm Hg, 96% SpO₂ on room air, and blood sugar 90 mg/dL (5 mmol/L).

The patient is moved to a stretcher.

The monitor shows a second-degree type II AV block.

Adult Bradycardia Algorithm

Instructor notes: The student should note the abnormal heart rate and hypotension. The bradycardia is narrow complex without ST changes.

The patient is unstable and given IV atropine (1 mg) twice without a change in heart rate or blood pressure.

What is the next action?

The patient is wheeled urgently to the hospital emergency department.

Adult Cardiac Arrest Algorithm (VF)

Instructor notes: The monitor demonstrates **VF**.

What is the action?

The patient has no pulse. CPR is started.

The student should follow the VF/pVT pathway. Shocks are delivered twice, and epinephrine and amiodarone are given. An advanced airway is placed.

A monitor check demonstrates asystole. No pulse or spontaneous respirations are confirmed.

Adult Cardiac Arrest Algorithm (Asystole and PEA)

Instructor notes: CPR is continued. Bag-mask ventilation with 100% oxygen is continued. Epinephrine is given (third dose). There is no change in her condition.

During the rhythm check, the monitor reveals a **narrow-complex tachycardia** with no pulse. The PEA pathway of the Adult Cardiac Arrest Algorithm is followed.

Post-Cardiac Arrest Care Algorithm

Instructor notes: The team continues high-quality chest compressions, the patient has ROSC, and the team initiates the Post-Cardiac Arrest Care Algorithm.

Megacode Testing Checklist: Scenario 12
Bradycardia → VF → Asystole/PEA → PCAC

Student Name _____ Date of Test _____

Critical Performance Steps						Check if done correctly
Team Leader						
Assigns team member roles						
Ensures high-quality CPR at all times	Compression rate 100-120/min ☐	Compression depth of ≥2 inches ☐	Chest compression fraction >80% ☐	Chest recoil (optional) ☐	Ventilation (optional) ☐	
Ensures that team members communicate well						
Bradycardia Management						
Starts oxygen if needed, places monitor, starts IV						
Places monitor leads in proper position						
Recognizes symptomatic bradycardia						
Administers correct dose of atropine						
Prepares for second-line treatment						
VF Management						
Recognizes VF						
Clears before analyze and shock						
Immediately resumes CPR after shocks						
Appropriate airway management						
Appropriate cycles of drug–rhythm check/shock–CPR						
Administers appropriate drug(s) and doses						
Asystole and PEA Management						
Recognizes asystole and PEA						
Verbalizes potential reversible causes of asystole and PEA (H's and T's)						
Administers appropriate drug(s) and doses						
Immediately resumes CPR after rhythm checks						
Post–Cardiac Arrest Care						
Identifies ROSC						
Ensures BP and 12-lead ECG are performed, O₂ saturation is monitored, verbalizes need for endotracheal intubation and waveform capnography, and orders laboratory tests						
Considers targeted temperature management						

STOP TEST

Test Results	Circle **PASS** or **NR** to indicate pass or needs remediation:	**PASS**	**NR**

Instructor Initials _____ Instructor Number _____ Date _____

Learning Station Competency
☐ Bradycardia ☐ Tachycardia ☐ Cardiac Arrest/Post–Cardiac Arrest Care ☐ Megacode Practice

Appendix B

Testing Checklists, Learning Station Checklists, and Other Tools

Advanced Cardiovascular Life Support
Adult High-Quality BLS
Skills Testing Checklist

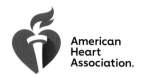
American Heart Association.

Student Name _____ Date of Test _____

Hospital Scenario: "You are working in a hospital or clinic, and you see a person who has suddenly collapsed in the hallway. You check that the scene is safe and then approach the patient. Demonstrate what you would do next."

Prehospital Scenario: "You arrive on the scene for a suspected cardiac arrest. No bystander CPR has been provided. You approach the scene and ensure that it is safe. Demonstrate what you would do next."

Assessment and Activation
- ☐ Checks responsiveness
- ☐ Checks breathing
- ☐ Shouts for help/Activates emergency response system/Sends for AED
- ☐ Checks pulse

Once student shouts for help, instructor says, "I am going to get the AED."

Compressions   *Audio/visual feedback device required for accuracy*
- ☐ Hand placement on lower half of sternum
- ☐ Perform continuous compressions for 2 minutes (100-120/min)
- ☐ Compresses at least 2 inches (5 cm)
- ☐ Complete chest recoil. (Optional, check if using a feedback device that measures chest recoil)

Rescuer 2 says, "Here is the AED. I'll take over compressions, and you use the AED."

AED (follows prompts of AED)
- ☐ Powers on AED
- ☐ Correctly attaches pads
- ☐ Clears for analysis
- ☐ Clears to safely deliver a shock
- ☐ Safely delivers a shock
- ☐ Shocks within 45 seconds of AED arrival

Resumes Compressions
- ☐ Ensures compressions are resumed immediately after shock delivery
  - Student directs instructor to resume compressions *or*
  - Second student resumes compressions

STOP TEST

Instructor Notes
• Place a check in the box next to each step the student completes successfully.
• If the student does not complete all steps successfully (as indicated by at least 1 blank check box), the student must receive remediation. Make a note here of which skills require remediation (refer to instructor manual for information about remediation).

Test Results	Circle **PASS** or **NR** to indicate pass or needs remediation:	**PASS**	**NR**

Instructor Initials _____   Instructor Number _____ Date _____

Airway Management
Skills Testing Checklist

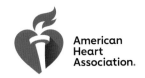

Student Name _____ Date of Test _____

Critical Performance Steps	Check if done correctly
BLS Assessment and Interventions	
Checks for responsiveness • Taps and shouts, "Are you OK?"	
Activates the emergency response system • Shouts for nearby help/Activates the emergency response system and gets the AED *or* • Directs second rescuer to activate the emergency response system and get the AED	
Checks breathing • Scans chest for movement (5-10 seconds)	
Checks pulse (5-10 seconds) **Breathing and pulse check can be done simultaneously** Notes that pulse is present and does not initiate chest compressions or attach AED	
Inserts oropharyngeal or nasopharyngeal airway	
Administers oxygen	
Performs effective bag-mask ventilation for 1 minute • Gives proper ventilation rate (once every 6 seconds) • Gives proper ventilation speed (over 1 second) • Gives proper ventilation volume (about half a bag)	

STOP TEST

Instructor Notes
- Place a check in the box next to each step the student completes successfully.
- If the student does not complete all steps successfully (as indicated by at least 1 blank check box), the student must receive remediation. Make a note here of which skills require remediation (refer to Instructor Manual for information about remediation).

Test Results	Circle **PASS** or **NR** to indicate pass or needs remediation:	**PASS**	**NR**

Instructor Initials _____ Instructor Number _____ Date _____

Megacode Testing Checklist: Scenarios 1/3/8
Bradycardia → Pulseless VT → PEA → PCAC

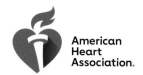

American Heart Association.

Student Name _____ Date of Test _____

Critical Performance Steps						Check if done correctly
Team Leader						
Assigns team member roles						
Ensures high-quality CPR at all times	Compression rate 100-120/min ☐	Compression depth of ≥2 inches ☐	Chest compression fraction >80% ☐	Chest recoil (optional) ☐	Ventilation (optional) ☐	
Ensures that team members communicate well						
Bradycardia Management						
Starts oxygen if needed, places monitor, starts IV						
Places monitor leads in proper position						
Recognizes symptomatic bradycardia						
Administers correct dose of atropine						
Prepares for second-line treatment						
Pulseless VT Management						
Recognizes pVT						
Clears before analyze and shock						
Immediately resumes CPR after shocks						
Appropriate airway management						
Appropriate cycles of drug–rhythm check/shock–CPR						
Administers appropriate drug(s) and doses						
PEA Management						
Recognizes PEA						
Verbalizes potential reversible causes of PEA (H's and T's)						
Administers appropriate drug(s) and doses						
Immediately resumes CPR after rhythm checks						
Post–Cardiac Arrest Care						
Identifies ROSC						
Ensures BP and 12-lead ECG are performed and O_2 saturation is monitored, verbalizes need for endotracheal intubation and waveform capnography, and orders laboratory tests						
Considers targeted temperature management						

STOP TEST

Test Results	Circle **PASS** or **NR** to indicate pass or needs remediation:	PASS	NR
Instructor Initials _____ Instructor Number _____ Date _____			

Learning Station Competency
☐ Bradycardia   ☐ Tachycardia   ☐ Cardiac Arrest/Post–Cardiac Arrest Care   ☐ Megacode Practice

Megacode Testing Checklist: Scenarios 2/5
Bradycardia → VF → Asystole → PCAC

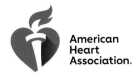

American Heart Association.

Student Name _____ Date of Test _____

Critical Performance Steps						Check if done correctly
Team Leader						
Assigns team member roles						
Ensures high-quality CPR at all times	Compression rate 100-120/min ☐	Compression depth of ≥2 inches ☐	Chest compression fraction >80% ☐	Chest recoil (optional) ☐	Ventilation (optional) ☐	
Ensures that team members communicate well						
Bradycardia Management						
Starts oxygen if needed, places monitor, starts IV						
Places monitor leads in proper position						
Recognizes symptomatic bradycardia						
Administers correct dose of atropine						
Prepares for second-line treatment						
VF Management						
Recognizes VF						
Clears before analyze and shock						
Immediately resumes CPR after shocks						
Appropriate airway management						
Appropriate cycles of drug–rhythm check/shock–CPR						
Administers appropriate drug(s) and doses						
Asystole Management						
Recognizes asystole						
Verbalizes potential reversible causes of asystole (H's and T's)						
Administers appropriate drug(s) and doses						
Immediately resumes CPR after rhythm checks						
Post–Cardiac Arrest Care						
Identifies ROSC						
Ensures BP and 12-lead ECG are performed and O_2 saturation is monitored, verbalizes need for endotracheal intubation and waveform capnography, and orders laboratory tests						
Considers targeted temperature management						

STOP TEST

Test Results	Circle **PASS** or **NR** to indicate pass or needs remediation:	**PASS**	**NR**
Instructor Initials _____ Instructor Number _____ Date _____			

Learning Station Competency
☐ Bradycardia ☐ Tachycardia ☐ Cardiac Arrest/Post–Cardiac Arrest Care ☐ Megacode Practice

Megacode Testing Checklist: Scenarios 4/7/10
Tachycardia → VF → PEA → PCAC

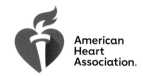
American Heart Association.

Student Name _____ Date of Test _____

Critical Performance Steps						Check if done correctly
Team Leader						
Assigns team member roles						
Ensures high-quality CPR at all times	Compression rate 100-120/min ☐	Compression depth of ≥2 inches ☐	Chest compression fraction >80% ☐	Chest recoil (optional) ☐	Ventilation (optional) ☐	
Ensures that team members communicate well						
Tachycardia Management						
Starts oxygen if needed, places monitor, starts IV						
Places monitor leads in proper position						
Recognizes unstable tachycardia						
Recognizes symptoms due to tachycardia						
Performs immediate synchronized cardioversion						
VF Management						
Recognizes VF						
Clears before analyze and shock						
Immediately resumes CPR after shocks						
Appropriate airway management						
Appropriate cycles of drug–rhythm check/shock–CPR						
Administers appropriate drug(s) and doses						
PEA Management						
Recognizes PEA						
Verbalizes potential reversible causes of PEA (H's and T's)						
Administers appropriate drug(s) and doses						
Immediately resumes CPR after rhythm checks						
Post–Cardiac Arrest Care						
Identifies ROSC						
Ensures BP and 12-lead ECG are performed and O$_2$ saturation is monitored, verbalizes need for endotracheal intubation and waveform capnography, and orders laboratory tests						
Considers targeted temperature management						

STOP TEST

Test Results	Circle **PASS** or **NR** to indicate pass or needs remediation:	**PASS**	**NR**
Instructor Initials _____ Instructor Number _____ Date _____			

Learning Station Competency
☐ Bradycardia   ☐ Tachycardia   ☐ Cardiac Arrest/Post–Cardiac Arrest Care   ☐ Megacode Practice

Megacode Testing Checklist: Scenarios 6/11
Bradycardia → VF → PEA → PCAC

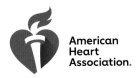
American Heart Association.

Student Name _____ Date of Test _____

Critical Performance Steps						Check if done correctly
Team Leader						
Assigns team member roles						
Ensures high-quality CPR at all times	Compression rate 100-120/min ☐	Compression depth of ≥2 inches ☐	Chest compression fraction >80% ☐	Chest recoil (optional) ☐	Ventilation (optional) ☐	
Ensures that team members communicate well						
Bradycardia Management						
Starts oxygen if needed, places monitor, starts IV						
Places monitor leads in proper position						
Recognizes symptomatic bradycardia						
Administers correct dose of atropine						
Prepares for second-line treatment						
VF Management						
Recognizes VF						
Clears before analyze and shock						
Immediately resumes CPR after shocks						
Appropriate airway management						
Appropriate cycles of drug–rhythm check/shock–CPR						
Administers appropriate drug(s) and doses						
PEA Management						
Recognizes PEA						
Verbalizes potential reversible causes of PEA (H's and T's)						
Administers appropriate drug(s) and doses						
Immediately resumes CPR after rhythm checks						
Post–Cardiac Arrest Care						
Identifies ROSC						
Ensures BP and 12-lead ECG are performed and O_2 saturation is monitored, verbalizes need for endotracheal intubation and waveform capnography, and orders laboratory tests						
Considers targeted temperature management						

STOP TEST

Test Results	Circle **PASS** or **NR** to indicate pass or needs remediation:	**PASS**	**NR**
Instructor Initials _____	Instructor Number _____	Date _____	

Learning Station Competency
☐ Bradycardia ☐ Tachycardia ☐ Cardiac Arrest/Post–Cardiac Arrest Care ☐ Megacode Practice

Megacode Testing Checklist: Scenario 9
Tachycardia → PEA → VF → PCAC

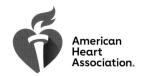
American Heart Association.

Student Name _____ Date of Test _____

Critical Performance Steps						Check if done correctly
Team Leader						
Assigns team member roles						
Ensures high-quality CPR at all times	Compression rate 100-120/min ☐	Compression depth of ≥2 inches ☐	Chest compression fraction >80% ☐	Chest recoil (optional) ☐	Ventilation (optional) ☐	
Ensures that team members communicate well						
Tachycardia Management						
Starts oxygen if needed, places monitor, starts IV						
Places monitor leads in proper position						
Recognizes tachycardia (specific diagnosis)						
Recognizes no symptoms due to tachycardia						
Considers appropriate initial drug therapy						
PEA Management						
Recognizes PEA						
Verbalizes potential reversible causes of PEA (H's and T's)						
Administers appropriate drug(s) and doses						
Immediately resumes CPR after rhythm check and pulse checks						
VF Management						
Recognizes VF						
Clears before analyze and shock						
Immediately resumes CPR after shocks						
Appropriate airway management						
Appropriate cycles of drug–rhythm check/shock–CPR						
Administers appropriate drug(s) and doses						
Post–Cardiac Arrest Care						
Identifies ROSC						
Ensures BP and 12-lead ECG are performed and O$_2$ saturation is monitored, verbalizes need for endotracheal intubation and waveform capnography, and orders laboratory tests						
Considers targeted temperature management						

STOP TEST

Test Results	Circle **PASS** or **NR** to indicate pass or needs remediation:	**PASS**	**NR**
Instructor Initials _____ Instructor Number _____ Date _____			

Learning Station Competency
☐ Bradycardia ☐ Tachycardia ☐ Cardiac Arrest/Post–Cardiac Arrest Care ☐ Megacode Practice

Megacode Testing Checklist: Scenario 12
Bradycardia → VF → Asystole/PEA → PCAC

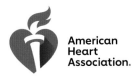
American Heart Association.

Student Name _____ Date of Test _____

Critical Performance Steps						Check if done correctly
Team Leader						
Assigns team member roles						
Ensures high-quality CPR at all times	Compression rate 100-120/min ☐	Compression depth of ≥2 inches ☐	Chest compression fraction >80% ☐	Chest recoil (optional) ☐	Ventilation (optional) ☐	
Ensures that team members communicate well						
Bradycardia Management						
Starts oxygen if needed, places monitor, starts IV						
Places monitor leads in proper position						
Recognizes symptomatic bradycardia						
Administers correct dose of atropine						
Prepares for second-line treatment						
VF Management						
Recognizes VF						
Clears before analyze and shock						
Immediately resumes CPR after shocks						
Appropriate airway management						
Appropriate cycles of drug–rhythm check/shock–CPR						
Administers appropriate drug(s) and doses						
Asystole and PEA Management						
Recognizes asystole and PEA						
Verbalizes potential reversible causes of asystole and PEA (H's and T's)						
Administers appropriate drug(s) and doses						
Immediately resumes CPR after rhythm checks						
Post–Cardiac Arrest Care						
Identifies ROSC						
Ensures BP and 12-lead ECG are performed and O$_2$ saturation is monitored, verbalizes need for endotracheal intubation and waveform capnography, and orders laboratory tests						
Considers targeted temperature management						

STOP TEST

Test Results	Circle **PASS** or **NR** to indicate pass or needs remediation:	**PASS**	**NR**
Instructor Initials _____	Instructor Number _____	Date _____	

Learning Station Competency
☐ Bradycardia   ☐ Tachycardia   ☐ Cardiac Arrest/Post–Cardiac Arrest Care   ☐ Megacode Practice

Adult Cardiac Arrest Learning Station Checklist (VF/pVT)

Adult Cardiac Arrest Algorithm (VF/pVT)

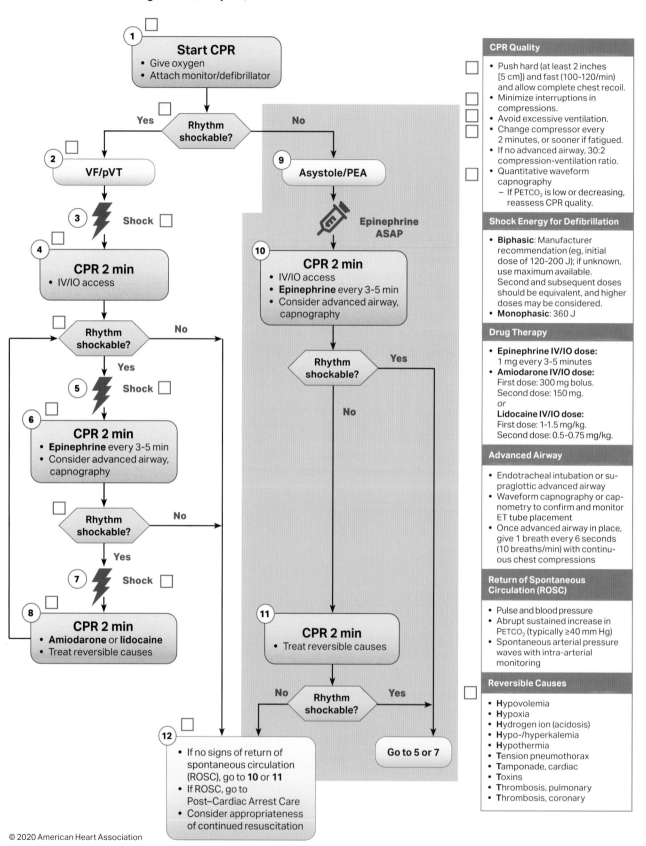

CPR Quality

- Push hard (at least 2 inches [5 cm]) and fast (100-120/min) and allow complete chest recoil.
- Minimize interruptions in compressions.
- Avoid excessive ventilation.
- Change compressor every 2 minutes, or sooner if fatigued.
- If no advanced airway, 30:2 compression-ventilation ratio.
- Quantitative waveform capnography
  - If PETCO$_2$ is low or decreasing, reassess CPR quality.

Shock Energy for Defibrillation

- **Biphasic**: Manufacturer recommendation (eg, initial dose of 120-200 J); if unknown, use maximum available. Second and subsequent doses should be equivalent, and higher doses may be considered.
- **Monophasic**: 360 J

Drug Therapy

- **Epinephrine IV/IO dose:** 1 mg every 3-5 minutes
- **Amiodarone IV/IO dose:** First dose: 300 mg bolus. Second dose: 150 mg.
  or
  Lidocaine IV/IO dose: First dose: 1-1.5 mg/kg. Second dose: 0.5-0.75 mg/kg.

Advanced Airway

- Endotracheal intubation or supraglottic advanced airway
- Waveform capnography or capnometry to confirm and monitor ET tube placement
- Once advanced airway in place, give 1 breath every 6 seconds (10 breaths/min) with continuous chest compressions

Return of Spontaneous Circulation (ROSC)

- Pulse and blood pressure
- Abrupt sustained increase in PETCO$_2$ (typically ≥40 mm Hg)
- Spontaneous arterial pressure waves with intra-arterial monitoring

Reversible Causes

- **H**ypovolemia
- **H**ypoxia
- **H**ydrogen ion (acidosis)
- **H**ypo-/hyperkalemia
- **H**ypothermia
- **T**ension pneumothorax
- **T**amponade, cardiac
- **T**oxins
- **T**hrombosis, pulmonary
- **T**hrombosis, coronary

Adult Cardiac Arrest Learning Station Checklist (Asystole/PEA)

Adult Cardiac Arrest Algorithm (Asystole/PEA)

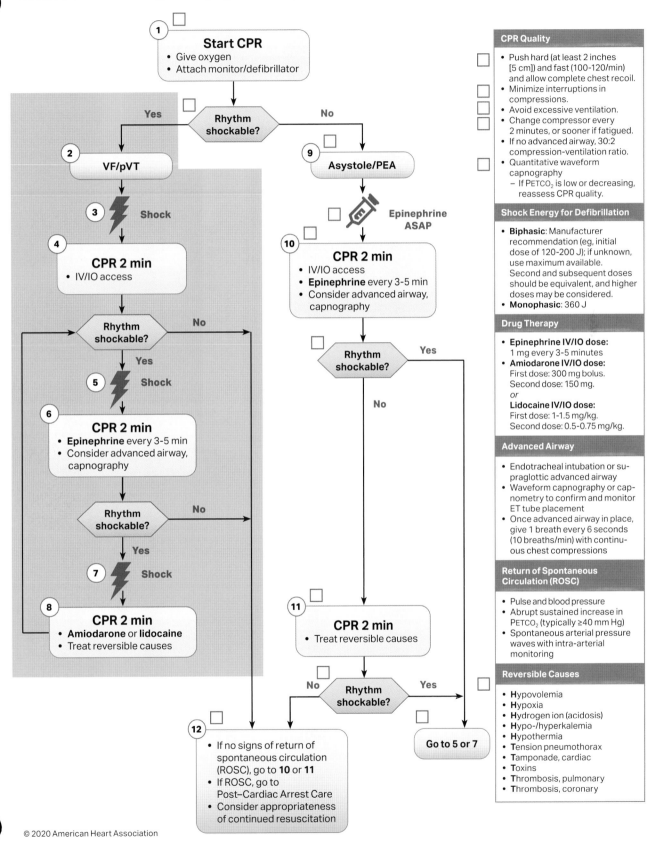

1 Start CPR
- Give oxygen
- Attach monitor/defibrillator

Rhythm shockable?

Yes

2 VF/pVT

3 Shock

4 CPR 2 min
- IV/IO access

Rhythm shockable? — No

Yes

5 Shock

6 CPR 2 min
- **Epinephrine** every 3-5 min
- Consider advanced airway, capnography

Rhythm shockable? — No

Yes

7 Shock

8 CPR 2 min
- **Amiodarone** or **lidocaine**
- Treat reversible causes

No

9 Asystole/PEA

Epinephrine ASAP

10 CPR 2 min
- IV/IO access
- **Epinephrine** every 3-5 min
- Consider advanced airway, capnography

Rhythm shockable? — Yes

No

11 CPR 2 min
- Treat reversible causes

Rhythm shockable? — No / Yes

Go to 5 or 7

12
- If no signs of return of spontaneous circulation (ROSC), go to **10** or **11**
- If ROSC, go to Post–Cardiac Arrest Care
- Consider appropriateness of continued resuscitation

CPR Quality
- Push hard (at least 2 inches [5 cm]) and fast (100-120/min) and allow complete chest recoil.
- Minimize interruptions in compressions.
- Avoid excessive ventilation.
- Change compressor every 2 minutes, or sooner if fatigued.
- If no advanced airway, 30:2 compression-ventilation ratio.
- Quantitative waveform capnography
  - If $PETCO_2$ is low or decreasing, reassess CPR quality.

Shock Energy for Defibrillation
- **Biphasic**: Manufacturer recommendation (eg, initial dose of 120-200 J); if unknown, use maximum available. Second and subsequent doses should be equivalent, and higher doses may be considered.
- **Monophasic**: 360 J

Drug Therapy
- **Epinephrine IV/IO dose:** 1 mg every 3-5 minutes
- **Amiodarone IV/IO dose:** First dose: 300 mg bolus. Second dose: 150 mg. *or* **Lidocaine IV/IO dose:** First dose: 1-1.5 mg/kg. Second dose: 0.5-0.75 mg/kg.

Advanced Airway
- Endotracheal intubation or supraglottic advanced airway
- Waveform capnography or capnometry to confirm and monitor ET tube placement
- Once advanced airway in place, give 1 breath every 6 seconds (10 breaths/min) with continuous chest compressions

Return of Spontaneous Circulation (ROSC)
- Pulse and blood pressure
- Abrupt sustained increase in $PETCO_2$ (typically ≥40 mm Hg)
- Spontaneous arterial pressure waves with intra-arterial monitoring

Reversible Causes
- **H**ypovolemia
- **H**ypoxia
- **H**ydrogen ion (acidosis)
- **H**ypo-/hyperkalemia
- **H**ypothermia
- **T**ension pneumothorax
- **T**amponade, cardiac
- **T**oxins
- **T**hrombosis, pulmonary
- **T**hrombosis, coronary

Adult Bradycardia Learning Station Checklist

Adult Bradycardia Algorithm

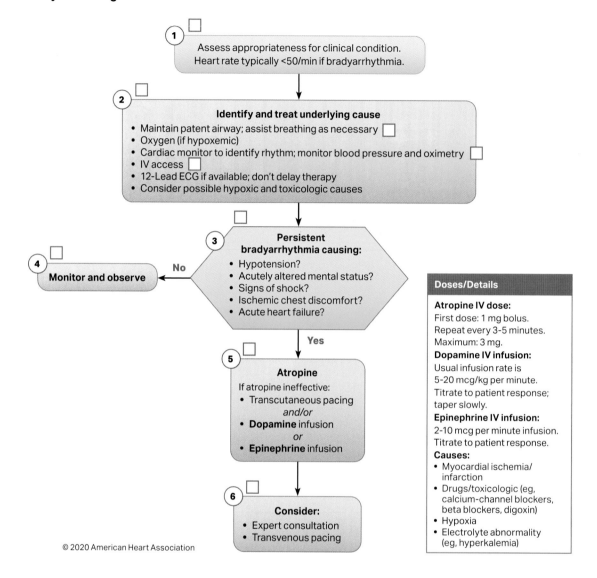

1 ☐ Assess appropriateness for clinical condition.
Heart rate typically <50/min if bradyarrhythmia.

2 ☐ **Identify and treat underlying cause**
- Maintain patent airway; assist breathing as necessary ☐
- Oxygen (if hypoxemic)
- Cardiac monitor to identify rhythm; monitor blood pressure and oximetry ☐
- IV access ☐
- 12-Lead ECG if available; don't delay therapy
- Consider possible hypoxic and toxicologic causes

3 ☐ **Persistent bradyarrhythmia causing:**
- Hypotension?
- Acutely altered mental status?
- Signs of shock?
- Ischemic chest discomfort?
- Acute heart failure?

No → **4** ☐ **Monitor and observe**

Yes ↓

5 ☐ **Atropine**
If atropine ineffective:
- Transcutaneous pacing
 and/or
- **Dopamine** infusion
 or
- **Epinephrine** infusion

6 ☐ **Consider:**
- Expert consultation
- Transvenous pacing

© 2020 American Heart Association

Doses/Details

Atropine IV dose:
First dose: 1 mg bolus.
Repeat every 3-5 minutes.
Maximum: 3 mg.

Dopamine IV infusion:
Usual infusion rate is
5-20 mcg/kg per minute.
Titrate to patient response;
taper slowly.

Epinephrine IV infusion:
2-10 mcg per minute infusion.
Titrate to patient response.

Causes:
- Myocardial ischemia/ infarction
- Drugs/toxicologic (eg, calcium-channel blockers, beta blockers, digoxin)
- Hypoxia
- Electrolyte abnormality (eg, hyperkalemia)

Adult Tachycardia With a Pulse Learning Station Checklist

Adult Tachycardia With a Pulse Algorithm

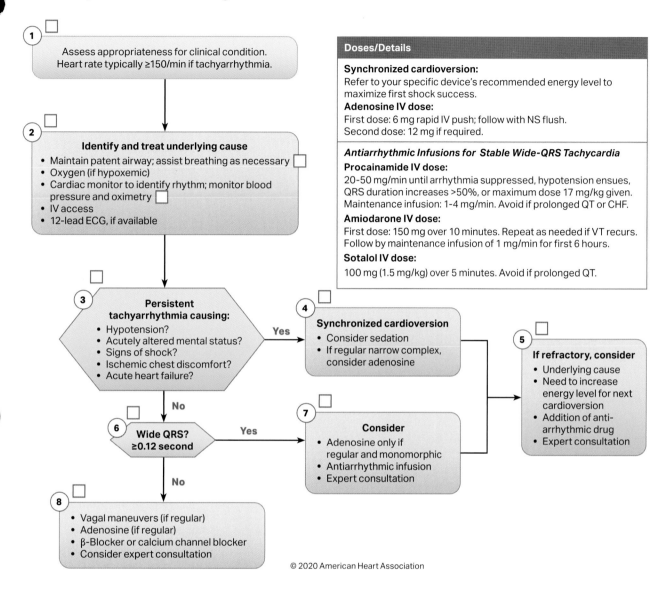

1 Assess appropriateness for clinical condition.
Heart rate typically ≥150/min if tachyarrhythmia.

2 **Identify and treat underlying cause**
- Maintain patent airway; assist breathing as necessary
- Oxygen (if hypoxemic)
- Cardiac monitor to identify rhythm; monitor blood pressure and oximetry
- IV access
- 12-lead ECG, if available

3 **Persistent tachyarrhythmia causing:**
- Hypotension?
- Acutely altered mental status?
- Signs of shock?
- Ischemic chest discomfort?
- Acute heart failure?

Yes →

4 **Synchronized cardioversion**
- Consider sedation
- If regular narrow complex, consider adenosine

5 **If refractory, consider**
- Underlying cause
- Need to increase energy level for next cardioversion
- Addition of anti-arrhythmic drug
- Expert consultation

No ↓

6 **Wide QRS?**
≥0.12 second

Yes →

7 **Consider**
- Adenosine only if regular and monomorphic
- Antiarrhythmic infusion
- Expert consultation

No ↓

8
- Vagal maneuvers (if regular)
- Adenosine (if regular)
- β-Blocker or calcium channel blocker
- Consider expert consultation

Doses/Details

Synchronized cardioversion:
Refer to your specific device's recommended energy level to maximize first shock success.

Adenosine IV dose:
First dose: 6 mg rapid IV push; follow with NS flush.
Second dose: 12 mg if required.

Antiarrhythmic Infusions for Stable Wide-QRS Tachycardia

Procainamide IV dose:
20-50 mg/min until arrhythmia suppressed, hypotension ensues, QRS duration increases >50%, or maximum dose 17 mg/kg given. Maintenance infusion: 1-4 mg/min. Avoid if prolonged QT or CHF.

Amiodarone IV dose:
First dose: 150 mg over 10 minutes. Repeat as needed if VT recurs. Follow by maintenance infusion of 1 mg/min for first 6 hours.

Sotalol IV dose:
100 mg (1.5 mg/kg) over 5 minutes. Avoid if prolonged QT.

Adult Post–Cardiac Arrest Care Learning Station Checklist

Adult Post–Cardiac Arrest Care Algorithm

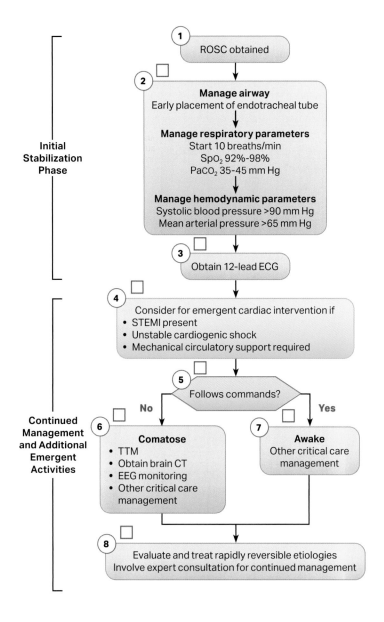

1 ROSC obtained

2 **Manage airway**
Early placement of endotracheal tube

Manage respiratory parameters
Start 10 breaths/min
SpO_2 92%-98%
$PaCO_2$ 35-45 mm Hg

Manage hemodynamic parameters
Systolic blood pressure >90 mm Hg
Mean arterial pressure >65 mm Hg

3 Obtain 12-lead ECG

4 Consider for emergent cardiac intervention if
• STEMI present
• Unstable cardiogenic shock
• Mechanical circulatory support required

5 Follows commands?

No — **6** **Comatose**
• TTM
• Obtain brain CT
• EEG monitoring
• Other critical care management

Yes — **7** **Awake**
Other critical care management

8 Evaluate and treat rapidly reversible etiologies
Involve expert consultation for continued management

Initial Stabilization Phase (bracket label)

Continued Management and Additional Emergent Activities (bracket label)

Initial Stabilization Phase

Resuscitation is ongoing during the post-ROSC phase, and many of these activities can occur concurrently. However, if prioritization is necessary, follow these steps:
• Airway management: Waveform capnography or capnometry to confirm and monitor endotracheal tube placement
• Manage respiratory parameters: Titrate FIO_2 for SpO_2 92%-98%; start at 10 breaths/min; titrate to $PaCO_2$ of 35-45 mm Hg
• Manage hemodynamic parameters: Administer crystalloid and/or vasopressor or inotrope for goal systolic blood pressure >90 mm Hg or mean arterial pressure >65 mm Hg

Continued Management and Additional Emergent Activities

These evaluations should be done concurrently so that decisions on targeted temperature management (TTM) receive high priority as cardiac interventions.
• Emergent cardiac intervention: Early evaluation of 12-lead electrocardiogram (ECG); consider hemodynamics for decision on cardiac intervention
• TTM: If patient is not following commands, start TTM as soon as possible; begin at 32-36°C for 24 hours by using a cooling device with feedback loop
• Other critical care management
  – Continuously monitor core temperature (esophageal, rectal, bladder)
  – Maintain normoxia, normocapnia, euglycemia
  – Provide continuous or intermittent electroencephalogram (EEG) monitoring
  – Provide lung-protective ventilation

H's and T's

Hypovolemia
Hypoxia
Hydrogen ion (acidosis)
Hypokalemia/**h**yperkalemia
Hypothermia
Tension pneumothorax
Tamponade, cardiac
Toxins
Thrombosis, pulmonary
Thrombosis, coronary

Adult Cardiac Arrest Learning Station Checklist (VF/pVT/Asystole/PEA)

Adult Cardiac Arrest Algorithm (VF/pVT/Asystole/PEA)

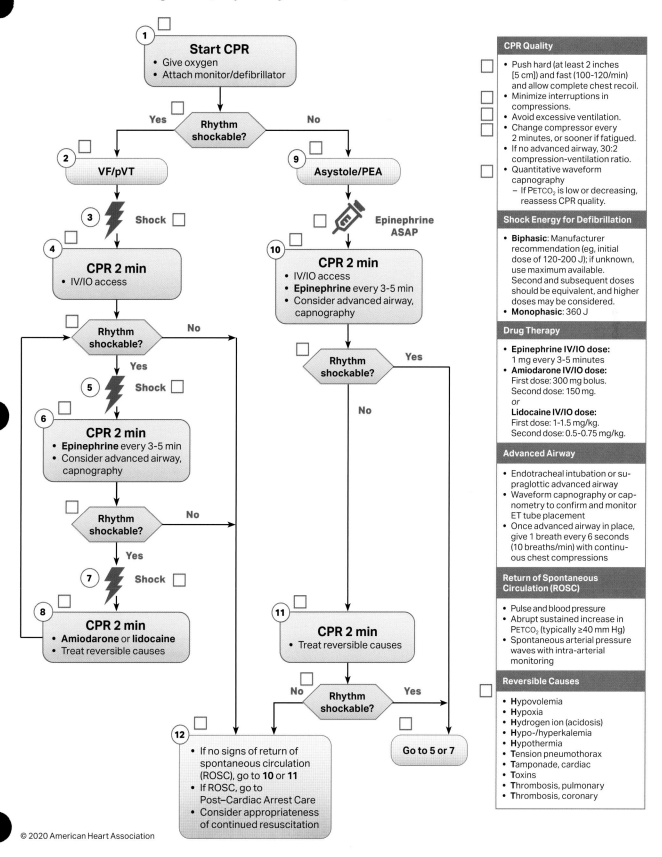

1 Start CPR
- Give oxygen
- Attach monitor/defibrillator

Rhythm shockable?

Yes → **2 VF/pVT**

No → **9 Asystole/PEA**

3 Shock

4 CPR 2 min
- IV/IO access

Rhythm shockable? — No →

Yes

5 Shock

6 CPR 2 min
- **Epinephrine** every 3-5 min
- Consider advanced airway, capnography

Rhythm shockable? — No →

Yes

7 Shock

8 CPR 2 min
- **Amiodarone** or **lidocaine**
- Treat reversible causes

Epinephrine ASAP

10 CPR 2 min
- IV/IO access
- **Epinephrine** every 3-5 min
- Consider advanced airway, capnography

Rhythm shockable? — Yes →

No

11 CPR 2 min
- Treat reversible causes

Rhythm shockable?

No → **12**

Yes → **Go to 5 or 7**

12
- If no signs of return of spontaneous circulation (ROSC), go to **10** or **11**
- If ROSC, go to Post–Cardiac Arrest Care
- Consider appropriateness of continued resuscitation

CPR Quality
- Push hard (at least 2 inches [5 cm]) and fast (100-120/min) and allow complete chest recoil.
- Minimize interruptions in compressions.
- Avoid excessive ventilation.
- Change compressor every 2 minutes, or sooner if fatigued.
- If no advanced airway, 30:2 compression-ventilation ratio
- Quantitative waveform capnography
  – If $PETCO_2$ is low or decreasing, reassess CPR quality.

Shock Energy for Defibrillation
- **Biphasic**: Manufacturer recommendation (eg, initial dose of 120-200 J); if unknown, use maximum available. Second and subsequent doses should be equivalent, and higher doses may be considered.
- **Monophasic**: 360 J

Drug Therapy
- **Epinephrine IV/IO dose:** 1 mg every 3-5 minutes
- **Amiodarone IV/IO dose:** First dose: 300 mg bolus. Second dose: 150 mg. *or* **Lidocaine IV/IO dose:** First dose: 1-1.5 mg/kg. Second dose: 0.5-0.75 mg/kg.

Advanced Airway
- Endotracheal intubation or supraglottic advanced airway
- Waveform capnography or capnometry to confirm and monitor ET tube placement
- Once advanced airway in place, give 1 breath every 6 seconds (10 breaths/min) with continuous chest compressions

Return of Spontaneous Circulation (ROSC)
- Pulse and blood pressure
- Abrupt sustained increase in $PETCO_2$ (typically ≥40 mm Hg)
- Spontaneous arterial pressure waves with intra-arterial monitoring

Reversible Causes
- **H**ypovolemia
- **H**ypoxia
- **H**ydrogen ion (acidosis)
- **H**ypo-/hyperkalemia
- **H**ypothermia
- **T**ension pneumothorax
- **T**amponade, cardiac
- **T**oxins
- **T**hrombosis, pulmonary
- **T**hrombosis, coronary

Cardiac Arrest in Pregnancy In-Hospital ACLS Learning Station Checklist

Cardiac Arrest in Pregnancy In-Hospital ACLS Algorithm

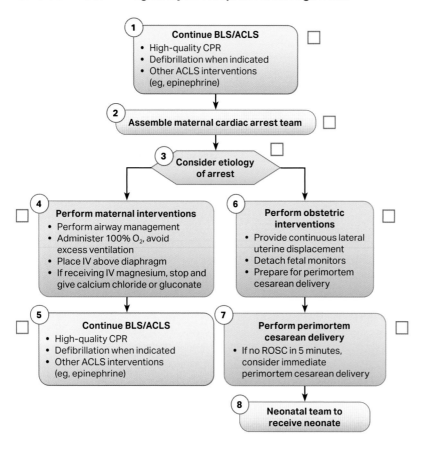

1 **Continue BLS/ACLS** ☐
- High-quality CPR
- Defibrillation when indicated
- Other ACLS interventions (eg, epinephrine)

2 Assemble maternal cardiac arrest team ☐

3 Consider etiology of arrest ☐

4 **Perform maternal interventions** ☐
- Perform airway management
- Administer 100% O_2, avoid excess ventilation
- Place IV above diaphragm
- If receiving IV magnesium, stop and give calcium chloride or gluconate

6 **Perform obstetric interventions** ☐
- Provide continuous lateral uterine displacement
- Detach fetal monitors
- Prepare for perimortem cesarean delivery

5 **Continue BLS/ACLS** ☐
- High-quality CPR
- Defibrillation when indicated
- Other ACLS interventions (eg, epinephrine)

7 **Perform perimortem cesarean delivery** ☐
- If no ROSC in 5 minutes, consider immediate perimortem cesarean delivery

8 Neonatal team to receive neonate

© 2020 American Heart Association

Maternal Cardiac Arrest
- Team planning should be done in collaboration with the obstetric, neonatal, emergency, anesthesiology, intensive care, and cardiac arrest services.
- Priorities for pregnant women in cardiac arrest should include provision of high-quality CPR and relief of aortocaval compression with lateral uterine displacement.
- The goal of perimortem cesarean delivery is to improve maternal and fetal outcomes.
- Ideally, perform perimortem cesarean delivery in 5 minutes, depending on provider resources and skill sets.

Advanced Airway
- In pregnancy, a difficult airway is common. Use the most experienced provider.
- Provide endotracheal intubation or supraglottic advanced airway.
- Perform waveform capnography or capnometry to confirm and monitor ET tube placement.
- Once advanced airway is in place, give 1 breath every 6 seconds (10 breaths/min) with continuous chest compressions.

Potential Etiology of Maternal Cardiac Arrest
A Anesthetic complications
B Bleeding
C Cardiovascular
D Drugs
E Embolic
F Fever
G General nonobstetric causes of cardiac arrest (H's and T's)
H Hypertension

Adult Ventricular Assist Device Learning Station Checklist

Adult Ventricular Assist Device Algorithm

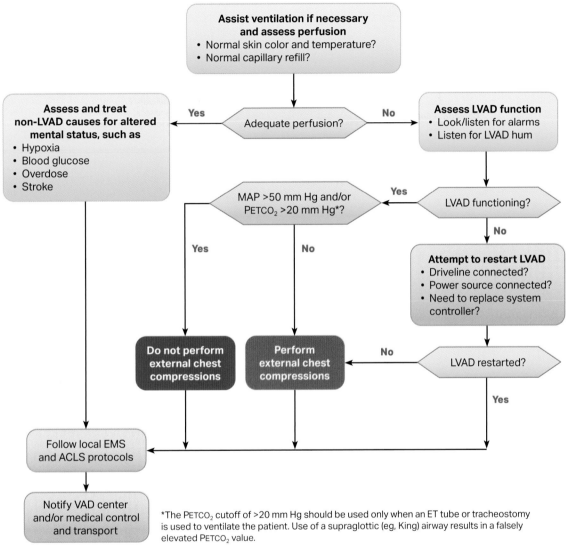

Assist ventilation if necessary and assess perfusion
- Normal skin color and temperature?
- Normal capillary refill?

Adequate perfusion?

Yes → **Assess and treat non-LVAD causes for altered mental status, such as**
- Hypoxia
- Blood glucose
- Overdose
- Stroke

No → **Assess LVAD function**
- Look/listen for alarms
- Listen for LVAD hum

LVAD functioning?

Yes → **MAP >50 mm Hg and/or PETCO₂ >20 mm Hg*?**

- Yes → **Do not perform external chest compressions**
- No → **Perform external chest compressions**

No → **Attempt to restart LVAD**
- Driveline connected?
- Power source connected?
- Need to replace system controller?

LVAD restarted?

No → **Perform external chest compressions**

Yes →

Follow local EMS and ACLS protocols

Notify VAD center and/or medical control and transport

*The PETCO₂ cutoff of >20 mm Hg should be used only when an ET tube or tracheostomy is used to ventilate the patient. Use of a supraglottic (eg, King) airway results in a falsely elevated PETCO₂ value.

© 2020 American Heart Association

237

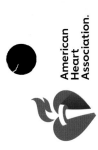

ACLS Code Timer/Recorder Sheet

American Heart Association.

Time team initiated action: _____

Time chest compressions started: _____

Time defibrillator applied: _____

First documented pulseless rhythm: _____

Time Compressor rotated: _____

Time	Quality CPR	Rhythm	Defibrillation (Joules)	Drug (name/dose)	Comments (ie, peripheral line placement, IO, vital signs, response to interventions)

Compression pause notes: _____

Chest compression fraction: _____ %

239

Atropine

1 mg

Dopamine

Epinephrine

1 mg

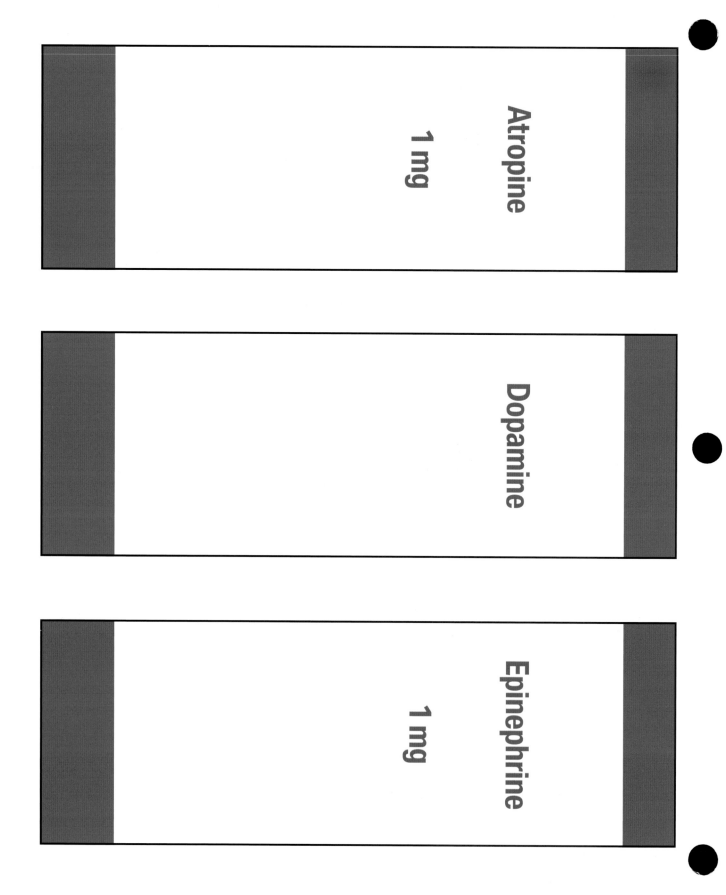

Atropine

1 mg

Dopamine

Epinephrine

1 mg

Lidocaine

Amiodarone

300 mg

Adenosine

6 mg

Lidocaine

Amiodarone

300 mg

Adenosine

6 mg

Amiodarone

150 mg

Adenosine

12 mg

Amiodarone

150 mg

Adenosine

12 mg

Science Summary Table

This table compares 2015 with 2020, providing a quick reference to what has changed and what is new in the science of advanced cardiovascular life support.

Table. Topical Comparison of 2015 and 2020 ACLS Science

ACLS topic	2015	2020
Ventilation	• 1 breath every 5 to 6 seconds for respiratory arrest, with a bag-mask device • 1 breath every 6 seconds for ventilation with an advanced airway in place	• 1 breath every 6 seconds for respiratory arrest with or without an advanced airway and also for cardiac arrest with an advanced airway (use this rate with a bag-mask device if your local protocol is continuous compressions and asynchronous ventilations for cardiac arrest)
Bradycardia	• Atropine dose: 0.5 mg • Dopamine dosing: 2 to 20 mcg/kg per minute	• Atropine dose: 1 mg • Dopamine dosing: 5 to 20 mcg/kg per minute

Tachycardia	• Synchronized cardioversion initial recommended doses:
	  – Narrow QRS complex, regular rhythm: 50 to 100 J
	  – Narrow QRS complex, irregular rhythm: 120 to 200 J
	  – Wide QRS complex, regular rhythm: 100 J
	• Wide QRS complex, irregular rhythm: defibrillation dose (not synchronized)
		• Follow your specific device's recommended energy level to maximize the success of the first shock
		• Wide QRS complex, irregular rhythm: defibrillation dose (not synchronized)

Post–Cardiac Arrest Care	• Titrate oxygen saturation to 94% or higher	• Titrate oxygen saturation to 92% to 98%
Adult Chain of Survival	• 5 links for both chains (in-hospital cardiac arrest and out-of-hospital cardiac arrest)	• 6 links for both chains (in-hospital cardiac arrest and out-of-hospital cardiac arrest): added a Recovery link to the end of both chains
IV/IO Access	• IV access and IO access are equivalent	• IV preferred over IO access, unless IV fails (then OK to proceed to IO)

ACLS topic	2020
Cardiac Arrest	• Epinephrine 1 mg every 3 to 5 minutes or every 4 minutes as a midrange (ie, every other 2-minute rhythm check) • Amiodarone and lidocaine are equivalent for treatment (ie, either may be used) • Added maternal cardiac arrest information and algorithms (in-hospital) • Added ventricular assist device information (left and right ventricular assist device) and algorithm • Added new prognostication diagram and information • Recommend using waveform capnography with a bag-mask device
Stroke	• Revised stroke algorithm • New stroke triage algorithm for EMS destination • Focus on large vessel occlusion for all healthcare providers • Endovascular therapy: treatment window up to 24 hours (previously up to 6 hours) • Both alteplase and endovascular therapy can be given/performed if time criteria and inclusion criteria are met • Consider having EMS bypass the emergency department and go straight to the imaging suite (computed tomography [CT]/magnetic resonance imaging); initial assessment can be performed there to save time • Titrate oxygen saturation to >94%

Part 6

ACLS Lesson Plans

Lessons are numbered only for labeling and convenience. Lessons 1 to 3 should be completed in order because they are the foundation of the course.

Precourse Preparation

Instructor Tips

- The time you invest in preparation is important. Prepare well, and anticipate questions and challenges
- Anticipate what could happen, and have a plan for possible challenges such as
  - Instructor does not arrive
  - Equipment fails/malfunctions
  - Batteries are dead (bring extras)

30 to 60 Days Before Class

- Determine course specifics
  - Target audience
  - Number of students
  - Special needs or equipment
- Review and reserve ACLS equipment
- Schedule the room(s) as soon as dates are determined
- Schedule additional instructors, if needed (Table 1)

Table 1. Class Size and Student-to-Instructor Ratios for Course Activities

Activity	Recommended size or ratio
Large-group interactions	The size of the group is limited by the size of the room and the number of video monitors or projection screens.
Learning stations and High-Performance Teams: Megacode Testing	6:1 up to a maximum of 8:1 The student-to-instructor ratio should be 6 students to 1 learning station, with 1 instructor for each station. In some cases, a maximum of 8 students to 1 instructor to 1 learning station may be used.

Optional

Instructors or Training Centers may consider offering an ACLS preparation course days or weeks before the ACLS Course to ensure that students understand

- ECGs (rhythm analysis)
- Pharmacology
- Airway management
- BLS skills

At Least 3 Weeks Before Class

- Confirm room reservations and setups
- Send students a precourse letter with student materials

- Ensure that students understand that precourse preparation is necessary for successful participation in the ACLS Course
- Provide students information on the precourse self-assessment and precourse work (interactive video lessons)
- Confirm additional instructors
- **Research local treatment protocols and prepare for discussion**

Day Before Class

- Set up the room
- Coordinate the plan with additional instructors, if needed for class size
- Use the Equipment List (found in Part 2 of this manual as well as in this lesson plan) as a checklist to ensure that all equipment is available and tested for operation (including feedback devices and their accessory devices, such as tablet computers and smartphones)
  - Have extra batteries on hand for equipment
- Check with your Training Center Coordinator to determine any Training Center–specific paperwork needed
- Ensure that all course paperwork is in order, such as
  - ACLS Course roster
  - Testing checklists
  - Learning station checklists

Day of Class

- Make sure all equipment is working
- Greet students as they arrive to help make them feel at ease
- Have students fill out the course roster. Rosters may vary between Training Centers; refer to the Instructor Network (**www.ahainstructornetwork.org**). Required: Make sure all students have passed the ACLS Precourse Self-Assessment and have completed all of the ACLS precourse work (except for the traditional course; see sample agenda) before entering the class

Equipment List

This table lists the equipment and supplies needed to optimally conduct this course. This includes a code cart for in-hospital providers and a jump kit and defibrillator unit for prehospital providers. The code cart or jump kit should contain the equipment and supplies listed in Table 2.

Table 2. Classroom Equipment and Supplies

Equipment and supplies	Quantity needed	Learning/testing station where equipment needed
Paperwork		
Course roster	1/class	Beginning of course
Listing of student groups	1/class	All
Name tags	1/student and instructor	All
Course agenda	1/student and instructor	All
Course completion card	1/student	End of course
ACLS Provider Manual	1/student and instructor	All
Handbook of ECC (optional)	1/student and instructor	All
ACLS posters	1 set/class	All
Precourse letter	1/student	Precourse
Airway Management Skills Testing Checklist	1/student	Airway Management
Adult High-Quality BLS Skills Testing Checklist	1/student	High-Quality BLS
High-Performance Teams: Megacode Testing Checklist	1/student	Megacode Testing
ACLS Provider Course exam (if not taking online)	1/student	Exam
Blank exam answer sheet (if not taking online)	1/student	Exam
Exam answer key (if not taking online)	1/class	Exam
ACLS Instructor Manual (including case scenarios) and ACLS Lesson Plans	1/instructor	All
Learning station checklists	1/student	High-Quality BLS; Airway Management; Preventing Arrest: Bradycardia; Preventing Arrest: Tachycardia (Stable and Unstable); High-Performance Teams: Cardiac Arrest and Post–Cardiac Arrest Care; and High-Performance Teams: Megacode Practice
Audiovisual Equipment		

(continued)

Equipment and supplies	Quantity needed	Learning/testing station where equipment needed
Course video: TV with DVD player or computer with internet access/streaming capability and projection screen	1/station	High-Performance Teams
CPR and AED Equipment		
Adult CPR manikin with shirt	1/every 3 students	High-Quality BLS
Adult airway manikin	1/every 3 students	Airway Management
Adult manikin (airway, CPR, and defibrillation capable)	1/every 6 students	Technology Review; Preventing Arrest: Bradycardia; Preventing Arrest: Tachycardia (Stable and Unstable); High-Performance Teams: Cardiac Arrest and Post–Cardiac Arrest Care; High-Performance Teams: Megacode Practice; and High-Performance Teams: Megacode Testing
CPR/short board	1/station	High-Quality BLS; High-Performance Teams: Cardiac Arrest and Post–Cardiac Arrest Care; High-Performance Teams: Megacode Practice; and High-Performance Teams: Megacode Testing
Code cart or jump kit	1/station	Technology Review; Bradycardia, Tachycardia; High-Performance Teams: Cardiac Arrest and Post–Cardiac Arrest Care; High-Performance Teams: Megacode Practice; and High-Performance Teams: Megacode Testing
Stopwatch/timing device (ventilation timing or CCF)	1/instructor	Airway Management; High-Performance Teams: Cardiac Arrest and Post–Cardiac Arrest Care; High-Performance Teams: Megacode Practice; and High-Performance Teams: Megacode Testing
Countdown timer	1/instructor	All
Feedback device (required)	1/station	High-Quality BLS; Airway Management; High-Performance Teams: Cardiac Arrest and Post–Cardiac Arrest Care; High-Performance Teams: Megacode Practice; and High-Performance Teams: Megacode Testing
AED trainer with adult AED training pads	1/every 3 students	High-Quality BLS

(continued)

Equipment and supplies	Quantity needed	Learning/testing station where equipment needed
Step stools to stand on for CPR	1/every 3 students	High-Quality BLS; High-Performance Teams: Cardiac Arrest and Post–Cardiac Arrest Care; High-Performance Teams: Megacode Practice; and High-Performance Teams: Megacode Testing
Ultrasound (optional)	1 every 6 students	High-Performance Teams: Cardiac Arrest and Post–Cardiac Arrest Care; High-Performance Teams: Megacode Practice; and High-Performance Teams: Megacode Testing
Airway and Ventilation		
Bag-mask device, reservoir, and tubing	1/every 3 students	All but High-Quality BLS; Preventing Arrest: Bradycardia; and Preventing Arrest: Tachycardia (Stable and Unstable)
Oral and nasal airways	1 set/station	All but High-Quality BLS; Preventing Arrest: Bradycardia; and Preventing Arrest: Tachycardia (Stable and Unstable)
Water-soluble lubricant	1/station	All but High-Quality BLS; Preventing Arrest: Bradycardia; and Preventing Arrest: Tachycardia (Stable and Unstable)
Nonrebreathing mask	1/every 3 students	All but High-quality BLS
Waveform capnography	1/station	Airway Management; High-Performance Teams: Cardiac Arrest and Post–Cardiac Arrest Care; High-Performance Teams: Megacode Practice; and High-Performance Teams: Megacode Testing
Rhythm Recognition and Electrical Therapy		
ECG simulator/rhythm generator	1/station	All but High-Quality BLS and Airway Management
Electrodes	1/station	All but High-Quality BLS and Airway Management
Monitor capable of defibrillation/ synchronized cardioversion, transcutaneous pacing	1/station	All but High-Quality BLS and Airway Management
Pacing pads, defibrillator pads, or defibrillator gel (if pads are not used)	1/station	All but High-Quality BLS and Airway Management
Spare batteries or power cord	1/station	All but High-Quality BLS and Airway Management

(continued)

Equipment and supplies	Quantity needed	Learning/testing station where equipment needed
Spare ECG paper	1/station	All but High-Quality BLS and Airway Management
Recommended Drugs, Drug Packages, or Drug Cards (Appendix)		
Epinephrine	1/station	Preventing Arrest: Bradycardia; High-Performance Teams: Cardiac Arrest and Post–Cardiac Arrest Care; High-Performance Teams: Megacode Practice; and High-Performance Teams: Megacode Testing
Atropine sulfate	1/station	Preventing Arrest: Bradycardia; High-Performance Teams: Cardiac Arrest and Post–Cardiac Arrest Care; High-Performance Teams: Megacode Practice; and High-Performance Teams: Megacode Testing
Amiodarone and/or lidocaine	1/station	Preventing Arrest: Bradycardia; Preventing Arrest: Tachycardia (Stable and Unstable); High-Performance Teams: Cardiac Arrest and Post–Cardiac Arrest Care; High-Performance Teams: Megacode Practice; and High-Performance Teams: Megacode Testing
Adenosine	1/station	Preventing Arrest: Tachycardia (Stable and Unstable); High-Performance Teams: Megacode Practice; and High-Performance Teams: Megacode Testing
Dopamine	1/station	Preventing Arrest: Bradycardia; High-Performance Teams: Cardiac Arrest and Post–Cardiac Arrest Care; High-Performance Teams: Megacode Practice; and High-Performance Teams: Megacode Testing
Saline fluid bags/bottles	1/station	All but ACS, Stroke, Airway Management, and High-Quality BLS
IV pole	1/station	All but High-Quality BLS and Airway Management
Safety		
Sharps container (if using real needles)	1/station	All but High-Quality BLS and Airway Management

(continued)

Equipment and supplies	Quantity needed	Learning/testing station where equipment needed
Advanced Airways (must choose endotracheal tube and at least 1 supraglottic device)		
Endotracheal tube and all equipment and supplies necessary for correct insertion	1/station	Airway Management; High-Performance Teams: Cardiac Arrest and Post–Cardiac Arrest Care; High-Performance Teams: Megacode Practice; and High-Performance Teams: Megacode Testing
Laryngeal tube and supplies necessary for correct insertion	1/station	Airway Management; High-Performance Teams: Cardiac Arrest and Post–Cardiac Arrest Care; High-Performance Teams: Megacode Practice; and High-Performance Teams: Megacode Testing
Laryngeal mask airway and supplies necessary for correct insertion	1/station	Airway Management; High-Performance Teams: Cardiac Arrest and Post–Cardiac Arrest Care; High-Performance Teams: Megacode Practice; and High-Performance Teams: Megacode Testing
Regionally available supraglottic airway and all equipment and supplies necessary for correct insertion	1/station	Airway Management; High-Performance Teams: Cardiac Arrest and Post–Cardiac Arrest Care; High-Performance Teams: Megacode Practice; and High-Performance Teams: Megacode Testing
Cleaning Supplies for Use Between Student Practice and After Every Class		
Manikin cleaning supplies	Varies	All

Note: Consider an emergency department or intensive care unit bed and/or stretcher to place manikins on for a more realistic case-based scenario during appropriate learning stations.

Lesson START
Welcome, Introductions, and
Course Administration

15 minutes

Instructor Tips

- Knowing what you want to communicate, why it's important, and what you want to have happen as a result is critical to the success of your presentation

- Be flexible: Be ready to adjust your lesson plan to students' needs and focus on what seems to be more productive rather than sticking to your original plan

- Introductions: Use a visual aid (flip chart, whiteboard) to display introduction requirements (name, occupation, specialty, place of practice)

Discussion

In a large group, with all students, do the following:

- Introduce yourself and additional instructors, if needed
- Invite students to introduce themselves and ask them to provide the following information:
  - Name
  - Occupation
  - Specialty
  - Place of practice
- As students are introducing themselves, document their occupation, specialty, etc. This information will help instructors tailor future case scenarios and lessons
- Explain that the course is interactive
  - Use of the provider manual, learning station checklists
  - Skills testing checklists
  - Hands-on learning stations
  - Explain the use of **feedback devices** (audiovisual) during the **learning and testing stations** with cardiac arrest or respiratory arrest. Also explain how **timing** is a critical component of the learning and testing stations
- Explain that parts of the course are somewhat physically strenuous
  - For example, Lesson 2 involves adult CPR, which will require students to perform 2 minutes of compressions, which could be physically strenuous
- Ask that anyone with a medical concern, such as knee or back problems, speak with one of the instructors
- Explain the layout of the building, including bathrooms and fire exits
- Advise students where an AED can be found in the building
- Tell students to silence cell phones
- If a call needs to be answered, tell students to answer it in the hallway
- Tell the students, "We are scheduled to end at _____"

Lesson 1
ACLS Course Overview and Organization   *10 minutes*

Instructor Tips

- Make sure to emphasize critical aspects of the course, such as the course agenda, design, and completion requirements

- Breaks: Think about how you want to manage breaks during this course. Making yourself available allows you to answer questions people might feel too embarrassed to ask in front of others. It also gives you time to create rapport and get feedback

- **In these lesson plans, items that are in boldface have greater importance**

 ## Discussion

In a large group, with all students, do the following:

- Present the course overview
- Discuss the course agenda, design, and completion requirements
- Be certain that students understand major course concepts
  - Importance of early high-quality CPR and early defibrillation to patient survival
  - Integration of effective BLS with ACLS interventions
  - The clinical signs of patient deterioration (preventing arrest)
  - The functioning of high-performance teams relative to patient survival
    - Timing, quality, coordination, and administration
- Discuss the importance of effective team interaction and communication during a resuscitation attempt. Explain the learning stations and rotations through the stations
  - Provide an overview of how the students will move through the stations
- Answer students' questions
- **Assign students to small groups for learning stations**
  - Limit the number of students to 6 (maximum of 8 per group)
- **Tell students that they will be using their provider manuals throughout the course**
- Explain the course completion requirements, including the mandatory use of an audiovisual feedback device for all CPR practice and testing. Students must
  - Pass the Adult High-Quality BLS Skills Test
  - Pass the Airway Management Skills Test
  - Demonstrate competency in learning station skills
  - Pass the Megacode Test
  - Pass the open-resource exam with a minimum score of 84% (does not apply to HeartCode students)
    - An open-resource exam allows students to use available resources, such as the Handbook of ECC and provider manual, posters, algorithms, etc, to process information analytically but also to think independently and creatively with curriculum content
  - You should issue a course completion card immediately after a student successfully completes the course but no later than 30 days after class

Lesson 2A
Learning/Testing Station:
High-Quality BLS Practice

45 minutes

Learning Objective

- Perform prompt, high-quality BLS, including prioritizing early chest compressions and integrating early AED use

Instructor Tips

- Students should rotate through the skills station

- Tell students that the skills testing portion will happen immediately after this lesson

- Monitor the rate and depth of chest compressions with a real-time audiovisual feedback device. If possible, monitor chest recoil as well

- The students should correct their own chest compressions in response to real-time output from the feedback device

- Use peer coaching to help with feedback and to allow students to feel comfortable correcting other providers

 ## Students Practice: Compressions

- Arrange students in groups with manikins (Figure 1)

    - 3 or fewer students per manikin

    - 1 instructor per 2 manikins

Figure 1. Positions for High-Quality BLS Learning Station with a CPR Coach.

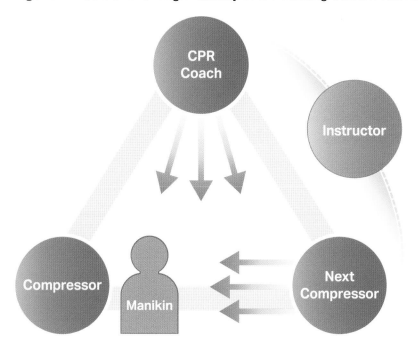

- Students rotate through continuous compressions practice for 2 minutes on manikins, adjusting their performance according to the real-time response of the feedback device and the CPR Coach (Table 3)
  - Summarize key points
    - High-quality BLS is the foundation of resuscitation
    - High-quality CPR is the primary component in influencing survival from cardiac arrest, but there is considerable variation in monitoring, implementation, and quality improvement
    - Target CPR performance metrics include the following:
      - Push hard: Compression depth of at least 2 inches (5 cm) in adults
      - Push fast: Compression rate of 100 to 120/min
      - Allow complete chest recoil after each compression
      - Ideally, achieve a chest compression fraction (CCF) greater than 80%
      - Switch providers about every 2 minutes to avoid fatigue
- Be sure that students perform correct chest compressions throughout the practice session
- Monitor the rate and depth of chest compressions with an audiovisual feedback device. If possible, monitor chest recoil as well
- Have peers coach other students on the basis of data from the feedback device
- Give feedback during practice to the Compressor and the CPR Coach

Table 3. Student Rotations for CPR Coaches and Compressors Learning Station

Round 1	Round 2	Round 3
Student 1: Compressor	Student 1: CPR Coach	Student 1: Next Compressor
Student 2: Next Compressor	Student 2: Compressor	Student 2: CPR Coach
Student 3: CPR Coach	Student 3: Next Compressor	Student 3: Compressor

Students Practice: Two-Rescuer BLS

- Assign student numbers
- Practice session (small groups around a manikin): practice 1- and 2-rescuer sequence according to the skills testing checklist
- Have the skills testing checklist available (*ACLS Provider Manual*, handout, etc)
- Use Table 4 to assign students for 2-rescuer practice

Table 4. Two-Rescuer Practice Student Number Assignments

Person assessing and compressing	Person with AED
Student 1	Student 2
Student 2	Student 3
Student 3	Student 1

Lesson 2B
Learning/Testing Station:
High-Quality BLS Testing—Testing Details

Instructor Tips

- Make sure you are familiar with how to use the skills testing checklist (refer to the instructor manual for information on how to use testing checklists)
- Complete a skills testing checklist for each student during this portion of the lesson
- Use an audiovisual feedback device to provide real-time feedback on compression quality

 ## Test Students One at a Time

- Tell students who are not being tested to practice on another manikin in another room
  - Test each student in a reasonably private environment
    - Each student must demonstrate the entire sequence of 2-rescuer BLS *without instructor prompting*
    - Fill out an Adult High-Quality BLS Skills Testing Checklist for each student
  - Carefully observe the student you are testing
    - Monitor the speed and depth of chest compressions with an audiovisual performance monitoring device. If possible, monitor chest recoil as well
- If a student is unsuccessful, refer them for immediate remediation
  - Each student may retest 1 additional time during this station
  - A student who remains unsuccessful may require additional remediation (refer to the sections titled Exam and Remediation in Part 1 of the instructor manual)
- Summarize the importance of high-quality CPR to patient survival

Lesson 3A
Learning/Testing Station:
Airway Management Practice

45 minutes

Learning Objectives

- Recognize respiratory arrest
- Perform early management of respiratory arrest

Instructor Tips

- **Use a stopwatch/timer or feedback device to make sure students are ventilating at appropriate rates and volumes**
- High-quality chest compressions and defibrillation are the highest priorities. As soon as enough personnel are available, initiate ventilation and oxygenation to support the resuscitation
- Make sure students are not ventilating too quickly or forcefully (about half-a-bag squeeze over 1 second)
- Healthcare providers often deliver excessive ventilation during CPR, particularly when an advanced airway is in place. Excessive ventilation is harmful because it
  - Increases intrathoracic pressure and impedes venous return and therefore decreases cardiac output, cerebral blood flow, and coronary perfusion
  - Causes air trapping, leading to increased end-expiratory lung volume
  - Increases the risk of regurgitation and aspiration in patients without an advanced airway
- For the *respiratory arrest* cases, you need to use only the lead-in and initial information to lead the student through the bag-mask ventilation and OPA/NPA skills testing. You may use the whole respiratory scenario if you want to go deeper into respiratory distress, respiratory failure, and respiratory arrest. However, to accommodate this approach, you will need to expand the airway management station

 ## Students Practice: Airway Management

- Assign student numbers
- Practice session (small groups around a manikin): **practice OPA and NPA insertion, discuss oxygen and suction, and practice 1- and 2-rescuer bag-mask ventilation**
- Students practice 1-rescuer bag-mask ventilation as in Figure 2
- Organize students for 2-rescuer bag-mask ventilation practice as in Table 5

Figure 2. Positions for Airway Management Learning and Testing Station with a CPR Coach.

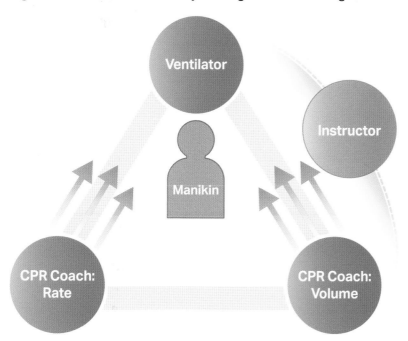

Table 5. Student Assignments for Airway Management Practice

Person squeezing the bag	Person holding the mask
Student 1	Student 2
Student 2	Student 3
Student 3	Student 1

Lesson 3B
Learning/Testing Station:
Airway Management Testing—Testing Details

Test Students One at a Time

- Advise students that they will be tested on bag-mask ventilation with OPA/NPA insertion skills
- Present the respiratory case scenario (case scenarios can be found in Appendix of the instructor manual or in the Instructor Reference Material)
- Each student manages a complete airway case (testing session)
  - Perform a full assessment
  - Begin ventilation without delay
  - Insert an OPA or an NPA
  - Connect the bag-mask device to oxygen and adjust the flow rate to the appropriate level
  - Give bag-mask ventilation with the OPA/NPA for 1 minute (skills test)
    - Rate (once every 6 seconds)
    - Speed (squeeze the bag for 1 second)
    - Volume (about half a bag)
  - Check off student's skills on the skills testing checklist as each student demonstrates adequate management of the respiratory case
  - **Monitor ventilation with a stopwatch/timer or feedback device** to make sure students are ventilating at appropriate rates and at appropriate volumes, if that information is available

Lesson 3C
Learning/Testing Station:
Airway Management—Student Practice Details (Optional)

Instructor Tips

- This portion of the lesson is optional
  - Whether or not you teach this lesson will depend on the makeup of your class. That is why it is important to ask students at the beginning of the class to introduce themselves and provide information about their occupations

Students Practice: Advanced Airway Insertion (Optional, Based on Students' Scope of Practice)

Students practice performing ventilations with a simulated advanced airway in place (depending on manikin limitations, instructors may use a standard manikin with a bag-mask device rather than a bag connected to a simulated airway tube)

- Rotate through all students performing ventilation
- Optional advanced airway device modules
  - Laryngeal Tube
  - Laryngeal Mask Airway
  - Endotracheal Tube

Lesson 4
Technology Review

Instructor Tips

- If there are 2 instructors, this activity can be done in 2 smaller groups. For 1 instructor, keep the class in 1 large group

- It is important that students get hands-on experience with the equipment they will be responsible for using during the learning stations and testing stations

- Ideally, equipment would be the same as would be used in a real emergency
  - Advise students that the equipment may be different in their workplace

Discussion

- **Demonstrate** and review monitor/defibrillator functions, buttons, and connections (features of your equipment may vary)
  - Power button
  - Transcutaneous pacing
  - Synchronized cardioversion
  - Blood pressure
  - P_{ETCO_2}
  - Pulse oximetry
  - Pad connections
  - ECG connections and lead placement (3-lead, 4-lead, 5-lead)
  - Optional 12-lead placement and right-sided 12-lead placement

- Review crash cart/jump kit supply locations

- Explain the use of **feedback devices** (audiovisual) during the **learning and testing stations** involving CPR and ventilations. Also explain how **timing** and objective measures are critical components of the learning and testing stations

Lesson 5A
Learning Station:
Preventing Arrest: Bradycardia
60 minutes

Instructor Tips

- Students often have difficulty differentiating between the heart block rhythms. Focus more on the treatments for stable vs unstable bradycardia than on detailed analysis of specific rhythms

- For in-hospital case scenarios only, students should request RRT/MET response

- When debriefing students:

  - Ask open-ended questions to engage group discussion and allow for greater detail

  - When answering a question, acknowledge the individual with eye contact, and then answer to the entire room, coming back to the questioner periodically

Optional: Play Bradycardia Algorithm Video

- Address what students will learn from the video

- Play the video

- Answer students' questions

Discussion

- Monitor/defibrillator technology review, if needed

  - Apply limb leads to patient so that pacing can be achieved through pacer pads

- Signs of clinical deterioration

- Stable vs unstable patients

- Definition of unstable signs and symptoms

- First-degree AV block

- Second-degree type I AV block

- Second-degree type II AV block

- Third-degree (complete block)

- Junctional rhythms (slow)

- Idioventricular rhythm

- H's and T's

- Local protocol

Lesson 5B
Learning Station:
Preventing Arrest: Bradycardia—Rotations

Instructor Tips

- This learning station is designed to allow 3 of the 6 students to be a Team Leader during this lesson and the other 3 to be a Team Leader in Lesson 6: Tachycardia

- When students have to rotate roles during practice, provide enough space for rotation to allow for effective observation and monitoring of student performance

- To ensure incorporation of knowledge into practice, make sure the students actually perform the skills of defibrillation, synchronized cardioversion, and transcutaneous pacing

Students Practice

Student Rotations in Learning Station Cases According to Team Roles

- The **Team Leader** will direct the actions of the other team members. For example, the Team Leader will coach the Airway team member if the performance of bag-mask ventilation is not making the chest rise

- **Team members** will perform interventions as directed by the Team Leader. This is an opportunity for students to practice skills and receive feedback from the Team Leader. Students will demonstrate effective team behaviors (eg, closed-loop communication, clear messages)

- **For bradycardia:** The **Timer/Recorder** will check off critical action boxes on the Bradycardia Learning Station Checklist

Students Practice

- Select 3 cases for 3 students to manage individually in this station (Table 6)

- Students will run scenarios (individually) and perform debriefing for all 3 cases (case scenarios can be found in the Appendix of the instructor manual or in the Instructor Reference Material)

Discussion

- Provide feedback on students' debriefing (Table 7)

  – Use the gather-analyze-summarize debriefing process described here

- What was challenging?

- What worked well in this case?

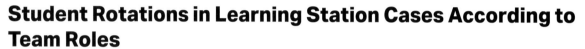

Table 6. Student Rotations for Bradycardia Learning Station

Team Role	Case 1 (10 minutes)	Case 2 (10 minutes)	Case 3 (10 minutes)
Team Leader	Student 6	Student 1	Student 2
Airway	Student 1	Student 2	Student 3
IV/IO/Medications	Student 2	Student 3	Student 4
Monitor/Defibrillator	Student 3	Student 4	Student 5
Compressor (if needed)	Student 4	Student 5	Student 6
Timer/Recorder	Student 5	Student 6	Student 1

Table 7. Structured and Supported Debriefing Process for Bradycardia Learning Station

Phase	Goal	Actions
Gather	Ask what happened during the case to develop a shared mental model of the events. Listen to students to understand what they think and how they feel about the simulation	• Request a narrative from the Team Leader • Request clarifying or supplementary information from the high-performance team
Analyze	Facilitate students' reflection on and analysis of their actions	• Review an accurate record of events • Report observations (both correct and incorrect steps) • Assist students in thoroughly reflecting on and examining their performance during the simulation as well as in reflecting on their perceptions during the debriefing • Direct and/or redirect students during the debriefing to ensure continuous focus on session objectives
Summarize	Facilitate identification and review of the lessons learned that can be taken into actual practice	• Summarize comments or statements from students • Have students identify positive aspects of their high-performance team or individual behaviors • Have students identify areas of their high-performance team or individual behaviors that require change or correction

Lesson 5C
Learning Station:
Preventing Arrest: Bradycardia—
Details for Case Rotations

 Students Practice

Use Table 8 to determine case rotations for this learning station.

Table 8. Timing and Tasks for Bradycardia Learning Station

Case rotations (3 rotations, 10 minutes each)	Directions for case rotations (Instructors must conduct the scenario in real time)

Start case scenario(s) (6 minutes)	• Review assigned team roles from the rotation chart for this case
	  – Ensure that students understand the expectations for their assigned roles (eg, "Your role is to use the bag-mask device to give ventilations that cause the chest to rise")
	• Introduce the case by reading the case scenario
	• Set the timer to 6 minutes
	• Ask the Team Leader to begin managing the case
	• Advise the Team Leader to observe and coach while being mindful of the case timing
	• Students may use the Handbook of ECC, pocket cards, or crash cart cards
	• Observe and coach
	  – Effective team performance
	  – Appropriate case management
	  – High-quality skills performance, including high-quality CPR, when needed, throughout the scenario
	• Guide the Team Leader through management of the case
	• Stop the case after 6 minutes

Case debriefing (4 minutes)	• Set the timer to 4 minutes
	• Conduct a debriefing at the end of the case (refer to Debriefing Tools in the instructor manual)
	• Ask the Team Leader to gather, analyze, and summarize the case, roles of team members, and areas for improvement
	• Ask the Timer/Recorder to critique the case
	• Give a summary of key concepts of the case
	  – Differentiating between signs and symptoms that are caused by the slow rate vs those that are unrelated
	  – Correctly recognizing the presence and type of AV block
	  – Using atropine as the drug intervention of first choice
	  – Deciding when to start transcutaneous pacing
	  – Deciding when to start epinephrine or dopamine to maintain heart rate and blood pressure
	  – Knowing when to call for expert consultation about complicated rhythm interpretation, drugs, or management decisions

Repeat for each of the remaining cases.

Lesson 6A
Learning Station:
Preventing Arrest: Tachycardia
(Stable and Unstable)

60 minutes

Learning Objectives

- Recognize tachycardias that may result in cardiac arrest or complicate resuscitation outcome
- Perform early management of tachycardias that may result in cardiac arrest or complicate resuscitation outcome

Instructor Tips

- Begin with the end in mind: knowing what you want to communicate, why it's important, and what you want to have happen as a result is critical to the success of your lesson
- Emphasize the need for rapid treatment (ie, electrical therapy) in patients with unstable tachycardia
- For in-hospital case scenarios only, students should request RRT/MET response
- To ensure incorporation of knowledge into practice, make sure the students actually perform the skills for defibrillation, synchronized cardioversion, and transcutaneous pacing

Optional: Play Tachycardia Algorithm Video

- Address what students will learn from the video
- Play the video
- Answer students' questions

Discussion

- Monitor/defibrillator technology review if needed
- Review tachycardias
  - Stable vs unstable patient
  - Sinus tachycardia
  - Reentry supraventricular tachycardia
  - Atrial fibrillation
  - Atrial flutter
  - Junctional rhythms (fast)
  - Monomorphic ventricular tachycardia (with pulse)
  - Polymorphic ventricular tachycardia (with pulse)
  - Torsades de pointes
  - Wide-complex tachycardia of uncertain type
  - Discuss local protocol

Lesson 6B
Learning Station:
Preventing Arrest: Tachycardia
(Stable and Unstable)—Rotations

Instructor Tips

- This learning station is designed to allow 3 of the 6 students to be a Team Leader during this lesson and the other 3 to be a Team Leader in Lesson 5: Bradycardia

- Other assigned student roles may vary depending on the number of students at the station

- Cases may be run in a different order, but assigned student roles should not be changed

- If students rotate roles during practice, provide enough space for rotation to allow for effective observation and monitoring of student performance

Students Practice

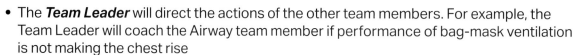

Student Rotations in Learning Station Cases According to Resuscitation Team Roles

- The *Team Leader* will direct the actions of the other team members. For example, the Team Leader will coach the Airway team member if performance of bag-mask ventilation is not making the chest rise

- *Team members* will perform interventions as directed by the Team Leader. This is an opportunity for students to practice skills and receive feedback from the Team Leader. Students will demonstrate effective team behaviors (eg, closed-loop communication, clear messages)

- The *Timer/Recorder* will check off critical action boxes on the Tachycardia Learning Station Checklist

Students Practice

- Select 3 cases for 3 students to manage individually in this station (Table 9)

- Run the scenario and perform the debriefing for all 3 cases (case scenarios can be found in the Appendix of the instructor manual or in the Instructor Reference Material)

Discussion

- Provide feedback on the students' debriefing

  - What was challenging?

  - What worked well in this case?

Table 9. Student Rotations for Tachycardia Learning Station

Team Role	Case 1 (10 minutes)	Case 2 (10 minutes)	Case 3 (10 minutes)
Team Leader	Student 3	Student 4	Student 5
Airway	Student 4	Student 5	Student 6
IV/IO/Medications	Student 5	Student 6	Student 1
Monitor/Defibrillator	Student 6	Student 1	Student 2
Compressor (if needed)	Student 1	Student 2	Student 3
Timer/Recorder	Student 2	Student 3	Student 4

Lesson 6C
Learning Station:
Preventing Arrest: Tachycardia
(Stable and Unstable)—Details for Case Rotations

 ## Students Practice

Use Table 10 to determine case rotations for this learning station.

Table 10. Timing and Tasks for Tachycardia Learning Station

Case rotations (3 rotations, 10 minutes each)	Directions for case rotations (Instructors must conduct the scenario in real time)

Start case scenario (6 minutes)	• Review assigned team roles from the rotation chart for this case
	   – Ensure that students understand the expectations for their assigned roles (eg, "Your role is to use the bag-mask device to give ventilations that cause the chest to rise")
	• Introduce the case by reading the case scenario
	• Set the timer to 6 minutes
	• Ask the Team Leader to begin managing the case
	• Students may use the Handbook of ECC, pocket cards, or crash cart cards
	• Observe and coach
	   – Effective team performance
	   – Appropriate case management
	   – High-quality skills performance
	   – Guide the Team Leader through management of the case
	• Stop the case after 6 minutes

Case debriefing (4 minutes)	• Set the timer to 4 minutes
	• Conduct a debriefing at the end of the case
	   – Refer to Debriefing Tools in the instructor manual
	• Ask the Team Leader to summarize the case, the roles of team members, and areas for improvement
	• Ask the Timer/Recorder to critique the case
	• Give a summary of key concepts of the case
	   – Begin with the end in mind: knowing what you want to communicate, why it's important, and what you want to have happen as a result is critical to the success of your lesson
	   – Discuss differentiating between signs and symptoms that are caused by a rapid rate vs those that are unrelated
	   – Emphasize the need for rapid treatment (ie, electrical therapy) in patients with unstable tachycardia
	   – For in-hospital case scenarios only, students should request RRT/MET response
	   – Discuss defibrillation, synchronized cardioversion, and transcutaneous pacing

Repeat for each of the remaining cases (Stable and Unstable Tachycardia).

Lesson 7
High-Performance Teams 30 minutes

Learning Objectives

- Model effective communication as a member or leader of a high-performance team
- Recognize the impact of team dynamics on overall team performance

Instructor Tips

- Clearly communicate the objectives of this lesson to help the students gain a better understanding of the lesson
- This team dynamics section is a great way to further engage the students
- Change the inflection in your voice and also change your pace to help change the energy level in the room

Play High-Performance Teams

Video (In-hospital, Out-of-Hospital, or Both)

- Ask students to open the *ACLS Provider Manual* to Part 3 (High-Performance Teams)
- Address what students will learn from the video
- Play the video

Discussion

- Ask students what questions they have about high-performance teams
  - What behaviors did they observe?
  - Discuss **timing** and **measurement** in relationship to impact on survival
  - Discuss the H's and T's that can help providers to arrive at a diagnosis in this case
  - Experienced providers may consider conducting an ultrasound analysis, although its usefulness has not been well established

Review/Summarize Key Points

- Team dynamics are critical during a code or resuscitation attempt
- The interaction among team members has a profound impact on the effectiveness of each individual as well as on the patient's overall survival
- The better you work as a team (timing, quality, coordination, and administration), the better the potential outcome for your patient
- That's why it's so important that you understand not just what to do in a resuscitation attempt but how to communicate and perform as an effective team, regardless of your role as team member or Team Leader

- The ability to follow and move through multiple algorithms is important
- Emphasize the importance of understanding the choreography of a resuscitation attempt as a team and the impact on timing
- Discuss the integration of high-quality BLS and ACLS care
- Remind students that they will be functioning as Team Leaders and as different members in the learning and testing stations and will need to apply these concepts
- Review critical aspects of high-performance teams (Figure 3)

Figure 3. Key areas of focus for high-performance teams to increase survival rates.

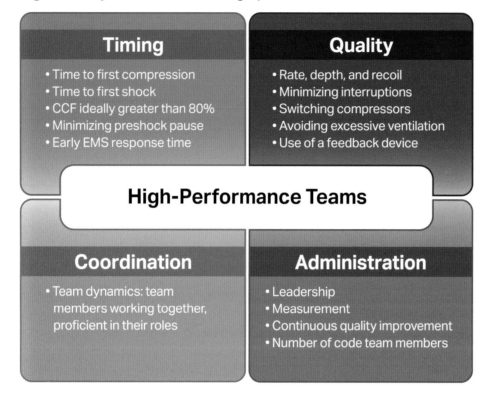

Timing
- Time to first compression
- Time to first shock
- CCF ideally greater than 80%
- Minimizing preshock pause
- Early EMS response time

Quality
- Rate, depth, and recoil
- Minimizing interruptions
- Switching compressors
- Avoiding excessive ventilation
- Use of a feedback device

High-Performance Teams

Coordination
- Team dynamics: team members working together, proficient in their roles

Administration
- Leadership
- Measurement
- Continuous quality improvement
- Number of code team members

Lesson 8A
Learning Station:
High-Performance Teams:
Cardiac Arrest and Post–Cardiac
Arrest Care
148 minutes

Learning Objectives

- Model effective communication as a member or leader of a high-performance team
- Recognize the impact of team dynamics on overall team performance
- Recognize cardiac arrest
- Perform early management of cardiac arrest until termination of resuscitation or transfer of care, including post–cardiac arrest care
- Evaluate resuscitative efforts during a cardiac arrest through continuous assessment of CPR quality, monitoring the patient's physiologic response, and delivering real-time feedback to the team

Instructor Tips

- This activity can be performed with 6 students and 1 instructor
  - If you have fewer than 6 students, you can assign multiple roles to individual students or substitute other instructors for those roles
- Transitional language: After showing the videos, be sure to provide a recap of what the video covered and what is next
- Encourage students to use their provider manual, pocket reference cards, or Handbook of ECC early on during the cases but to become less reliant on those resources as the cases progress
- The instructor should have working knowledge of all vasopressors associated with the students' workplace
- Conduct **prebriefing** before starting the case
  - Team should discuss the plan for managing each case including **objective timing goals**
- **Conduct learning station cases in real time**
- If possible, use real equipment in a realistic setting for your students
- Monitor rate and depth of chest compressions along with CCF by using an audiovisual feedback device with real-time feedback. In addition, monitor chest recoil if possible and ventilations
- High-quality CPR should be performed with real-time feedback throughout the cardiac arrest case-based scenario
- When debriefing students:
  - Ask open-ended questions to engage group discussion and allow for greater details
  - Discuss **prebriefing** goals (eg, CCF 82%,) vs actual results, with reflection on how they can perform better for the next case
  - When answering a question, acknowledge the individual with eye contact, and then answer to the entire room, coming back to the questioner periodically

Optional: Play Cardiac Arrest Algorithm Video and Post–Cardiac Arrest Algorithm Video

- Address what students will learn from the video
- Play the video
- Answer students' questions

Discussion

- Monitor/defibrillator technology review if needed
- Review team roles, responsibilities, and assignments for each case (refer to Lesson Plans 8B and 8C)
  - Case scenarios can be found in the Appendix of the instructor manual or in the Instructor Reference Material
- Students may use the Handbook of ECC, pocket reference cards, posters, or crash cart cards
- To show the continuum of care, all VF case scenarios must achieve ROSC
- 4 cases will be VF/pVT resulting in ROSC (post–cardiac arrest care)
- 2 cases will be split between PEA and asystole
- Ask students to recall the post–cardiac arrest care priorities
  - Maximize oxygenation and ventilation
  - Maximize hemodynamics
  - Obtain a 12-lead ECG; move to the cath lab if ST-segment elevation myocardial infarction (STEMI) is present
  - Implement targeted temperature management
- For post–cardiac arrest care, ensure that students address
  - Oxygenation and ventilation
  - Hemodynamic optimization (blood pressure, 12-lead, glycemic control)
  - Targeted temperature management
  - Criteria for percutaneous coronary intervention
- Advise that students will perform debriefing
  - Refer to Debriefing Tools in the instructor manual
- Select cases for each student to demonstrate appropriate management
- Discuss local protocol
- Highlight effective patient management through the Adult Post–Cardiac Arrest Care Algorithm

Lesson 8B
Learning Station: High-Performance Teams: Cardiac Arrest and Post–Cardiac Arrest Care—Rotations

Instructor Tips

It is important that every student have a role in each case

- Student role assignments may vary depending on the number of students at the station. However, every student must function as the Team Leader for 1 case

- Cases may be run in a different order, but ensure that no single student always goes first in subsequent learning stations

- Any additional students may be given roles as additional recorders

Students Practice

Student Rotations in Learning Station Cases According to Resuscitation Team Roles

- The **Team Leader** will direct the actions of the other team members. For example, the Team Leader will coach the Airway team member if performance of bag-mask ventilation is not making the chest rise.

- **Team members** will perform interventions as directed by the Team Leader. This is an opportunity for students to practice skills and receive feedback from the Team Leader. Students will demonstrate effective team behaviors (eg, closed-loop communication, clear messages)

- The **Timer/Recorder** will use a stopwatch to time 2-minute intervals for case management, announce each 2-minute interval for switching roles, and record critical action times on the ACLS Code Timer/Recorder Sheet (in the Appendix of the instructor manual or in the Instructor Reference Material) or on a whiteboard

Students Practice

- Select the cases for the students to manage individually in this station (Table 11)

- Run the scenario and perform the debriefing for all cases (case scenarios can be found in the Appendix of the instructor manual or in the Instructor Reference Material)

Discussion

- Provide feedback on the students' debriefing (Table 12)

  - What was challenging?

  - What worked well in this case?

Table 11. Student Rotations for Cardiac Arrest and Post–Cardiac Arrest Care Learning Station

Team role	Case 1	Case 2	Case 3	Case 4	Case 5	Case 6
Team Leader	Student 1	Student 2	Student 3	Student 4	Student 5	Student 6
Airway	Student 2	Student 3	Student 4	Student 5	Student 6	Student 1
IV/IO/Medications	Student 3	Student 4	Student 5	Student 6	Student 1	Student 2
Monitor/ Defibrillator/ CPR Coach	Student 4	Student 5	Student 6	Student 1	Student 2	Student 3
Compressor	Student 5	Student 6	Student 1	Student 2	Student 3	Student 4
Timer/Recorder	Student 6	Student 1	Student 2	Student 3	Student 4	Student 5

Table 12. Structured and Supported Debriefing Process for Cardiac Arrest and Post–Cardiac Arrest Care Learning Station

Phase	Goal	Actions
Gather	Ask what happened during the case, to develop a shared mental model of the events. Listen to students to understand what they think and how they feel about the simulation	• Request a narrative from the Team Leader • Request clarifying or supplementary information from the high-performance team
Analyze	Facilitate students' reflection on and analysis of their actions	• Review an accurate record of events • Report observations (both correct and incorrect steps) • Assist students in thoroughly reflecting on and examining performance during the simulation as well as in reflecting on their perceptions during the debriefing • Direct and/or redirect students during the debriefing to ensure continuous focus on session objectives
Summarize	Facilitate identification and review of the lessons learned that can be taken into actual practice	• Summarize comments or statements from students • Have students identify positive aspects of their high-performance team or individual behaviors • Have students identify areas of their high-performance team or individual behaviors that require change or correction

Lesson 8C
Learning Station: High-Performance Teams: Cardiac Arrest and Post–Cardiac Arrest Care— Details for Case Rotations

 Students Practice

Use Table 13 to determine case rotations for this learning station

Table 13. Timing and Tasks for Cardiac Arrest and Post–Cardiac Arrest Care Learning Station

Case rotation (6 rotations, 25 minutes each)	Directions for case rotations (Instructors must conduct the scenario in real time)
Case prebriefing (Figure 4) (5 minutes)	• Set timer to 5 minutes • Set case plan and goals including objective timing goals

Start case scenario (10 minutes)	• Review assigned team roles from the rotation chart for this case
	   – Ensure that students understand the expectations for their assigned roles (eg, "Your role is to use the bag-mask device to give ventilations that cause the chest to rise")
	• Introduce the case by reading the case scenario
	• Set the timer to 10 minutes
	• Ask the Team Leader to begin managing the case
	• Observe and coach
	   – Effective team performance
	   – Appropriate case management
	   – High-quality skills performance, including high-quality CPR in real time throughout the scenario with real time audiovisual feedback on CPR quality
	• Guide the Team Leader through management of the case
	• Stop the case after 10 minutes

Case debriefing (10 minutes)	• Set the timer to 10 minutes • Conduct a team debriefing at the end of the case – Refer to Debriefing Tools in the instructor manual

Repeat for each of the remaining 5 cases.

Figure 4. Prebriefing and structured debriefing tasks: a flow chart.

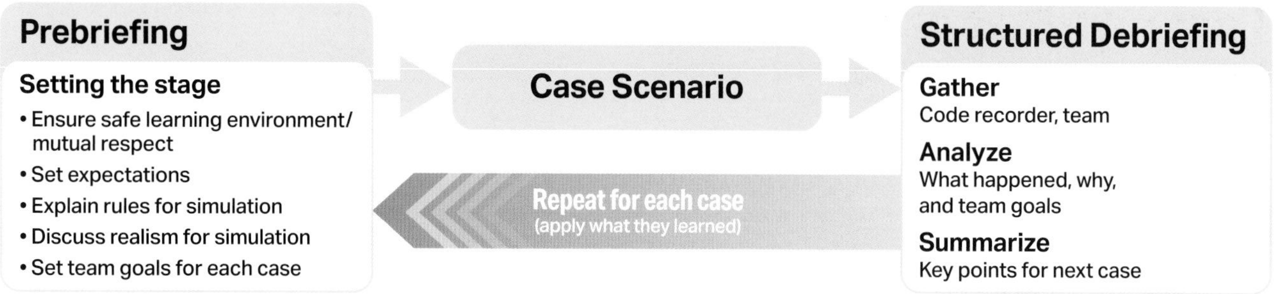

Prebriefing

Setting the stage
- Ensure safe learning environment/ mutual respect
- Set expectations
- Explain rules for simulation
- Discuss realism for simulation
- Set team goals for each case

Case Scenario

Repeat for each case
(apply what they learned)

Structured Debriefing

Gather
Code recorder, team

Analyze
What happened, why, and team goals

Summarize
Key points for next case

Lesson 9A
Learning Station: High-Performance Teams: Megacode Practice

138 minutes

Instructor Tips

- Organize into stations of 6 students each, with 1 instructor per station
- **Conduct learning station cases in real time (do not skip through the case)**
- Each scenario should last 10 minutes, with prebriefing lasting 5 minutes and debriefing should take place for 10 minutes
- Learning can be achieved just as effectively during structured debriefing as during the scenario

Discussion

- Highlight effective patient management through several algorithms
- **Demonstrate a Megacode case as a Team Leader**
- Review team roles, responsibilities, and assignments for each case (refer to Lesson Plans 9C and 9D)
  - Case scenarios can be found in the Appendix of the instructor manual or in the Instructor Reference Material
- Present a Megacode practice case for each student to manage (refer to Lesson Plan 9C)
- Students may use the Handbook of ECC, pocket reference cards, or crash cart cards
- Conduct **prebriefing** before starting the case
  - Team should discuss the plan for managing each case including **objective timing goals**
- If possible, use real equipment in a realistic setting for your students
- Monitor the rate and depth of chest compressions along with CCF by using an audiovisual feedback device with real time feedback. In addition, monitor chest recoil if possible and ventilations
- High-quality CPR should be performed with feedback throughout the cardiac arrest case-based scenario
- Advise students that they will perform **structured debriefing**

Lesson 9B
Learning/Testing Station: High-Performance Teams: Megacode Practice—Instructor Demo

Instructor Tips

When debriefing students:

- Ask your audience open-ended questions that focus on their perspectives to engage their minds and increase energy focus

- When answering a question, acknowledge the individual with eye contact, and then answer to the entire room, coming back to the questioner periodically

 Students Practice

Use Table 14 to determine timing and tasks for this learning station

Table 14. Timing and Tasks for Instructor Case Scenario Demonstration

Demonstrate a case scenario with you as Team Leader and students playing team roles	
Case prebriefing (5 minutes)	• Set timer to 5 minutes • Set case plan and goals, including objective timing goals

Start demonstration of a case scenario (10 minutes)	• Introduce the case
	• Assign a Team Leader
	• Assign team member roles to students
	• Set the timer to 10 minutes
	• Begin the case
	• Students should demonstrate case management, showing
	  – Effective team performance
	  – Appropriate application of algorithm
	  – High-quality skills performance, including high-quality CPR in real time throughout the scenario
	• Stop the case after 10 minutes

Case debriefing (10 minutes) **Total time for case demonstration: 25 minutes**	• Set the timer to 10 minutes • Go over the Megacode Practice Learning Station Checklist • Discuss prebriefing goals vs actual results • Discuss applying learning to the next case • Summarize the case, emphasizing proper roles of Team Leader and team members

Lesson 9C
Learning Station: High-Performance Teams: Megacode Practice—Practice Cases

Instructor Tips

- **Make sure students understand their roles and responsibilities in managing a Megacode case**
- This is the last opportunity to facilitate learning before the Megacode Testing. Use this time to address critical areas where students may still be weak

Students Practice

Present Megacode practice cases for each student, one at a time, 25 minutes each (5-minute prebriefing, 10-minute case, 10-minute debriefing)

- Determine the Team Leader for the first case (refer to rotations on the next lesson plan)
- Team Leader organizes other students into team roles
- Perform case prebriefing: set goals for the case, including objective timing goals
- Provide the team with an individual case
- Students may use the Handbook of ECC, pocket reference cards, or emergency crash cart cards
- Team Leader assigns and directs the team through the entire Megacode case
- Rotate through all students practicing as Team Leader for remaining 5 cases, depending on the number of students
- Timer/Recorder announces 2-minute intervals and checks off critical actions on the Megacode Testing Checklist
- Give feedback and answer questions
- Perform structured debriefing and have students apply learning to the next case

Lesson 9D
Learning Station: High-Performance Teams: Megacode Practice—Rotations

Instructor Tips

- Cases may be run in a different order, but assigned Team Leader roles should not be changed
- Each student must have the opportunity to run a complete Megacode case as a Team Leader
- When students have to rotate roles during practice, be sure to designate areas of the room to which students can move to have more space during practice and that allow the instructor to clearly observe and monitor student performance

 Students Practice

Use Table 15 to determine case rotations for this learning station

Table 15. Student Rotations for High-Performance Teams Learning Station

Team role	Case 1	Case 2	Case 3	Case 4	Case 5	Case 6
Team Leader	Student 2	Student 3	Student 4	Student 5	Student 6	Student 1
Airway						
IV/IO/Medications						
Monitor/Defibrillator/ CPR Coach			Team Leader assigns other students to each team role			
Compressor						
Timer/Recorder						

Testing Details and Testing Station Setups (T1)

Instructor Tips

- Organize students into 2 groups of 6 for the Megacode Testing Stations, depending on the number of students and instructors in the class
- In this station, the focus changes from facilitating learning to evaluating student performance. Students must perform the test from beginning to end. Do not interrupt students while they are completing the test. Address any deficiencies during remediation
- **Conduct testing station cases in real time**

Megacode Testing Stations and Exam (Open-Resource Exam)

- Explain the testing rotation for the Megacode Test and exam
- Remind students that the passing grade for the open-resource exam is 84%

Recommended Testing Station Setup

- 2 Megacode stations, 2 instructors, 6 students each (consider 2 instructors per station to optimize student assessment)
- Other testing setups are permissible as long as
  - The open-resource exam is proctored and secure
  - The open-resource exam is not interrupted to move a student to the Megacode Test

High-Performance Teams: Megacode Testing and Megacode Testing Details (T2-T4)

12 to 75 minutes

 Megacode Testing Stations

- Provide Megacode case scenario
- Use the Megacode Testing Checklist to test the team until they pass
- **You must conduct the scenario in *real time***
- **Monitor CPR quality with audiovisual feedback device(s) with real-time feedback**
- Students may use the Handbook of ECC, pocket reference cards, or emergency crash carts, with restrictions (refer to the instructor manual)
- Timer/Recorder announces 2-minute intervals
- Take no longer than 10 minutes to test and give students feedback on their performance (pass or fail)
- Do not give hints or provide coaching during the test
- Refer students for remediation as needed

Megacode Test Rotations

Use Table 16 to determine case rotations for this test, if needed.

Table 16. Student Rotations for High-Performance Teams Testing

Team role	Case 1	Case 2	Case 3	Case 4	Case 5	Case 6
Team Leader	Student 5	Student 6	Student 1	Student 2	Student 3	Student 4
Airway						
IV/IO/Medications						
Monitor/Defibrillator/ CPR Coach		Team Leader assigns other students to each team role				
Compressor						
Timer/Recorder						

Exam and Exam Details
(T5, T6)

Exam

- Exams are administered online, though there may be an occasional need to administer a paper exam. Refer to the Instructor Network for more information about delivering exams
- Collect and score any paper exams
- Review the answers with the students

Exam Details

- The exam is an open-resource exam
  - Resources could include the provider manual, either in printed form or as an eBook on a personal device, any notes the student took during class, the Handbook of ECC, the latest *AHA Guidelines for CPR and ECC*, posters, etc. Open resource does not mean open discussion with other students or the instructor
- Students may not talk to each other during the exam
- When a student completes the paper exam, grade the exam
- Refer to the annotated answer key to discuss questions answered incorrectly
- Answer any questions
- Students who scored less than 84% need immediate remediation
  - Make sure the student understands the errors and corrects the answers
  - Give a second test or have the student orally go over each item that he or she answered incorrectly, showing understanding of those incorrect items

Do not interrupt the exam to have a student go to the Megacode Testing Station

Remediation (REM)

Instructor Tip

- For Megacode retesting, the instructor may play multiple team member roles, or other available students may be team members

 ## Exam

The information below applies primarily to online and paper exams and does not apply to HeartCode students.

- Review course material for each student who needs remediation
- Retest students as necessary
- Give feedback
- Evaluate competency

Lesson VAS
Learning Station: Vascular Access (Optional)

Instructor Tip

- Participation in this lesson is not required to complete the ACLS Course

Play Intraosseous Access Video

- Address what students will learn from the video
- Play the video
- Answer students' questions

Students Practice

- Have students practice IO insertion skills on appropriate manikins
- Ensure that each student can prepare equipment to administer an IO bolus rapidly
- Have students verbalize the correct adult drug dose
- Ensure that each student can perform IO access correctly and confirm when the needle has reached the marrow cavity
- Ensure that each student can prepare equipment to administer an IO bolus, including 3-way stopcock and syringes
- Observe each student; provide corrective feedback

Lesson COP
Learning Station: Coping With Death (Optional)

Instructor Tips

- Remind students that if they have recently experienced the loss of a loved one, this video might be difficult to view
- **Participation in this lesson is not required to complete the ACLS Course**
- Students may choose not to view this video, at their discretion

Play Coping With Death Video

- Address what students will learn from the video
- Play the video (video will automatically pause)
- Answer students' questions

Discussion

- Discuss how the news of the death of the patient could be delivered more effectively
  - Family was not allowed in the room during the resuscitation attempt
  - Family was not informed that they had a choice about whether to stay in the room
  - News was delivered in the hallway, with no privacy
  - Vague terms were used to describe the death
  - The words *dead* or *died* were never used
  - Physician left family for "another emergency"
  - Physician left family with no support and no one to answer their questions
- Ask if there are any questions

Resume Coping With Death Video

- Play the video
- Answer students' questions

Lesson ACLS-HeartCode P1
Learning Station: HeartCode ACLS Practice   198 minutes

Instructor Tips

- This is a time where you can bridge the gap for students who have taken the HeartCode ACLS Course and help them develop their skills

- Make sure to set aside enough time to allow these students to practice on the manikins

- The use of required feedback devices should help students improve the quality of their compressions

- Make sure that each student has been offered adequate practice to feel comfortable testing

- **Conduct learning station cases in real time (do not fast-forward the video)**

Students Practice

- High-quality BLS: Follow ACLS Lessons 2A and 2B

- Airway management with OPA/NPA insertion: Follow ACLS Lessons 3A and 3B

- Megacode practice: Follow ACLS Lessons 9A through 9D

Lesson ACLS-HeartCode T1
Testing Station: HeartCode ACLS
Competency Testing

12 to 75 minutes

Instructor Tips

- This section provides a great way to further engage the students
- Change the inflection in your voice and also change your pace to help change the energy level in the room
- Allow students to work together, and be prepared to answer questions
- Make sure that each student has successfully mastered all of the skills before you move forward with the skills test
- **Conduct testing station cases in real time (do not skip the case scenario)**

Skills Test

- Conduct high-quality BLS skills testing, airway management with OPA/NPA insertion skills testing, and Megacode Testing
- Follow ACLS Lesson Plans T2 through T4
- Testing details:
  - Test each student on high-quality BLS and airway management with OPA/NPA insertion
  - Test each student with a team (at least 3 students) for Megacode
  - Each student must demonstrate the entire sequence for high-quality BLS, airway management with OPA/NPA insertion, and Megacode without instructor prompting
  - Carefully observe the student during testing
  - Do not coach or give hints during the test
  - Fill out the Adult High-Quality BLS and Airway Management Skills Testing Checklists and the Megacode Testing Checklist
  - Refer the student for remediation if the test is unsuccessful
- If necessary, retest student(s) 1 additional time; if a student does not pass the test the second time, refer them for remediation

Lesson ACLS-Traditional 2*
Systems of Care

10 minutes

Instructor Tips

- Ask students to use the provider manual in this section to help further engage them and help with retention of information

- Make sure not to interrupt the video if you have any comments to add; write them down and discuss them at the end of the video. Students do not learn well when they are trying to listen to 2 things at once

Play Systems of Care Video

- Ask students to open the provider manual to Part 1

- Play the video

Discussion

- Answer students' questions from the video

- Review and define Systems of Care

  - Discuss benefits and ways to improve

- Discuss the AHA Chain of Survival in relation to local protocol

- Highlight that a victim's survival depends on the entire systems of care working together in a timely fashion.

*Optional lesson plans for use with the Sample Agenda for ACLS Traditional Course. **These lessons must be added if using the ACLS Traditional Course agenda.**

Lesson ACLS-Traditional 3
Learning Station:
The Science of Resuscitation

15 minutes

This video lesson focuses on the key science that drives increased patient survival

Instructor Tips

- Transitional language: After showing the video, be sure to provide language that helps students with the transition back to teaching, such as a recap of what the video covered and what is next

- When reviewing the material presented in the video with students, ask leading questions to help facilitate discussion; avoid lecturing

Play Science of Resuscitation Video

In a large group or small groups:

- Introduce the video The Science of Resuscitation

- Play the video

- Discuss high-quality BLS and feedback devices

- Answer questions

- Review/summarize key points

Lesson ACLS-Traditional 4
Systematic Approach

15 minutes

Instructor Tips

- Ask students to use the provider manual in this section to help further engage them and help with retention of information

- Make sure not to interrupt the video if you have any comments to add; write them down and discuss them at the end of the video. Students do not learn well when they are trying to listen to 2 things at once

Play Systematic Approach Video

- Ask students to open the provider manual to Part 1

- Play the video

Discussion

- Answer students' questions from the video

- Remind students that they will be functioning as Team Leader and different members as they rotate through the learning and testing stations

- Review and summarize key points (See Tables 17 and 18)

Table 17. BLS Assessment

Assessment	Assessment technique and action
Check for responsiveness.	• Tap and shout, "Are you OK?"
Shout for nearby help/activate the emergency response system and get the AED/defibrillator.	• Shout for nearby help. • Activate the emergency response system. • Get an AED if one is available, or send someone to activate the emergency response system and get an AED or defibrillator.
Check breathing and pulse.	• **To check for absent or abnormal breathing** (no breathing or only gasping), **scan the chest for rise and fall** for at least 5 but no more than 10 seconds. • Check the pulse for at least 5 but no more than 10 seconds. • Perform the pulse check simultaneously with the breathing check **within 10 seconds** to minimize delaying CPR. • If you find no breathing and no pulse within 10 seconds, start CPR, beginning with chest compressions. • If you find a pulse, start rescue breathing at 1 breath every 6 seconds. Check pulse about every 2 minutes.
Defibrillate.	• If pulse is not felt, check for a shockable rhythm with an AED/defibrillator as soon as it arrives. • Provide shocks as indicated. • Follow each shock immediately with CPR, beginning with compressions.

Table 18. Primary Assessment

Assessment	Assessment technique and action

Airway
• Is the patient's airway patent?
• Is an advanced airway indicated?
• Have you confirmed proper placement of the airway device?
• Is the tube secured, and are you reconfirming placement frequently and with every transition?
	• Maintain an open airway in unconscious patients by using a head tilt–chin lift, an oropharyngeal airway, or a nasopharyngeal airway.
	• Use advanced airway management if needed (eg, laryngeal mask airway, laryngeal tube, endotracheal tube).
	  – Weigh the benefits of placing an advanced airway against the adverse effects of interrupting chest compressions. If bag-mask ventilation is adequate, you may defer inserting an advanced airway until the patient does not respond to initial CPR and defibrillation or until ROSC. Advanced airway devices such as a laryngeal mask airway, a laryngeal tube, or an esophageal-tracheal tube can be placed while chest compressions continue.
	  – If using advanced airway devices:
	    ▪ Confirm the proper integration of CPR and ventilation
	    ▪ Confirm the proper placement of advanced airway devices by physical examination and quantitative waveform capnography
	    ▪ Secure the device to prevent dislodgment
	    ▪ Monitor airway placement, effectiveness of CPR, and ROSC with continuous quantitative waveform capnography

Assessment	Assessment technique and action

Breathing
• Are ventilation and oxygenation adequate?
• Are quantitative waveform capnography and oxyhemoglobin saturation monitored?
	• Give supplemental oxygen when indicated.
	  – For cardiac arrest patients, administer 100% oxygen.
	  – For others, adjust the oxygen administration to achieve oxygen saturation of 95% to 98% by pulse oximetry (90% for ACS and 92% to 98% for post–cardiac arrest care).
	• Monitor the adequacy of ventilation and oxygenation by
	  – Clinical criteria (chest rise and cyanosis)
	  – Quantitative waveform capnography
	  – Oxygen saturation
	  – Avoid excessive ventilation

Circulation
• Are chest compressions effective?
• What is the cardiac rhythm?
• Is defibrillation or cardioversion indicated?
• Has intravenous (IV)/ intraosseous (IO) access been established?
• Is ROSC present?
• Is the patient with a pulse unstable?
• Are medications needed for rhythm or blood pressure?
• Does the patient need volume (fluid) for resuscitation?
	• Monitor CPR quality.
	  – Quantitative waveform capnography (if the partial pressure of CO_2 in exhaled air at the end of the exhalation phase, or P_{ETCO_2}, is less than 10 mm Hg, attempt to improve CPR quality). Waveform capnography should be as high as possible with improved CPR quality. Continuous quantitative waveform capnography provides an indirect measure of cardiac output during chest compressions because the amount of carbon dioxide exhaled is associated with the amount of blood that passes through the lungs. An $ETCO_2$ less than 10 mm Hg during chest compressions rarely results in ROSC.
	  – A sudden increase in $ETCO_2$ to more than 25 mm Hg may indicate ROSC.
	  – Intra-arterial pressure (if relaxation phase [diastolic] pressure is less than 20 mm Hg, attempt to improve CPR quality). Inter-arterial pressure should be as high as possible with improved CPR quality. If intra-arterial pressure monitoring is available, strive to optimize blood pressure. Relaxation phase (diastolic) pressures less than 20 during chest compressions rarely results in ROSC.
	• Attach monitor/defibrillator for arrhythmias or cardiac arrest rhythms (eg, VF, pVT, asystole, PEA).
	• Provide defibrillation/cardioversion.
	• Obtain IV/IO access.
	• Give appropriate drugs to manage rhythm and blood pressure.
	• Give IV/IO fluids if needed.
	• Check glucose and temperature.
	• Check perfusion issues.

Disability	• Check for neurologic function. • Quickly assess for responsiveness, levels of consciousness, and pupil dilation. • AVPU: Alert, Voice, Painful, Unresponsive
Exposure	• Remove clothing to perform a physical examination. • Look for obvious signs of trauma, bleeding, burns, unusual markings, or medical alert bracelets.

Secondary Assessment

• Focused medical history (SAMPLE)

• H's and T's

Lesson ACLS-Traditional 5
CPR Coach

10 minutes

Instructor Tips

- Ask students to use the provider manual in this section to help further engage them and help with retention of information

- Make sure not to interrupt the video if you have any comments to add; write them down and discuss them at the end of the video. Students do not learn well when they are trying to listen to 2 things at once

Play CPR Coach Video

- Ask students to open the provider manual to Part 3

- Play the video

Discussion

- Answer students' questions from the video

- Remind students that they will be functioning as a CPR Coach during the CPR and Airway Management stations throughout the class

- Review and summarize key points (See *ACLS Provider Manual*)

Lesson ACLS-Traditional 6
Learning Station: Recognition:
Signs of Clinical Deterioration

10 minutes

This video lesson focuses on preventing arrest

Instructor Tips

- Transitional language: After showing the video, be sure to provide language that helps students with the transition back to teaching, such as a recap of what the video covered and what is next

- When reviewing the material presented in the video with students, ask leading questions to help facilitate discussion; avoid lecturing

Play Recognition: Signs of Clinical Deterioration

In a large group or small groups:

- Introduce the video Recognition: Signs of Clinical Deterioration

- Play the video

Discussion

- Review and define MET/RRT for in-hospital cardiac arrest (optional for EMS)

- Answer questions

- Review/summarize key points

Lesson ACLS-Traditional 7A
Learning Station: Acute Coronary Syndromes—
Video Discussion 1
30 minutes

Learning Objective

- Discuss early recognition and management of acute coronary syndromes, including appropriate disposition

Instructor Tips

- Allow students to work together to answer questions and allow for self-discovery

- When summarizing what the video has covered, be sure to allow students to lead this discussion at times by asking for what they observed/learned during the video segment

- Students are often hesitant to answer questions at first. Before this lesson, write down additional leading questions to help prompt discussion. These video-based lessons are designed to allow you to challenge students, whether they are novice or experienced providers. Adjust the difficulty of your questions based on the knowledge level of the students in the course

Play ACS Video

- Address what students will learn from the video

- Play the video (automatically pauses)

  - Address pause 1 questions 1, 2, and 3

- Refer to Part 2 of the provider manual

- Lead the discussion with the group

Discussion

- Advise students to refer to Part 2, ACS in the *ACLS Provider Manual*. Capture key concepts from the discussion

Pause 1

1. **What is the difference between stable angina, unstable angina, and myocardial infarction?**

Angina is a tightness or discomfort (not a sharp pain) in the center of the chest and/or the surrounding area. The onset of discomfort associated with stable angina is often predictable; in many cases, it begins during exertion or with strong emotions. It is a symptom, not a diagnosis of coronary artery disease or acute ischemic symptoms. While often associated with myocardial ischemia, chest discomfort may have other causes. In the presence of coronary disease, the most common cause of angina is an obstructing or disrupted coronary plaque.

Angina may be stable and predictably produced by exertion or emotion. At rest, a fixed coronary plaque generally allows enough blood supply. However, blood flow is insufficient during stress. When a plaque becomes unstable, ACS occurs. Due to a sudden reduction in the cross-sectional area of the blood vessel, blood flow is insufficient. This causes a clinical presentation called *unstable angina,* which is characterized by prolonged anginal pain that occurs at rest or with minimal effort. When the lack of blood flow is severe enough to cause damage to the heart muscle, a myocardial infarction is said to occur. This event often correlates with angina episodes of 15 minutes or longer.

2. This patient is having chest discomfort. What are the possible causes of chest discomfort that may be life threatening?

Although most *life-threatening* chest discomfort is due to ACS, the initial emergency diagnosis may include several other disorders. When a diagnosis of ACS is uncertain, the following possible diagnoses should be considered in the initial evaluation as well as the continuing assessment:

- Aortic dissection
- Pulmonary embolism
- Acute pericarditis with effusion and tamponade
- Spontaneous pneumothorax
- Esophageal rupture

3. What are the classic symptoms of acute ischemic chest discomfort?

The predominant symptom in most patients with ischemic syndromes is chest discomfort. This discomfort is often not described as a pain. Brief episodes of chest discomfort may be due to ischemia and may or may not progress to infarction. However, when symptoms are constant (ie, last for more than 15 to 20 minutes), myocardial infarction may be present. Symptoms suggestive of ACS include

- Uncomfortable pressure, fullness, squeezing, or pain in the center of the chest lasting several minutes (infarction: usually more than 15 minutes)
- Pain spreading to the shoulders, neck, arms, or jaw, or pain in the back or between the shoulder blades
- Chest discomfort with light-headedness, fainting, sweating, or nausea
- Shortness of breath with or without chest discomfort
- Denial that they are having chest pain/discomfort and minimizing severity

Lesson ACLS-Traditional 7B
Learning Station: Acute Coronary Syndromes— Video Discussion 2

Play ACS Video

- Address what students will learn from the video
- Play the video (automatically pauses)
  - Address pause 2 questions 1, 2, and 3
- Refer to Part 2 in the provider manual
- Lead the discussion with the group

Discussion

- Advise students to refer to Part 2, ACS in the *ACLS Provider Manual*. Capture key concepts from the discussion

Pause 2

1. Half of ACS patients do not arrive at the hospital by EMS.

Why is early EMS dispatch important for patients with ACS?

Patients with a STEMI have a complete occlusion of a coronary artery. Early opening of the artery reduces mortality and the size of infarction. In many cases, EMS can begin symptom-stabilizing care before the patient arrives at the hospital, which will permit earlier reperfusion therapy. *Early opening of the artery reduces mortality and the size of infarction.* Patients arriving by EMS receive earlier reperfusion. EMS providers should consider the risk of VF in the early hours after a STEMI.

What are the most important components of a community ACS recognition program?

ACS is the most common cause of cardiac arrest in adults. Every community should develop a program to respond to cardiac arrest and identify patients with possible ACS. Components of this program include

- Recognizing symptoms of ACS
- Activating the EMS system
- Providing early CPR
- Providing defibrillation with AEDs available through lay rescuer CPR and defibrillation programs

2. What are the goals of therapy for patients with ACS?

Improving systems of care enables early initiation of reperfusion therapy for patients with possible ACS and increases the likelihood of target goal achievement. These goals (discussed in detail in the ACS video) are

- Relief of ischemic chest discomfort
- Prevention of major adverse cardiac events, such as death, nonfatal myocardial infarction (MI), and the need for postinfarction urgent revascularization

- Treatment of acute, life-threatening complications of ACS, such as VF/pulseless VT, symptomatic bradycardia, and unstable tachycardia

Reperfusion therapy opens an occluded coronary artery with either drugs or mechanical means. "Clot buster" drugs are called *fibrinolytics*—a more accurate term than *thrombolytics*. Percutaneous coronary intervention (PCI) is a procedure used to open blocked or narrowed coronary (heart) arteries. PCI, performed in the heart catheterization suite following coronary angiography, allows balloon dilation and/or stent placement for an occluded coronary artery. PCI performed as the initial reperfusion method is called primary PCI.

3. What role does aspirin play in ACS? What are the indications and contraindications?

The most common cause of ACS is the rupture of a lipid-laden plaque with a thin cap. After rupture, a monolayer of platelets covers the surface of the ruptured plaque (platelet adhesion). Additional platelets are recruited (platelet aggregation) and activated. Aspirin irreversibly binds to platelets and partially inhibits platelet function.

Studies have shown that aspirin reduces mortality during MI. The recommended dose is 162 to 325 mg. Aspirin is indicated in all patients with possible ACS.

Contraindications include true aspirin allergy and recent or active gastrointestinal bleeding.

Lesson ACLS-Traditional 7C
Learning Station: Acute Coronary Syndromes—
Video Discussion 3

Play ACS Video

- Address what students will learn from the video
- Play the video (automatically pauses)
  - Address pause 3 questions 1, 2, and 3
- Refer to Part 2 in the provider manual
- Lead the discussion with the group

Discussion

- Advise students to refer to Part 2, ACS in the *ACLS Provider Manual*. Capture key concepts from the discussion

Pause 3

1. **Let's review. What is the initial drug therapy for ACS? We have already discussed aspirin.**

Other initial agents may include oxygen (to keep the saturation 90% or greater), nitroglycerin, and opiates (eg, morphine).

What are the doses and indications/contraindications/cautions for nitroglycerin?

Nitroglycerin is administered via the sublingual route, either in a tablet or spray form. Three doses may be administered after repeating assessments of blood pressure and heart rate. Conditions where nitroglycerin administration should be used with caution or withheld in patients with ACS include

- **Inferior MI and right ventricular (RV) infarction:** Use nitroglycerin with caution in patients with known inferior wall STEMI. For these patients, perform a right-sided ECG to assess the degree of RV involvement. If RV infarction is confirmed by right-sided precordial leads or clinical findings by an experienced provider, nitroglycerin and other vasodilators (morphine) or volume-depleting drugs (diuretics) are contraindicated. Patients with acute RV infarction are very dependent on RV-filling pressures (preload) to maintain cardiac output and blood pressure.

- **Hypotension, bradycardia, or tachycardia:** Avoid use of nitroglycerin in patients with hypotension (systolic blood pressure less than 90 mm Hg), extreme bradycardia (less than 50/min), or marked tachycardia.

- **Recent use of phosphodiesterase inhibitor (often used for erectile dysfunction):** If the patient has recently taken a phosphodiesterase inhibitor (eg, sildenafil or vardenafil within 24 hours; tadalafil within 48 hours), nitrates may cause severe hypotension refractory to vasopressor agents.

2. **What are the possible ECG groups that help triage initial ACS? What are they called?**

Analysis of the ECG ST segment allows triage of ACS patients into 1 of 2 diagnostic and treatment groups: STEMI and NSTE-ACS (high-risk unstable angina/non–ST-segment elevation MI and normal or nondiagnostic ECG). (Refer to the ACS Algorithm.)

Why is it recommended that EMS send advance notification of the ECG to the receiving facility?

Time is a critical factor in producing a positive outcome for an ACS patient, especially for STEMI patients. The American Heart Association recommends that EMS systems implement 12-lead ECG programs to assist in the early recognition of those patients who could benefit most from treatment at a specialty cardiac center. EMS providers who lack training in advanced ECG interpretation can still acquire and transmit the 12-lead ECG to the emergency department for interpretation there. With an ECG diagnostic for STEMI, EMS providers should activate the local STEMI response plan at the earliest opportunity.

Early ECG interpretation and notification of the receiving hospital speeds the time to reperfusion therapy, saves heart muscle, and may reduce mortality.

3. Why is STEMI special and the focus of this case?

Reperfusion therapy for STEMI is perhaps the most important advance in the treatment of cardiovascular disease in cardiovascular therapy. Early fibrinolytic therapy or direct catheter-based reperfusion has been established as a standard of care for patients with acute myocardial infarction.

Reperfusion therapy reduces mortality and saves heart muscle. The shorter the time to reperfusion, the greater the benefit. For example, a 47% reduction in mortality was noted when fibrinolytic therapy was provided in the first hour after onset of symptoms.

Guidelines have set goals for first medical contact to balloon inflation within *90 minutes*. STEMI systems of care (EMS systems and emergency department initial triage) have a major impact on these goals.

Learning Objectives

- Discuss early recognition and management of stroke, including appropriate disposition

Instructor Tips

- Allow students to work together to answer questions and allow for self-discovery
  - Encourage student-to-student interaction
- These video-based lessons are designed to allow you to challenge students, whether they are novice or experienced providers. Adjust the difficulty of your questions based on the knowledge level of the students in the course

Play Stroke Video

- Address what students will learn from the video
- Play the video (automatically pauses)
  - Address pause 1 questions 1, 2, and 3
- Refer to Part 2 in the provider manual
- Lead the discussion with the group

Discussion

- Advise students to refer to Part 2, Acute Stroke in the *ACLS Provider Manual*. Capture key concepts from the discussion

Pause 1

1. What signs and symptoms is this patient having?

Students should recognize that the patient is having difficulty speaking and moving. These are some of the warning signs of stroke. Ask students what some other warning signs or symptoms of stroke are.

How are they typical of stroke?

The signs and symptoms of a stroke may be subtle. They can include

- Sudden weakness or numbness of the face, arm, or leg, especially on one side of the body
- Sudden confusion
- Trouble speaking or understanding
- Sudden trouble seeing in one or both eyes
- Sudden trouble walking
- Dizziness or loss of balance or coordination
- Sudden severe headache with no known cause

2. What are the major types of stroke?

The major types of stroke are

- **Ischemic stroke:** Accounts for 87% of all strokes and is usually caused by an occlusion of an artery to a region of the brain
- **Hemorrhagic stroke:** Accounts for 13% of all strokes and occurs when a blood vessel in the brain suddenly ruptures into the surrounding tissue. Fibrinolytics are contraindicated in this type of stroke

In addition:

- **Transient ischemic attack:** Transient ischemic attack is a transient episode of neurologic dysfunction caused by focal brain, spinal cord, or retinal ischemia, without acute infarction

Is there any treatment that can reduce disability?

Stroke is a general term. It refers to acute neurologic impairment that follows interruption in blood supply to a specific area of the brain. Although expeditious care for stroke is important for all patients, this case emphasizes reperfusion therapy for acute *ischemic* stroke because rapid therapy with a fibrinolytic agent can reduce the disability from stroke.

3. If this patient is having a stroke, what are some goals for stroke care?

The goal of stroke care is to minimize brain injury and maximize the patient's recovery. The Stroke Chain of Survival described by the AHA and the American Stroke Association is similar to the Chain of Survival for sudden cardiac arrest. It links actions to be taken by patients, family members, and healthcare providers to maximize stroke recovery. These links are

- Rapid recognition and reaction to stroke warning signs
- Rapid activation of the EMS system
- Rapid EMS-system transport to and prearrival notification of the receiving hospital
- Rapid diagnosis and treatment in the hospital

Lesson ACLS-Traditional 8B
Learning Station: Acute Stroke—Video Discussion 2

Play Stroke Video

- Address what students will learn from the video
- Play the video (automatically pauses)
  - Address pause 2 questions 1, 2, and 3
- Refer to Part 2 in the provider manual
- Lead the discussion with the group

Discussion

- Advise students to refer to Part 2, Acute Stroke in the *ACLS Provider Manual*. Capture key concepts from the discussion

Pause 2

1. What are the critical EMS assessments and actions to provide the best outcome for this patient with a potential stroke?

- **Identify signs:** Define and recognize the signs of transient ischemic attack and stroke.

- **Assess ABCs:** Administer oxygen if the oxygen saturation is 94% or less or the oxygen saturation is unknown.

- **Complete stroke assessment:** Perform a rapid out-of-hospital stroke assessment and stroke severity score.

- **Establish time:** Determine when the patient was last known to be at neurologic baseline. This represents time zero. If the patient wakes from sleep and is found with symptoms of stroke, time zero is the last time the patient was seen to be normal.

- **Transport:** Transport the patient to a stroke center on the basis of stroke assessment, stroke severity score, and local stroke protocols. Consider bringing a witness, family member, or caregiver with the patient to confirm time of onset of stroke symptoms.

- **Alert hospital:** Provide prehospital notification to the receiving hospital so they can activate their stroke team.

- **Check glucose:** During transport, support cardiopulmonary function, monitor neurologic status, and, if authorized by medical control, check blood glucose.

2. What type of hospital is appropriate for this patient?

A stroke center has the capability to rapidly triage and treat patients by using a multidisciplinary approach.

Why is advance notification so important?

Evidence indicates a favorable benefit when stroke patients are triaged directly to designated stroke-prepared centers (primary/comprehensive centers).

Advance notification allows activation of the facility stroke plan and team, minimizing delay in evaluation and treatment.

3. What stroke screen was used in the video?

Cincinnati Prehospital Stroke Scale (CPSS)

What are the 3 important physical findings?

The CPSS identifies stroke on the basis of 3 physical findings:

- Facial droop (have the patient smile or try to show teeth)
- Arm drift (have the patient close eyes and hold both arms out)
- Abnormal speech (have the patient say, "You can't teach an old dog new tricks")

Using the CPSS, medical personnel can evaluate the patient in less than 1 minute.

The presence of 1 finding on the CPSS indicates a 72% probability of stroke.

The presence of all 3 findings indicates that the probability of stroke is greater than 85%.

Play Stroke Video

- Address what students will learn from the video
- Play the video
  - Address pause 3 questions 1, 2, and 3
- Lead the discussion with the group

Discussion

- Advise students to refer to Part 2, Acute Stroke in the *ACLS Provider Manual*. Capture key concepts from the discussion

Pause 3

1. Let's review. What is the initial emergency department assessment and stabilization?

- **Assess ABCDs:** Assess the ABCDs and evaluate baseline vital signs.

- **Provide oxygen:** Provide supplemental oxygen if the patient is hypoxemic, ie, oxygen saturation is 94% or less , or in patients with an unknown oxygen saturation value.

- **Establish IV access and obtain blood samples:** Establish IV access and obtain blood samples for baseline blood count, coagulation studies, and blood glucose, but do not let this delay obtaining a CT scan of the brain.

- **Check glucose:** Promptly treat hypoglycemia.

- **Perform neurologic screening:** National Institutes of Health Stroke Scale or Canadian Neurological Scale.

- **Activate stroke team:** Activate the stroke team or arrange consultation with a stroke expert.

- **Order CT brain scan:** Order an emergent CT scan of the brain and have it read promptly by a radiologist.

- **Obtain 12-lead ECG:** Obtain a 12-lead ECG, which may identify a recent acute myocardial infarction or arrhythmias (eg, atrial fibrillation) as a cause of embolic stroke. Life-threatening arrhythmias can follow or accompany stroke, particularly intracerebral hemorrhage. If the patient is hemodynamically stable, treatment of non–life-threatening arrhythmias (bradycardia, VT, and atrioventricular conduction blocks) may not be necessary. This should not delay getting the CT scan of the brain.

2. What are the possible outcomes of the CT scan?

Emergent CT or magnetic resonance imaging scans of patients with suspected stroke should be promptly interpreted by an expert. The presence of hemorrhage versus no hemorrhage determines the next steps in treatment and whether the patient is a candidate for fibrinolytic therapy.

Which test result makes the patient a candidate for fibrinolytic therapy?

No, hemorrhage is not present.

If the CT scan shows no evidence of hemorrhage, the patient may be a candidate for fibrinolytic therapy.

Yes, hemorrhage is present.

If hemorrhage is noted on the CT scan, the patient is **not** a candidate for fibrinolytics. Consult a neurologist or neurosurgeon and consider transfer for appropriate care.

3. What does fibrinolytic therapy do for patients with ischemic stroke?

Several studies have demonstrated a higher likelihood of good-to-excellent functional outcome when alteplase was given to adults with acute ischemic stroke within 3 hours of symptom onset. These results occurred only when alteplase was given by physicians in hospitals with a stroke protocol that rigorously adhered to the eligibility criteria and therapeutic regimen of the National Institute of Neurological Disorders and Stroke protocol. Evidence from prospective randomized studies in adults also documents a greater likelihood of benefit when treatment begins earlier.

Studies have also shown improved clinical outcome in carefully selected patients when fibrinolytic administration occurred between 3 and 4.5 hours after symptom onset, although the degree of benefit was smaller than seen in the group receiving treatment at 3 hours or more.

Lesson ACLS-Traditional 8D
Learning Station: Acute Stroke—Review of 8 D's

Instructor Tip

- Advise students to refer to Part 2 in the *ACLS Provider Manual*. Capture key concepts from the discussion

 ## Discussion

In a large group, with all students, discuss the following:

- Patients with acute ischemic stroke have a time-dependent benefit for fibrinolytic therapy similar to that of patients with ST-segment elevation MI, but this time-dependent benefit is much shorter

- The critical time period for administration of IV fibrinolytic therapy begins with the onset of symptoms

  - **D**etection: Rapid recognition of stroke signs and symptoms

  - **D**ispatch: Early activation and dispatch of EMS by phoning 9-1-1

  - **D**elivery: Rapid EMS stroke identification, management, triage, transport, and prehospital notification

  - **D**oor: Urgent emergency department triage to a high-acuity area and immediate assessment by the stroke team

  - **D**ata: Rapid clinical evaluation, laboratory testing, and brain imaging

  - **D**ecision: Establishing stroke diagnosis and determining optimal therapy selection

  - **D**rug/**D**evice: Administration of fibrinolytic and/or endovascular therapy if eligible

  - **D**isposition: Rapid admission to the stroke unit or critical care unit, or emergency interfacility transfer for endovascular therapy